DICTIONARY OF HEALTH ECONOMICS AND FINANCE

Dr. David Edward Marcinko

MBA, CFP©, CMP©

Editor-in-Chief

Hope Rachel Hetico

RN, MSHA, CPHQ, CMP©

Managing Editor

SPRINGER PUBLISHING COMPANY
New York

The *Dictionary of Health Economics and Finance* is dedicated to Lieutenant William Pentin (*retired*), an electrical engineer from the Michigan Technological University and an MBA from the Harvard Graduate School of Business Administration Class of 1949, who served in the U.S. Army from 1943 to 1945; and to Mackenzie Hope Marcinko, an internationally accomplished brown-belt martial-arts student in Taido Karate, who is emerging as all a young woman should be as she moves toward her teen years. They constantly reminded us to present concepts as simply as possible, as we endeavored to create a comprehensive *Dictionary* relevant to the entire health care industrial complex.

Copyright © 2007 Springer Publishing Company, LLC

All rights reserved.

No part of this publication may be reproduced, stored in a retrieval system, or transmitted in any form or by any means, electronic, mechanical, photocopying, recording, or otherwise, without the prior permission of Springer Publishing Company, LLC.

Springer Publishing Company, LLC
11 West 42nd Street
New York, NY 10036

Acquisitions Editor: Sheri W. Sussman
Production Editor: Emily Johnston
Cover design: Mimi Flow
Composition: Apex Publishing

07 08 09 10/ 5 4 3 2 1

Library of Congress Cataloging-in-Publication Data

Dictionary of health economics and finance / David Edward Marcinko,
    editor-in-chief ; Hope Rachel Hetico, managing editor.
        p. ;   cm.
    Includes bibliographical references and index.
    ISBN 0–8261–0254–9
    1. Medical economics—Dictionaries.   I. Marcinko, David E. (David
Edward)   II. Hetico, Hope R.
    [DNLM: 1. Economics, Medical—Dictionary—English.   2. Health
Care Sector—Dictionary—English.   W 13 D55716 2006]
    RA410.A3D53 2006
    338.4′7362103—dc22   2006018586

Printed in the United States of America by Electronic Printing Inc.

Contents

iii

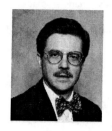

Dr. David Edward Marcinko, MBA, CFP©, CMP©, is a health economist, lexicographer, and board certified surgical fellow from Temple University in Philadelphia. In the past, he edited four practice-management books, three medical texts in two languages, six financial planning books, and two CD-ROMs for physicians, hospitals, financial advisors, accountants, attorneys, and health care business consultants. Internationally recognized for his work, he provides litigation support and expert witness testimony in State and Federal Court, with clinical publications archived in the Library of Congress and the Library of Medicine at the National Institute of Health. His thought leadership essays have been cited in journals such as: *Managed Care Executives, Healthcare Informatics, Medical Interface, Plastic Surgery Products, Teaching and Learning in Medicine, Orthodontics Today, Chiropractic Products, Podiatry Today, Investment Advisor Magazine, Registered Representative, Financial Advisor Magazine, CFP© Biz (Journal of Financial Planning), Journal of the American Medical Association (JAMA. ama-assn.org), The Business Journal for Physicians,* and *Physicians Money Digest;* by professional organizations such as the Medical Group Management Association (MGMA), American College of Medical Practice Executives (ACMPE), American College of Physician Executives (ACPE), American College of Emergency Room Physicians (ACEP), Health Care Management Associates (HMA), and PhysiciansPractice.com; and by academic institutions such as the Northern University College of Business, Creighton University, UCLA School of Medicine, Medical College of Wisconsin, Washington University School of Medicine, University of North Texas Health Science Center, University of Pennsylvania Medical and Dental Libraries, Southern Illinois College of Medicine, University at Buffalo Health Sciences Library, University of Michigan Dental Library, University of Medicine and Dentistry of New Jersey, Emory University School of Medicine, and the Goizueta School of Business at Emory University, among others.

Dr. Marcinko also has numerous editorial and reviewing roles to his credit. His most recent offering from Springer Publishing Company is: *Dictionary of Health Insurance and Managed Care.* A favorite on the lecture circuit often quoted in the media, he speaks frequently to medical and financial societies throughout the country in an entertaining and witty fashion.

Dr. Marcinko received his undergraduate degree from Loyola University (Baltimore), completed his internship and residency training at Atlanta Hospital and Medical Center, earned his business degree from the Keller

Graduate School of Management (Chicago), and his financial planning diploma from Oglethorpe University (Atlanta). He is a licensee of the Certified Financial Planner© Board of Standards (Denver) and holds the Certified Medical Planner© designation (CMP©). He obtained Series #7 (general securities), Series #63 (uniform securities state law), and Series #65 (investment advisory) licenses from the National Association of Securities Dealers (NASD) and a life, health, disability, variable annuity, and property-casualty license from the State of Georgia. Dr. Marcinko was also a cofounder of an ambulatory surgery center that was sold to a publicly traded company, a Certified Physician in Healthcare Quality (CPHQ); a certified American Board of Quality Assurance and Utilization Review Physician (ABQAURP); a medical-staff vice president of a general hospital; an assistant residency director; a founder of a computer-based testing firm for doctors; a president of a regional physician practice-management corporation in the Midwest; a member of the American Health Economics Association (AHEA) and the International Health Economics Association (IHEA); and a member of the U.S. Microsoft Partners Program, and both the Microsoft Professional Accountant's Program (MPAN) and Microsoft Health User's Group (MS-HUG).

Currently, Dr. Marcinko is Chief Executive Officer and Academic Provost for the Institute of Medical Business Advisors©, Inc. The firm is headquartered in Atlanta, has offices in five states and Europe, and works with a diverse list of individual and corporate clients. It sponsors the professional Certified Medical Planner© charter designation program. As a national educational resource center and referral alliance, the *i*MBA and its network of independent professionals provide solutions and managerial peace of mind to medical professionals, emerging health care organizations, and their consulting business advisors.

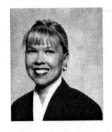

Hope Rachel Hetico, RN, MSHA, CPHQ, CMP©, received her nursing degree (RN) from Valpariso University, and Master's of Science Degree in Healthcare Administration (MSHA) from the University of St. Francis, in Joliette, Illinois. She is authors and editor of a dozen major textbooks and a nationally known expert in managed medical care, medical reimbursement, case management, health insurance, security and risk management, utilization review, HIPPAA, NACQA, HEDIS, and JCAHO rules and regulations.

Initially, a devotee of pedagogy, Ms. Hetico became an apostle of adult-learning using the andragogic principles of *i*MBA for corporate, professional, and practitioner audiences. She continually recruits and hosts a think tank of talented thought-leadership visionaries, essayists, and experts for the firm.

With this documented history of identifying innovations in education and accelerating their adoption by the medical and financial services industries, she is frequently quoted in the health care business media and brings a decade of entrepreneurship and creative leadership skills to the *i*MBA National Network© of independent advisors.

Prior to joining the *i*MBA as Chief Operating Officer, Ms. Hetico was a hospital executive, financial advisor, insurance agent, Certified Professional in Healthcare Quality, and distinguished visiting instructor of Healthcare Administration for the University of Phoenix, Graduate School of Business and Management. She was also national corporate Director for Medical Quality Improvement at Apria Health Care, a public company in Costa Mesa, California.

Currently, a Senior Linguistic Docent© for *i*MBA, and devotee of econometric heutagogy and andragogy, Ms. Hetico is responsible for leading www.MedicalBusinessAdvisors.com to the top of the exploding adult educational marketplace, expanding the online and on-ground Certified Medical Planner© charter designation program, and continuing to nurture the company's rapidly growing list of financial services colleagues and medical and institutional clients (www.CertifiedMedicalPlanner.com).

Preface

The emergence of health economics as a distinct field and separate financial discipline may be traced back to Nobel Laureate Kenneth J. Arrow's seminal work, *Uncertainty and the Welfare Economics of Medical Care*, in 1963.

New financial and economic concepts are common now, 45 years later, and so is its innovative jargon. Just consider the tortuous contorted term, *incurred but not reported* (IBNR), which may be defined as: "a potential floating-type accounting system entry that provides reserves in a health care account, for monies resulting from the liability of recognized medical services rendered but not currently reported in a capitated, fixed contractual or prospective health insurance payment system."

Medical economics and finance, however, is more than verbal chicanery; it is an integral component of the protean health care industrial complex. Its language is a diverse and broad-based concept covering many other industries: accounting, insurance, mathematics and statistics, public health, provider recruitment and retention, Medicare, utilization and cost accounting, health policy, forecasting, transactions costs and contracting, aging and long-term care, labor force trends, national health accounts and the impact of technology on health care spending, are all comingled arenas.

Even seemingly "non-health care" terms from the financial investing markets and Wall Street are also common because of their centrality to the personal and business-enterprise process of involved participants. The discipline is not contained in a single space, and its language needs to be codified to avoid confusion. But, the field is rapidly changing in our cost-constrained environment. More terms have reached the health care economics marketplace in the last few years than in all previous decades.

The use of words from other professions is even more rapid as we consider the impact from cost accountants, capitation actuaries, and forensic auditors; managed care's prospective payment system of capitation, reverse-capitation and risk pools; the Balanced Budget Agreement, Sarbanes-Oxley and the Patriot Acts; merger and acquisition fervor, financial advisors and international markets, the Asian contagion and currency exchanges; and the options and synthetic derivatives of day traders to name a few more verbiage generators. Moreover, with its quixotic efforts, the U.S. Department of Health and Human Services, along with the private insurance underwriting sector, has created a labyrinth of new economic programs with confusing financial terminology. For example, terms such as accretion, absorbed costs, deductible corridors, percentage of claims, geometric mean average length of stay, medical savings accounts, deletes and retrodeletes, kurtosis, and homo- or heteroskedasticity did not exist in the vernacular just a decade ago. Eponyms such as the Ho-Lee option model, Herfindahl-Hirschman Index, Kondratief wave, *i*MBA Index, and Laffer curve were similarly absent as were slang expressions such as channeling, gunslinger, doughnut-hole, people-pill, or buffing, while Latin phrases such as *qui-tam, ceteris paribus, ex-gratia payments, per diem,* and *ultra-vires* no longer seem like linguistic novelties.

And so, the *Dictionary of Health Economics and Finance* was conceived as an essential tool for doctors, nurses and clinicians, benefits managers, executives and health care administrators; endowment fund managers, lawyers and business consultants; accountants, fiduciaries and actuaries; HMOs, PPOs, and commercial insurance companies; as well as medical, dental, business and health care administration graduate students and patients.

With more than 5,000 definitions, 3,000 whimsical abbreviations and acronyms, and a 2,000 item oeuvre of resources, readings, and nomenclature derivatives, the *Dictionary* is really a 3-in-1 reference. It contains more than 10,000 entries that cover the financial and economics language of every health care industry sector: (a) layman, purchaser, and benefits manager; (b) physician, provider, and health care facility; and (c) payer, intermediary, and financial professional. We highlight new terminology and current definitions and include a list of confusing acronyms and alphabetical abbreviations. The *Dictionary* also contains offerings of the recent past that are still in colloquial use. These definitions are contemporaneously expanded where appropriate with simple examples, cross-references to research various other definitions, or to pursue relevant and/or related terms.

Of course, by its very nature, the *Dictionary of Health Economics and Finance* is ripe for periodic updates by engaged readers working in the fluctuating health care economics milieu. It will be periodically updated and edited to reflect the changing lexicon of terms, as older words are retired, and newer ones are continually created. Accordingly, if you have any comments, suggestions, or would like to contribute substantive unlisted abbreviations, acronyms, eponyms, or definitions to a future edition, or to nominate an expert, please contact us. We are flexible, market responsive, and committed to making this encyclopedic tool a valuable resource of the future.

REFERENCE

Arrow, K., J. (1963). Uncertainty and the welfare economics of medical care. *American Economic Review, 53,* 941–973.

David Edward Marcinko
Hope Rachel Hetico
Institute of Medical Business Advisors, Inc.
www.MedicalBusinessAdvisors.com
www.CertifiedMedicalPlanner.com
www.HealthDictionarySeries.com

Foreword

Why the *Dictionary of Health Economics and Finance*?

Every business and health care administration student I've ever taught over the last three decades has struggled to decipher the alphabet soup of medical economics (e.g., OPHCOO, ALOS, DRG, RBRVS, behavioral health, acuity, etc.), while those coming from clinical medicine struggled to internalize the lingo of finance (e.g., call premium, cost benefit ratios, IGARCH, AACPD, IBNR, ABCM, internal rate of return, accounts receivable days outstanding, etc.). Until we have a common language however, medical and business professionals cannot possess a shared vision, nor can we communicate successfully to create health care entities that provide quality care to patients and reasonable profits to medical practitioners. Of course, no single tool can meet all needs, and there are many fine books on health care economics and finance, along with a legion of consulting firms, management associations, and university programs. Yet, to effectively use these resources, one needs to have the right words, and to use seemingly everyday terms in a way that economists and health care financial experts speak.

Unfortunately, health care service costs continued to rise more rapidly than wages during the last decade, and consumed an ever larger share of Gross Domestic Product (GDP), creating hardships for both employers and employees. For example, health spending accounted for 15.3% of the nation's economy or $2.05 trillion in 2006, averaging $6,175 for every American. Health insurance premiums rose 8.8% to more than $14,500 for family coverage, and by 2013, the U.S. government forecasts health spending will reach 18.4% of GDP. It is no wonder that controlling costs is the top concern of fringe benefit specialists, according to Deloitte Consulting and the International Society of Certified Employee Benefit Specialists (Gawande, 2005). More than one-third of the rise was due to a 13.6% increase in outpatient spending. Higher utilization rates accounted for 43% of the increase, fueled by increased demand, more intense medical treatment and defensive medicine, according to Pricewaterhouse Cooper. And, let us not forget that one in seven Americans lack health insurance; that's 46 million people or 15.7% (Armstrong, 2005).

At the same time, medical professionals struggled to maintain adequate income levels. While some specialties flourished, others such as primary care barely moved forward, not even incrementally keeping up with inflation. In the words of Atul Gawande, MD, a surgical resident at Brigham and Women's Hospital in Boston, and one of the best young medical writers in America, "Doctors quickly learn that how much they make has little to do with how good they are. It largely depends on how they handle the business side of their practice" (2005).

Increasingly, some physicians have become more aggressive in seeking out business opportunities. For example, Neurosurgeon Larry Teuber, MD, built a specialty hospital in Rapid City, SD, and earned $9 million dollars in a single year (2006). While investors also became wealthy, the hospital where he previously practiced and some former colleagues were not so fortunate or happy, even suggesting that he stepped over the line. While it is difficult to fully understand a complex situation from a brief overview, it is vital for medical professionals to have definitions that clarify the so-called line and for businesses to define the forces and implicit understandings that underlie medical ethics. Alas, the *Dictionary of Health Economics and Finance* cannot solve these problems, just as the rule-of-law cannot answer the question of whether or not Dr. Teuber did the right thing. What the *Dictionary* can do, however, is set the context and clarify the terms of debate.

Consumers also need to know what these terms and conditions mean. If this was not evident until now, passage of Medicare Part D has made it painfully obvious that clarity is needed, and that continuing education in the economic and financial terminology of health care is a lifetime task. Once drug co-payments, corridor deductibles, and exclusions are mastered, one can begin to sort out the limits on long-term care insurance, homecare and hospice benefits, and the ever-changing levels of hospital and physician reimbursement dictated by sustainable growth adjustments (SGA) . . . and there is still much more to study and learn.

It takes knowledge to practice medicine and to earn capital, assume risk, and invest in emerging health care entities. And, none of us can escape the responsibility of knowing what the terms of engagement are. In times of great flux, such as the revolution in reimbursement and payment systems occurring today, codified information protects us all. The *Dictionary of Health Economics and Finance* provides that protection by bringing stability to the nomenclature of health care fiscal and economic concerns. With 10,000 definitions, acronyms, illustrations, cliometric equations, and industry notables, the *Dictionary* is an authoritative and comprehensive guide to better health care administration transactions.

Dr. David Edward Marcinko, Academic Provost for the *Institute* of Medical Business Advisors, Inc. and a Certified Medical Planner©, should be complimented for conceiving and completing this ambitious project. The *Dictionary of Health Economics and Finance* spells out the terms of reference and the principle players in the contemporaneous health care industrial complex. Having such a compendium readily at hand and sharing it with others is a way for patients, accountants, financial planners and insurance agents, medical practitioners, nurse managers, and health care executives to improve economic efficiency and clinical quality. Of course, it may even help restore fiscal enterprise-wide sanity, as well.

Simply put, my suggestion is to read, recommend, and refer to the *Dictionary of Health Economics and Finance* frequently, and "reap."

REFERENCES

Armstrong, David. (2005, August 2). "Skillful operation: A surgeon earns riches, enmity by plucking profitable patients." *Wall Street Journal*, 1.

Gawande, Atul. (2005, April 4). "Piecework: Medicine's money problem," *The New Yorker*, 47.

Thomas E. Getzen, PhD
Executive Director, International Health Economics
Association (iHEA)
Professor of Risk, Insurance and Health Care Management
The Fox School of Business—Temple University
www.HealthEconomics.org

Acknowledgments

Creating the *Dictionary of Health Economics and Finance* was a significant effort that involved all members of our firm. Major source materials include those publications, journals, and books listed as references, as well as personal communication with experts in accounting, wealth management and related fields.

Over the past year, we interfaced with public resources such as various State Governments, the Federal Government, Federal Register (FR), Centers for Disease Control and Prevention (CDC), the Centers for Medicare and Medicaid (CMS), Institute of Medicine (IOM), National Research Council (NRC), and the U.S. Department of Health and Human Services (HHS), as well as numerous private firms and professionals to discuss contents of this book. Although impossible to acknowledge every person that played a role in its production, there are several people we wish to thank for their moral support and extraordinary input.

Among these are: Timothy Alexander, MS, vice president of Library Research, and Robert James Cimasi, MHA, ASA, CBA, AVA, FHBI, CMP©, president and founder, Health Capital Consultants, LLC, St. Louis, MO; Dr. Michael J. Burry, Scion Capital, LLC, San Jose, CA; the late Russell Coile Jr., Senior Vice President, Superior Consultant Co., Southfield, MI; Jeffrey S. Coons, PhD, CFA©, and Christopher J. Cummings, CFA©, CFP©, Manning & Napier Advisors, Inc., Rochester, NY; Joseph M. Fabiszak, CPA, Managing Partner of Fabiszak & Kuczak, Baltimore, MD; J. Wayne Firebaugh, Jr., CPA, CLU, CFP©, CMP© of Firebaugh Capital Management, Roanoke, VA; Richard Frye, PhD, Forte Information Resources, LLC, Denver, CO; Professor Gregory O. Ginn, PhD, CPA, MBA, MEd, Department of Health Care Administration, University of Las Vegas, NV; Thomas A. Muldowney, MSFS, CLU, CFP©, CMP©, Managing Director for Savant Capital Management, Inc., Rockford, IL; Hugh O'Neill, Vice President, Integrated Health Care Markets, Sanofi-Aventis Pharmaceuticals, Bridgewater, NJ; Dr. Kenneth Shubin-Stein, CFA©, Spencer Capital Management, New York, NY; Dr. Dimitri Sogoloff, MBA, Alexandra Investment Management, LLC, New York, NY; Patricia A. Trites, PhD, MPA, CHBC, CHCO, CMP: (*Hon*), CEO: Health Care Compliance Resources, Augusta, MI; Karen White, PhD, MSE, Vice President: Superior Consultant Company, Inc., Ann Arbor, MI; Calvin W. Wiese, MBA, CPA, CMA, former Vice President, Superior Consultant Company, Inc., Ann Arbor, MI; and Ted Nardin CEO, Sara Yoo, production editor, and Sheri W. Sussman, Senior Vice-President, Editorial, of Springer Publishing Company, New York, NY, who directed the publishing cycle from conception to release.

Instructions for Use

Alphabetization

Entries in the *Dictionary* are alphabetized word by word. Alphanumeric definitions and unusual terminology are listed phonetically. Charts, graphs, tables, equations, lists, and other visual items are included to enhance reading, understanding and interest.

Cross-References, Synonyms, and Variations

Contrasting or related terms, as well as synonyms and variations, may be included in the *Dictionary* to enhance reader understanding. Once an entry has been fully defined by another term, a synergistic term may also be suggested (e.g., health maintenance organization; managed care organization). Colloquial slang terms are listed when appropriate, along with more than 200 notable *movers and shakers* in public and private health care economics and finance (e.g., Kongstvedt, Herzlinger, Clark, Enthoven, Reinhardt, Nash, Helppie and Ellwood, etc.).

Definitions

Because many academic and real-world words have distinctly different meanings depending on their context, it is left up to the reader to determine their relevant purpose. And, although health care economic and finance terms may be sparsely included elsewhere in nonmedical terms, or as a brief glossary in a specific text, it may be difficult to quickly return to a portion of the book containing the desired terms. Therefore, the *Dictionary* offers an expanded presentation of terms and definitions from many perspectives and sources. Yet, it is realized that one person's definitional diatribe may be another's parsimony. Moreover, the various meanings of a term have been listed in the *Dictionary* by bullets or functional subheading for convenience. Older mature terms still in colloquial use are also noted (e.g., HCFA), as well as contemporaneous new items (e.g., CMS), in order to help better appreciate the growing spectrum of economics and finance relationships within the health care industry. Eponyms and health care legislative acts are included, and Latin phrases and some foreign terms are defined as they become part of the global health care administration language. *See* Unusual Definitions.

Disciplines

The meanings of various words and phrases are given multiple utility according to their field of use, and there are few fields more immersed in the cross-pollination of concepts than health care administration. Accordingly, professional definitions from the disciplines of accounting, mathematics, taxation, statistics, insurance and risk management, benefits, retirement and estate planning, actuarial and legal sciences, as well as various new investment instruments, futures and options exchange mechanisms, and contracted insurance products are all included as they integrate with our core focus on health care economics and finance.

Disclaimer

All definitions, abbreviations, eponyms, acronyms, variations and synonyms, and information listed in the *Dictionary* are intended for general understanding, and do not represent the thoughts, ideas, or opinions of the *Institute* of Medical Business Advisors, Inc.© Care has been taken to confirm information accuracy, but we offer no warranties, expressed or implied, regarding currency and are not responsible for errors, omissions, or for any consequences from the application of this information. Furthermore, some terms are not complete because many are written in simplest form. The health care economics, finance, business, and accounting industry is evolving rapidly, and all information should be considered time sensitive.

Italics

Italic type may be used to highlight the fact that a word has a special meaning to the health care industry (i.e., *modifier, Medicare + Choice, International Classification of Diseases, Tenth Edition, Clinical Modification*). It is also used for the titles of publications, books, and journals referenced in the *Dictionary*.

Unusual Definitions

Unique trade or industry terms that play an active role in the field of health care economics and finance are included in the *Dictionary* along with a brief explanation, as needed (i.e., Aunt Millie, Roth 401(k), 403(b), *Bowie Bonds*, green-shoes, etc.). For related health insurance, Medicare, Medicaid, long-term care, disability, worker's compensation, and other managed care definitions, please review the companion work: *Dictionary of Health Insurance and Managed Care*, by Springer Publishing Company, New York.

Use

Beyond the health care administration space, the *Dictionary* can be used as a handy quick reference source and supplement to sales literature for insurance agents, stockbrokers, financial planners, and benefits managers; to answer prospect sales questions as well as inquiries about product servicing (fast, succinct, and technically accurate responses to such questions can sometimes mean the difference between closing and not closing a sale); negotiating a favorable health care insurance contract, or reducing costs when purchasing a health-related financial product or service. And, let us not forget about savvy consumers who will find the *Dictionary of Health Economics and Finance* a wealth of information in readily understood language. Astonishingly, the accounting, finance, and health insurance product purchase decision is often made directly by the layperson without sufficient basic knowledge of acronyms, financial definitions, and economic policy explanations!

Terminology: A–Z

Acronyms, Abbreviations, and Eponyms

Abbreviations with multiple meanings are included in the *Dictionary* because the industry does not possess a body of standardized acronyms, eponyms, and abbreviations.

Bibliography

Collated printed readings, electronic references, and organizations from a variety of sources allow further research into specific subjects of interest, as well as an opportunity to perform critical comparisons not possible without other narrative periodicals or publications. Information on physician reimbursement is included, too.

- Print Media Textbooks
- Print Media Publications
- Print Media Journals
- Electronic Internet Media
- Associations and Organizations
- Securities Exchange Commission
- Physician Compensation
- Related Titles

  - *The Advanced Business of Medical Practice: Advanced Profit Maximization Techniques for Savvy Doctors,* 2nd edition, Springer Publishing Company.

TERMINOLOGY: A–Z

Jargon is the verbal sleight of hand that makes the old-hat, seem newly fashionable.

—*David Lehman, American poet*

A

A FORTIORI: Latin phrase for "even stronger"; used to compare two economic theorems or proofs. It is interpreted to mean "in the same way."

A&L MANAGEMENT: The analysis and management of a health care entity's assets and liabilities and/or financial statements; especially the balance sheet.

ABANDONMENT: To willfully give up all rights and claims to assets.

ABATEMENT: Removal of an amount due (usually a tax or penalty within a governing agency).

ABILITY TO PAY PRINCIPLE: The philosophy that those with more affluence should be taxed more than those with less; for the public good.

ABSOLUTE ADVANTAGE: The advantage a health care entity has over another similar health care entity if it can produce more health care units over a certain period of time, all inputs being equal.

ABSOLUTE VOLATILITY: The true volatility of an investment or asset.

ABSORBED: A health care cost that is treated as an expense rather than transferred to a patient, MHO, or third party payer.

ABSORPTION COSTING: Cost accounting method that assigns both variable and fixed costs to health care products, goods, and services.

ABSTRACT: A hospital or health care discharge summary.

ABSTRACTION: The elimination of extraneous or irrelevant facts in order to derive a valid health care economic principle.

ABSTRACTOR: One who selects and redacts financial, economic, statistical, or other information from a medical record for data mining purposes.

ACCELERATED COST RECOVERY SYSTEM (ACRS): The predecessor of modified ACRS (MACRS). A depreciation method in which the cost of tangible property, such as a MRI machine or CT scanner, is recovered over a determined period of time. The approach disregards salvage value, imposes a period of cost recovery that depends on the classification of the asset into one of various recovery periods, and determines the applicable percentage of cost that can be deducted each year.

ACCELERATED DEPRECIATION: A method of loss recovery in which larger portions of depreciation are taken in the beginning periods of asset life and smaller portions taken in later periods.

ACCELERATED DEPRECIATION ALLOWANCE: The deduction from pretax health care business entity income that is allowed when the company purchases new plants or equipment.

ACCELERATED PAYMENT: The partial advancement of funds to temporarily pay for delayed health care claims, human resource payrolls, or other business or corporate claims.

ACCELERATION CLAUSE: Any clause, term, or condition on a bond, debt, or loan that allows immediate principal payment on-demand if other agreements are not met.

ACCEPT ASSIGNMENT: Physician or medical facility agreement to accept the fees allowed by an insurance plan, HMO, prospective payment system, or by Medicare, and so on.

ACCESS FEE: A managed care or health care insurance plan fee (surcharge) necessary to access its panel of member medical providers or facilities.

ACCIDENTAL DEATH BENEFIT: An extra benefit that generally equals the face value of a life, health insurance or managed care contract, or a principal sum payable in addition to other insurance benefits in the event of death as the result of an accident.

ACCIDENTAL DEATH AND DISMEMBERMENT BENEFIT: An insurance policy provision that pays a stated benefit in case of death or the loss of limbs or sight as a result of an accident.

ACCIDENTAL MEANS DEATH BENEFIT: An optionally available health or life insurance benefit providing for the payment of a multiple (usually double) of the face amount of the policy in case of death by accidental means. The benefit usually covers death resulting from bodily injury affected solely through external, violent, and accidental means, independently and exclusively of all other causes, and within 90 days after such injury.

ACCOUNT: A detailed record of the changes in assets, liabilities, and equity for a given period; a contractual relationship between a seller (health care provider) and buyer (patient, third party, insurance company), and so on.

ACCOUNT BALANCE: A statement net of credits and debits at the end of an accounting reporting period.

ACCOUNT EXECUTIVE (AE): The party who acts as a financial agent for a patient, a company, or another, and so on.

ACCOUNT RECONCILIATION: Adjusting a balance to match a bank statement.

ACCOUNT STATEMENT: Invoice showing an investor's investment, insurance, bank, or financial company services position at a given time. It may include a variety of information, including performance and transactions; personal or corporate.

ACCOUNTABILITY: Subject to accounting, civil and legal responsibilities, and liabilities for: Generally Accepted Accounting Principles (GAAP), American

Institute of Certified Public Accountants (AICPA) and/or other rules of conduct.

ACCOUNTANT'S OPINION: Signed statement by an independent accountant that describes the nature, purpose, scope and outcome of an examination of a health care or other entity's books, taxes, and financial records.

ACCOUNTANT'S REPORT: Formal document that communicates an independent accountant's: (1) expression of limited assurance on financial statements as a result of performing inquiry and analytic procedures; (2) results of procedures performed as agreed on for project scope; (3) nonexpression of opinion or any form of assurance in the form of financial statements information that is the representation of management in compilation report; or (4) opinion on an assertion made by management in accordance with the Statements on Standards for Attestation Engagements (SSAE). An accountants' report is not an audit.

ACCOUNTING: A formal professional system that gathers processes and presents financial information in report form to corporate management, and/or state and federal tax authorities, as needed.

ACCOUNTING CHANGE: Alterations in (1) an accounting principle, (2) an accounting estimate, or (3) the reporting entity that necessitates disclosures in published financial reports.

ACCOUNTING COST: A measure of health care or other entity operating input costs; the explicit costs of operating a business.

ACCOUNTING CYCLE: The process by which financial statements are produced for a given period.

ACCOUNTING EQUATION: Assets equal liabilities plus owner's (stockholder's) equity.

ACCOUNTING PERIOD: A calendar month, quarter, cycle, or year between accounting periods.

ACCOUNTING PERSPECTIVES: Opinions and thoughts underlying decisions on which categories of goods and services to include as costs or benefits in an analysis

ACCOUNTING PRINCIPLES BOARD (APB): Board of the American Institute of Certified Public Accountants (AICPA), which issued what is traditionally known as Generally Accepted Accounting Principles (GAAP) from 1959 to 1973. The APB was replaced by the Financial Accounting Standards Board (FASB) in 1973.

ACCOUNTS PAYABLE (AP): The amount of money a health care or other organization is obligated to pay vendors. A liability backed by general reputation and credit of the debtor.

ACCOUNTS RECEIVABLE (AR): The amount of money a health care or other organization is due from insured patients, payers, vendors, or other sources.

ACCOUNTS RECEIVABLE INSURANCE (ARI): Insurance coverage for uncollected accounts, plus the expenses of record reconstruction and various other collection fees, but sans physical, paper or electronic devices, computer disks, CDs, tapes, or memory sticks.

ACCOUNTS RECEIVABLE TURNOVER (ART): The speed in which accounts receivable are converted to cash. The ratio of net credit sales to average net accounts receivable.

ACCREDITED INVESTOR: Rule 501 of Regulation D of the Securities Act of 1933 requires a natural person whose individual net worth, or joint net worth together with a spouse, exceeds $1,000,000. Alternatively, under the same rule, an accredited investor is a natural person with an individual income in excess of $200,000 in each of the two most recent years or joint income with a spouse in excess of $300,000 in each of those years and has a reasonable expectation of reaching the same income level in the current year. Such investors are often used in private placements for health care facility bonds and equipment securities.

ACCRETE: Medicare term for the addition of new enrollees in a health care plan.

ACCRETION: Difference between a bond price at original discount purchase and current par value; asset value increase through internal growth and expansion.

ACCRETION OF A DISCOUNT: Accounting process by which the book value of a security purchased at a discount from par is increased during the security's holding period. The accretion reflects the increase in the security's holding value as it approaches the redemption date. Under a "straight line" accretion method, the yearly accretion is the same for all years and is equal to the product of the total amount of the discount divided by the number of years to redemption.

ACCRUAL: An amount of money that is set aside to cover a medical benefit plan or other expenses. Accrual is the best estimate of what expenses are and is based on a combination of input data, lag factor, and IBNR.

ACCRUAL BASIS OF ACCOUNTING: Method of accounting that attempts to match health entity or other revenues with expenses and claims by recognizing revenue when a service is rendered and expense when the liability is incurred irrespective of the receipt or disbursement of cash.

ACCRUAL BONDS: Zero coupon bonds void of regular interest payments until all are due at maturity.

ACCRUE: To accumulate, as in debt or revenue.

ACCRUED ASSETS AND LIABILITIES: The accumulation of both assets and liabilities.

ACCRUED EXPENSES: Incurred, but not yet paid, expenses.

ACCRUED INTEREST: Interest earned, but not received, when a buyer purchases a hospital or other bond (debt) from a bondholder (creditor). The buyer owes the bondholder interest for the period of time the bondholder held the bond. Because interest is paid semiannually, the period of time that has elapsed is known as the accrual period.

ACCRUED REVENUE: Revenue earned by a health care or other business entity but not yet received in cash.

ACCUMULATED DEPRECIATION: The total accumulated amount of depreciation recognized as an asset by a health care or other organization, since purchase. For example, assume that a computerized blood storage machine costs $5,000 and has an expected life of 5 years, with no residual value. After 3 years the accumulated depreciation would be $3,000 (3 × $1,000 annual depreciation).

ACCUMULATED DIVIDEND: Dividends due on cumulative preferred stock not yet paid out.

ACCUMULATION: Total utilized services per dollar, of covered health care, medical services, or other benefits.

ACCUMULATION ACCOUNT (AA): An account established by the sponsor of a unit investment trust (UIT) into which securities purchased for the trust portfolio are formally deposited.

ACCUMULATION PERIOD (AP): Specific time period for incurred expenses that are at least equal to the deductible or similar amount, in order to begin a managed care or health insurance benefit period.

ACCUMULATION PLAN (AP): Investor arrangement for the regular and automatic purchase of large or small asset amounts.

ACCUMULATION STAGE: Period when monetary contributions are made to an annuity account.

ACCUMULATION UNIT: A unit used to measure the value of the separate account of an annuity during the pay-in (accumulation phase). An AA is similar to a mutual fund share. It is the value of one unit (i.e., share) in the annuity separate account. Usually valued on a daily basis, it will fluctuate in value based on the performance of the investments chosen or directed into the separate account.

ACID TEST: A health care or other business liquidity financial test that measures how much cash and marketable securities are available to pay all current liabilities of the organization.

ACID TEST RATIO: A liquidity percentage that measures how much cash and marketable securities are available to pay all current liabilities of a health care or other business organization (i.e., cash and marketable securities/ current liabilities).

ACQUIRED SURPLUS: Uncapitalized net worth in a pooling-of-interests situation.

ACQUISITION: A corporate merger or gain process that takes controlling interest in another company, in either a friendly or unfriendly manner.

ACQUISITION COST: The cost of soliciting and acquiring patients, managed care insurance contracts, and/or other business interests.

ACTIVE INVESTMENT MANAGEMENT: An investment approach that involves the active trading of securities while attempting to outperform markets.

ACTIVE MARKET: Heavy volume trading in a particular securities or commodities market.

ACTIVE MONEY: Currency that is in circulation.

ACTIVITY RATIOS: Financial percentages that measure how effectively a business or health care organization is using its assets to produce revenues.

ACTIVITY-BASED COSTING (ABC): A process that defines costs in terms of a health care or other organization's processes or activities and determines costs associated with significant activities or events. ABC relies on the following three step process: (1) activity mapping, which involves mapping activities in an illustrated sequence; (2) activity analysis, which involves defining and assigning a time value to activities; and (3) bill of activities, which involves generating a cost for each main activity. *See also* activity-based management.

ACTIVITY-BASED MANAGEMENT (ABM): Supports health entity operations by focusing on the causes of costs and how costs can be reduced. It assesses cost drivers that directly affect the cost of a product or service, and uses performance measures to evaluate the financial or nonfinancial benefit an activity provides. By identifying each cost driver and assessing the value the element adds to the health care enterprise, ABM provides a basis for selecting areas that can be changed to reduce costs. *See also* activity-based costing.

ACTUAL: Real or reported price, data, or event. It compares to the theoretical, implied, or hypothetical price, data, or event. The actual or observed data describe or define the underlying process or condition. For example, real patient revenues rather than pro forma estimates of patient revenue.

ACTUAL ACQUISITION COST: Net payment after expenses for provided products, care, or health services.

ACTUAL BUDGET: The amount of money spent in the health care industrial complex, less the amount collected from private patients, third parties, or federal and state health care program payers. The money cannot be used to determine if the health care industrial complex is producing a contracting or expanding economic policy.

ACTUAL CHARGE: The amount of money a medical provider or health care facility submits to a health insurance carrier or insurance company for payment. It is usually more than received.

ACTUAL DEFICIT: The size of the health care industrial complex deficit or surplus actually benchmarked or recorded in any given year.

ACTUAL HEDGING: A bona fide long or short position that is involved in an offsetting transaction, usually in the derivatives market.

ACTUAL INVESTMENT: The amount that the health care industrial complex actually invests in society. It equals planned health care investments plus unplanned investments.

ACTUALS: Real or underlying assets for a derivative medical product or health care commodity market.

ACTUARIAL: Refers to the mathematical and statistical calculations used to determine rates, prices, fee schedules, and/or premiums charged to patients or insurance companies based on projections of health care utilization and cost for a defined population, segment, or cohort.

ACTUARIAL ASSUMPTIONS: Estimate a health care entity uses in establishing premiums, fees, rates, charges, scheduling policy provisions, and projecting future cost increases. The most important assumptions are based on probabilities of illness, accident, and/or death and assumptions about interest and capital gains, as well as sales commissions and other related expenses.

ACTUARIAL COST: A cost derived through the use of actuarial present values estimations.

ACTUARIAL DEFICIT: A negative actuarial balance; a loss.

ACTUARIAL FACTORS: The nomenclature for actuarial assumptions used by the Centers for Medicare and Medicaid Services (CMS).

ACTUARIAL PRESENT VALUE: The current worth of an account payable (AP) or account receivable (AR) in the future, is where each amount is discounted at an assumed rate of interest and adjusted for the probability of its payment or receipt.

ACTUARIAL SOUNDNESS: The requirement that the development of capitation and insurance rates meet common principles and rules.

ACTUARIALLY FAIR: Health insurance plan that is expected to pay out in benefits an amount equal to the premiums paid by patient beneficiaries.

ACTUARY: A mathematician or professional person who determines health insurance policy rates, reserves, and dividends, as well as conducts various other statistical studies.

ACUTE CARE HOSPITAL: A health care organization or "anchor hospital" in which a patient is treated for an acute (immediate and severe) episode of illness or the subsequent treatment of injuries related to an accident or trauma, or during recovery from surgery. Specialized personnel using complex and sophisticated technical equipment and materials usually render acute professional care in a hospital setting. Unlike chronic care, acute care is often necessary for only a short time. Financial and economic measures of acute health care utilization are represented by three separate rates:

- rate of admissions per 1,000 patients,
- average length of stay per admission, and
- total days of care per 1,000 patients.

ADAPTIVE EXPECTATIONS THEORY: The concept that patients determine their personal health care and medical care expectations based on past experiences and change them as events concurrently unfold.

ADDITIONAL BENEFITS: Health care services not covered by Medicare and reductions in premiums or cost sharing for Medicare-covered services. Additional benefits are specified and are offered to Medicare beneficiaries at no additional premium. Those benefits must be at least equal in value to the adjusted excess amount calculated in the adjusted community rating (ACR). An excess amount is created when the average payment rate exceeds the adjusted community rate (as reduced by the actuarial value of coinsurance, co-payments, and deductibles under Parts A and B of Medicare). The excess amount is then adjusted for any contributions to a stabilization fund. The remainder is the adjusted excess, which will be used to pay for services not covered by Medicare or to reduce charges otherwise allowed for Medicare-covered services.

ADDITIONAL BONDS TEST: The earnings test that must be satisfied under the provisions of a hospital or other revenue-type bond contract before bonds of an additional issue having the same lien on a pledged revenue source can be issued. Typically, the test would require that historical revenues plus future estimated revenues (in some cases) exceed projected debt service requirements for both the existing issue and the proposed issue by a certain ratio.

ADDITIONAL PAID-IN CAPITAL: Common stock plus donated capital or paid-in capital excess of par value. It includes other amounts paid by stockholders and charged to equity accounts or capital stock.

ADEQUATE DISCLOSURE: The inclusion of material items in consolidated or other financial statements.

ADJUDICATION: To formally judge or economically review a medical or other claim for payment processing.

ADJUSTABLE RATE: An interest rate that changes according to some defined index (average).

ADJUSTED AVERAGE CHARGE PER DAY (AACPD): The average charge billed by hospitals for one day of care, which is adjusted total charges (ATC) divided by total days of care.

ADJUSTED AVERAGE CHARGE PER DISCHARGE (AACPD): The average charge billed by hospitals for an inpatient stay (from the day of admission to the day of discharge), which is adjusted total charges (ATC) divided by number of discharges.

ADJUSTED AVERAGE PER CAPITA COST (AAPCC): (1) Actuarial projections of per capita Medicare spending for enrollees in fee-for-service Medicare. Separate AAPCCs are calculated, usually at the county level, for Part A services and Part B services for the aged, disabled, and people with End State Renal Disease (ESRD). Medicare pays risk plans by applying adjustment factors to 95% of the Part A and Part B AAPCCs. The adjustment factors reflect differences in Medicare per capita fee-for-service spending related to age, sex, institutional status, Medicaid status, and employment status. (2) A county-level estimate of the average cost incurred by Medicare for each beneficiary in fee for service. Adjustments are made so that the AAPCC represents the level of spending that would occur if each county contained the same mix of beneficiaries. Medicare pays health plans 95% of the AAPCC, adjusted for the characteristics of the enrollees in each plan.

ADJUSTED BASIS: The difference between asset purchase and sale price if any, which determines capital gains profit or loss. After a taxpayer's basis in medical office real estate or property is determined, it must be adjusted upward to include any additions of capital to the property and reduced by any returns of capital to the taxpayer. Additions might include improvements to the property, and subtractions may include depreciation or depletion. The adjusted basis in property is deducted from the amount realized to find the gain or loss on sale or disposition.

ADJUSTED BOOK VALUE METHOD (ABVM): Asset approach business-valuation method where all assets and liabilities are reworked to fair market value (FMV). It is the book value that results after one or more asset or liability amounts are added, deleted, or changed from the respective book (accounting) amounts of the health care or other business entity.

ADJUSTED COVERAGE PER CAPITA COST: Estimate of average monthly health care benefits cost, after certain adjustments.

ADJUSTED DEBIT BALANCE: Margin account determination formula, used and required under Regulation T of the Securities Exchange Commission (SEC).

ADJUSTED EARNINGS: Net earnings from health care operations, plus the estimated value of additional fees, charges, or subscriptions or earnings.

ADJUSTED ENTRIES: End-period accounting entries that assign revenues and expenses to the periods earned and incurred.

ADJUSTED GROSS INCOME (AGI): An important subtotal that serves as the basis for computing percentage limitations on certain itemized personal deductions (e.g., medical and dental expenses, casualty and theft losses, and miscellaneous itemized deductions). The subtotal consists of all income less adjustments to gross income, which is reduced by business and other specified expenses of individual taxpayers. It is also an important figure in the basis of other individual financial planning issues as well as a key line item on the IRS form 1040 and required state forms.

ADJUSTED NET GAIN FROM OPERATIONS: The net gain from health care or other business operations, plus the estimated value of increases in the amount of fees and/or the growth in charges or prices during the year.

ADJUSTED NET WORTH: The worth of a managed care, health insurance. or other company, consisting of capital and surplus, plus an estimated value for the business on the company's books.

ADJUSTED PAYMENT RATE (APR): A Medicare capitated payment to risk-contract HMOs. For a given plan, the APR is determined by adjusting county-level adjusted annual per capita cost (AAPCC) to reflect the relative risks of the health plan's enrollees.

ADJUSTED TOTAL CHARGES: Because OSHPD regulations require that hospitals report charges for the last 365 days of a stay, only total charges for a patient who stays more than one year must be adjusted upward (increased) to reflect the entire stay. Thus, for patients staying longer than one year, the average daily charge for the last year of the stay is calculated and applied to the entire stay. The formula is: (Total Charges ÷ 365 = Charge per Day) × Length of Stay = Adjusted Total Charges.

ADJUSTED TRIAL BALANCE: A list of adjusted balances in ledger accounts, which is used in financial statement preparation.

ADJUSTING JOURNAL ENTRY: Accounting entry made into a subsidiary ledger or General Journal to account for changes, omissions, and/or other financial data required to be reported "in the books" but not usually posted to the journal. This entry is posted to the general ledger accounts usually by number, date, and explanation. Example: MD#1: 12–31–2006, debit cash in bank $3,000. Credit interest income $3,000, to record interest income on medical practice bank account at year end, not recorded in cash receipts journal but credited by the bank.

ADJUSTMENT: A change made to an insurance claim, medical invoice, or other bill.

ADJUSTMENT REASONS: A schedule of insurance code information to explain medical bill or fee schedule changes.

ADJUSTMENTS FOR AGI: Deductions from income to arrive at AGI. These are *"above-the-line"* deductions. This includes ordinary and necessary expenses incurred in a trade or business, half of self-employment tax paid, all alimony paid, certain payments to an IRA, moving expenses, penalty on early withdrawal of savings, Keogh retirement plan and self-employed SEP deductions, and health insurance deduction for self-employed taxpayers. There are no above-the-line deductions for health care or other corporations.

ADJUSTMENTS TO PAYMENT: Difference between actual and estimated number of health plan members determined for advanced payment calculations.

ADMINISTRATIVE COST CENTERS: Health care organizational support units responsible for their own costs.

ADMINISTRATIVE COSTS: All expenses related to utilization review, insurance marketing, medical underwriting, agents' commissions, premium collection, claims processing, insurer profit, quality assurance programs, and risk management. Administrative costs include the costs assumed by a health care entity for administrative services such as billing and overhead costs.

ADMINISTRATIVE LOADING: Usually excessive health care management costs, fees, or sales charges.

ADMINISTRATIVE PROFIT CENTERS: Health care organizational support units responsible for their own profits or fundraising.

ADV: A two-part form filed by investment advisors who register with the Securities and Exchange Commission (SEC), as required under the Investment Advisers Act. ADV Part II information must be provided to potential investors and made available to current investors.

AD-VALOREM: *"According to value"*; a Latin phrase.

AD-VALOREM TAX: A direct tax calculated *"according to value"* of property. Such tax is based on an assigned valuation (market or assessed) of real property and, in certain cases, on a valuation of tangible or intangible personal property. In virtually all jurisdictions, the tax is a lien on the property enforceable by seizure and sale of the property. An ad-valorem tax is normally the one substantial tax that may be raised or lowered by a local governing body without the sanction of superior levels of government (although general restrictions, such as rate limitations, may exist on the exercise of this right). Hence, ad-valorem taxes often function as the balancing element in local budgets.

ADVANCE CHECK: Payment sent to a health care facility or medical provider that precedes the filing of a health insurance claim.

ADVANCE/DECLINE RATIO (A/D RATIO): The number of stocks that have advanced divided by the number that declined over a certain time period. Ratios plotted one after another show the direction of the market, and the steepness of the line shows the strength of that direction.

ADVANCE/DECLINE THEORY: A stock market theory that uses the relative number of advances versus declines in relation to total issues traded on the New York Stock Exchange (NYSE) to make buying and/or selling decisions. This theory measures the breadth of the market.

ADVANCED BENEFICIARY NOTICE (ABN): Notice from a medical provider, health care facility, or DME vendors that informs patients that charges for certain products or medical services may not be covered by Medicare. A signature may indicate patient payment responsibility.

ADVANCED REFUNDING: A procedure where outstanding securities are refinanced by a new issue of securities prior to the date on which the outstanding securities become due, or are callable. Accordingly, for a period of time, both the issue being refunded and the refunding issue are outstanding. The proceeds of the refunding securities are generally invested in U.S. Government or federal agency securities (although other instruments such as bank certificates of deposit are occasionally used), with principal and interest from these securities being used to pay principal and interest on the refunded securities (or, in some cases, interest on the refunding securities and subsequently principal on the refunded securities). Securities are escrowed to maturity when the proceeds of the refunding securities are deposited in escrow for investment in an amount sufficient to pay the principal of and interest on the issue being refunded on the original interest payment and maturity dates. Securities are considered pre-refunded when the refunding issue's proceeds are escrowed only until a call date or dates on the refunded issue, with the refunded issue redeemed at that time.

ADVERSE ACTION: Under HIPAA, adverse actions include:

- civil judgments, such as malpractice suits;
- federal or state criminal convictions;
- license revocation or suspension;
- reprimand, censure, or probation from health plans or hospital medical staff;
- exclusion from participation in any federal or state health programs;
- any adjudicated actions as determined by the Department of Health and Human Services (HHS) regulations; or
- any other federal or state agency negative actions or finding that is publicly available.

ADVERSE OPINION: Auditor's opinion that a firm's financial statements do not accurately reflect its current financial position, operating condition, and/or cash flows in conformity with GAAP.

ADVISOR: A registered individual (registered representative or stockbroker) or organization that is employed by a health care entity, other business, or private individual to give professional advice on its investments and management of its assets and/or endowment funds.

ADVISORY FEE: A fee charged by a financial advisor or services company to a mutual fund, investment account, clinic, medical practice, hospital endowment, and others, based on the average assets. This fee may also be known as a management fee.

ADVISORY LETTER: A written offer of financial, economic, or accounting advice.

AFFIDAVIT: Written statement made under oath before an authorized person such as an attorney or notary public.

AFFILIATED COMPANY: A firm in which there is indirect or direct ownership of 5% or more of outstanding and voting shares.

AFFILIATED PERSON: Anyone in a position to influence decisions made in a health care or other corporation, including officers, directors, principal stockholders, and members of their immediate families. Shares are often referred to as "Control Stock."

AFFILIATION: The legally separate status of a firm within another organization.

AFTER HOURS: Securities trading after regular hours on a stock exchange.

AFTER MARKET: A market for a security either over-the-counter (OTC) or on an exchange after an initial public offering has been made.

AFTER-TAX BASIS: Ratio of pre- to post-tax returns (a 10% taxable asset would have an after-tax return of 6.5% for one in a 35% tax bracket).

AGAINST ACTUALS: A commodity market transaction where futures are exchanged or transferred against a cash position.

AGAINST-THE-BOX: A short securities sale by the owner of a long (owned) securities position.

AGE OF ACCOUNTS: Accounts receivable (AR) or accounts payable (AP) accounting recognition time lapse.

AGE-OF-PLANT RATIO: The average number of years a health care or other entity has owned its own plant and/or equipment (accumulated depreciation / depreciated expense).

AGE REPORTING: Cycle time documentation for health care economic administrative processes, such as claims turnaround time, accounts receivable, reimbursement adjustments, and so forth.

AGENCIES: A colloquial term for securities issued by one of the federal agencies.

AGENCY FUND: Assets fund where the holder agrees to remit the assets, income from the assets, or both, to a specified beneficiary at a specified time.

AGENT: The role of a broker/dealer firm when it acts as an intermediary or broker between its customer and a market maker or contrabroker. For this service the firm receives a stated commission or fee. Also an insurance agent or securities salesperson (stockbroker), or other nonfiduciary.

AGENT'S COMMISSION: The payment of a percentage of the premium generated from a securities sale, insurance policy, or asset sale to the agent/broker by a company.

AGGREGATE: Broad totals of health care or other economic variables such as medical production units, staffing, facility over- or under-capacity, or nurse unemployment.

AGGREGATE AMOUNT: The maximum for which a health plan member is insured for any single incident.

AGGREGATE DEMAND: The ratio between the quantity of a health care good or service demanded, and its price level.

AGGREGATE DEMAND-SUPPLY HEALTH CARE MODEL: The macroeconomic health care model that uses aggregate health care demand, and aggregate health care supply, to explain medical cost pricing levels.

AGGREGATE EXPENDITURES: The total amount spent for final health care products, goods, and services in the domestic economy.

AGGREGATE HEALTH CARE DEBT: The purchasing power of money outstanding that domestic households have borrowed for health care products and services and are obligated to repay.

AGGREGATE HEALTH CARE DEMAND CURVE: An illustrative model of total domestic health care production demanded, measured by real GDP, which varies with price level.

AGGREGATE HEALTH CARE EXPENDITURE: The sum of health care consumption expenditures, investment expenditures, purchases, and net exports during a fiscal year.

AGGREGATE HEALTH CARE PURCHASES: The market value of health care goods, products, and services purchased at any level of income.

AGGREGATE HEALTH CARE QUANTITY DEMANDED: The quantity of final health care goods, products, and services that patients or buyers are willing and able to purchase at a given price.

AGGREGATE HEALTH CARE QUANTITY SUPPLIED: The quantity of final health care goods, products, and services supplied by doctors, hospitals, clinics, facilities, medical care producers, and vendors at a given price.

AGGREGATE HEALTH CARE SUPPLY: The total quantity of health care products, goods, and services supplied or produced at different pricing levels.

AGGREGATE INDEMNITY: Maximum dollar amount collected for a physical disability or period of insurance disability.

AGGREGATE INDEMNITIES: The sum total that can be collected under all health insurance policies applicable to the covered loss.

AGGREGATE LIMIT: Maximum dollar amount of coverage in force under a health insurance policy.

AGGREGATE MARGIN: A margin that compares revenues to expenses for a group of hospitals, rather than a single hospital. The margin is computed by subtracting the sum of expenses for all hospitals in the group from the sum of revenues and dividing by the sum of revenues.

AGGREGATE PPS OPERATING MARGIN/AGGREGATE TOTAL MARGIN: A prospective payment system operating margin, or total margin, that compares revenue to expenses for a group of hospitals, rather than a single hospital. The margin is computed by subtracting the sum of expenses for all hospitals in the group from the sum of revenues and dividing by the sum of revenues.

AGGREGATE REAL INCOME: The real or nominal money income of a nation, industry, health care facility, insurance company, or cohort, adjusted for inflation.

AGGREGATE STOP LOSS: The form of excess health insurance risk coverage that provides protection for the employer against accumulation of claims exceeding a certain level. This is protection against abnormal frequency of claims in total, rather than abnormal severity of a single claim.

AGGREGATE SUPPLY: The relationship between health care price levels and the total quantity of health care goods, products, and services supplied.

AGGREGATE SUPPLY CURVE: An illustration of how the aggregate quantity of goods, products, and services supplied changes with various price levels, all things being equal.

AGGRESSIVE FINANCIAL STRATEGY: Attempt to maximize profit by investing in riskier products or services to obtain higher financial returns.

AGING: Concept where a newly issued health care or other entity debt tends to prepay slower than older or seasoned loans. This aging refers to the underlying collateral and not the securities created upon that collateral or health care entity assets.

AGING REPORT: A schedule of claims processing cycle time, or turnaround time.

AGING SCHEDULE: Method of classifying accounts receivable by the time they were recognized and/or forgiven as a bad-debt expense.

AGREEMENT AMONG UNDERWRITERS: An agreement among members of an underwriting syndicate (investment bankers) specifying securities sales and distribution duties and privileges, among other terms and conditions.

AGREEMENT OF LIMITED PARTNERSHIP: Contractual agreement between limited and general partner(s).

AGWUNOBI, ANDREW, MD, MBA: Former President and CEO of Grady Health System in Atlanta, Georgia.

AIR POCKET: A security that quickly drops in price due to bad internal (non-systemic) corporate news.

AKAIKE'S CRITERION (AC): Useful for selecting among nested health care or other economic models; a number associated with each model: $AIC = \ln(sm^2) + 2m/T$, where m is the number of parameters in the model, and sm^2 is (in an AR(m) example) the estimated residual variance: $sm^2 = $ (sum of squared residuals for model m)/T; the average squared residual for model m.

AKERLOF, GEORGE A.: Koshland Professor of Economics at the University of California, Berkeley, and 2001 Nobel Laureate in Economics. He studied "near rational wage and price setting and the optimal rates of inflation and unemployment."

ALIEN CORPORATION: Company incorporated in a foreign country regardless of where it operates.

ALIGNMENT OF INCENTIVES: The economic arrangement between medical providers in health facilities that allows the sharing of fiscal risks and rewards of patient treatment, care, and intervention.

ALL PAYER RATE SETTING: Older State of Maryland health care cost-containment system that established maximum target payment rates for Medicare, Medicaid, and commercial insurance payers.

ALL PAYER SYSTEM: A system by which all payers of health care bills, such as the government, private insurers, big companies, and individuals, pay the same rates, set by the government, for the same medical service. This system does not allow for cost shifting.

ALL-CLAUSE DEDUCTIBLE: A single deductible to cover patient expenses as the result of the same or similar health insurance clauses within a given time period.

ALL-OR-NONE (AON) OFFERING: A "best-efforts" offering of newly issued securities in which the corporation instructs the investment banker to cancel the entire offering (sold and unsold) if all cannot be distributed.

ALL-OR-NONE (AON) ORDER: An order to buy or sell more than one round lot of securities at one time, and at a designated price or better. It must not be executed until both of these conditions are satisfied simultaneously.

ALLIED MEMBER: A voting member of the New York Stock Exchange (NYSE) who is not a personal member.

ALLIGATOR SPREAD: High commission costs in the options market.

ALLOCATED BENEFITS: Payments for a specific covered medical purpose, up to a set maximum, such as an x-ray, casts, blood test, and so forth.

ALLOCATION BASE: Costing diversification statistic or starting point. It is the determination of corporate costs based on causal relationships.

ALLOCATIVE EFFICIENCY: The condition that exists when health care resources are divided in ways that allow maximum net benefit for their use.

ALLOCATIVE FACTOR: The ability of the health care industrial complex to divide and redivide resources to achieve annual growth that current input supply factors make available.

ALLOTMENT: Portion of securities assigned to each underwriting syndicate (investment banker).

ALLOWABLE CHARGE: The maximum fee that a third party will reimburse a medical provider or health care entity for a given health care product or service.

ALLOWABLE COSTS: Items or elements of a health care institution's costs reimbursable under a payment formula. Allowable costs may exclude, for example, uncovered services, luxury accommodations, costs that are not reasonable, and expenditures that are unnecessary. It is a type of retrospective payment that determines reimbursement rates after all nonmedically necessary expenses and costs.

ALLOWANCE: Deduction from the total value of a health care invoice or bill, as noted on an Explanation of Benefits (EOB) statement.

ALLOWANCE CONTRACTUAL DEDUCTIONS: Accounting method that illustrates the difference between actual health care charges and the influence of third party discounts, prospective payments, and so forth.

ALLOWANCE METHOD: The recording of losses on the basis of estimates, rather than the final actual outcome.

ALLOWANCE FOR UNCOLLECTIBLE ACCOUNTS: Balance sheet entry that lists the total number of accounts that likely will not be collected. These are also known as bad debt expenses (BDEs).

ALLOWANCE UNCOLLECTIBLES: Balance sheet account that estimates a medical provider or health care organization's total amount of patient or vendor accounts receivable (ARs) that likely will not be collected.

ALLOWED AMOUNT: Maximum dollar amount assigned for a medical service or procedure based on various pricing mechanisms. This is also known as a maximum allowable fee.

ALLOWED CHARGE: The reimbursement Medicare approves for physician payment. Typically, Medicare pays 80% of the approved charge, and the beneficiary pays the remaining 20%. The allowed charge for a nonparticipating physician is 95% of that for a participating physician. Nonparticipating physicians may bill beneficiaries for an additional amount above the allowed charge.

ALLOWED EXPENSE: The maximum dollar amount for covered health care expenses that a third party will reimburse for a service or item when a claim is made.

ALPHA: The measure of the amount of a stock's expected return that is not related to the stock's sensitivity to market volatility. It measures the residual nonmarket influences that contribute to a securities risk unique to each security. Alpha uses beta as a measure of risk, a benchmark and a risk-free rate of return (usually T-bills) to compare actual performance with expected performance. For example, a fund with a beta of 0.80 in a market that rises 10% is expected to rise 8%. If the risk-free return is 3%, the alpha would be -0.6%, calculated as follows:

$$(\text{Fund return} - \text{Risk-free return}) - (\text{Beta} \times \text{Excess return})$$
$$= \text{Alpha} (8\% - 3\%) - [0.8 \times (10\% - 3\%)] = -0.6\%$$

A positive alpha indicates outperformance while a negative alpha means underperformance.

ALPHABET STOCK: Common stock categories associated with certain subsidiaries created by restructurings or corporate acquisitions.

ALTERNATE VALUATION: The value of all property, with exceptions, includable in a decedent's gross estate 6 months after the decedent's date of death. If an asset is sold or distributed, its sale price or value on the date of distribution is the alternate value. In either case, the sale or distribution must occur within 6 months of death.

ALTERNATE VALUATION DATE: Six months from the date of death.

ALTERNATIVE COST: An older term for economic opportunity cost.

ALTERNATIVE INVESTMENTS: Investments other than mutual funds, certificates of deposit, or direct investments in equities and bonds, which might comprise a hospital or health care endowment's portfolio. Some alternatives are: art, collectibles, commodities, commodity funds, commodity pools, derivatives, foreign exchange, hedge funds, oil and gas, precious metals, and real estate ventures.

ALTERNATIVE MINIMUM TAX (AMT): An additional federal tax (26–28%) for taxpayers who benefit from the tax laws that allow special treatment to some types of income and special deductions to some types of expenses.

ALTERNATIVE MINIMUM TAX (AMT) BOND: Certain private purpose municipal hospital bonds pay tax-exempt interest that is subject to the AMT. These are called private purpose rather than public purpose because 10% or more of the proceeds goes to private activities. Examples are bonds used to fund large ASCs and public or private hospitals. The Municipal Securities Rulemaking Board (MSRB) rules require that confirmations indicate if the bond is subject to the AMT.

ALTERNATIVE ORDER: Securities order given to a stockbroker between two courses of action, either or, but never both.

ALTMAN, DREW: President and CEO of the Henry J. Kaiser Family Foundation in Menlo Park, California.

AMBAC (AMBAC INDEMNITY CORPORATION): A wholly owned subsidiary of the Mortgage Guarantee Investment Corporation (MGIC) which offers noncancelable insurance contracts by which it agrees to pay a security holder all, or any part, of scheduled principal and interest payments on the securities as they become due and payable, in the event that the issuer is unable to pay. Hospital bonds insured by AMBAC are currently granted a Standard & Poor's rating of AAA.

AMBULANCE LEVY: A tax for free emergency ambulance transport between hospitals at the discretion of the ambulance service.

AMBULATORY PATIENT GROUP/CLASS: (APG/C): Similar or like class of patients receiving ambulatory health care services, goods, or products that are homogenous in nature, diagnosis, treatments, or other demographic benchmarks. Originally called ambulatory payment groups (APGs), they are a set of Medicare payment regulations that were implemented in 2000. Ambulatory patient classes (APCs) replaced previous cost-based and cost plus reimbursement contracts for all outpatient services. The federal government and the Health Care Financing Administration (HCFA), now CMS, planned this shift to prospective payments through the Outpatient Prospective Payment System (OPPS) for more than a decade, as a result of the Omnibus Budget Reconciliation Act of 1986 (OBRA). The APC system is designed to explain the amount and type of resources used in outpatient visits. Each APC consists of patients with similar characteristics and resource usage and includes only the facility portion of the visit, with no impact on providers who will continue to be paid from the traditional CPT-4 fee schedule and modifier system. The APC system will effectively eliminate separate payments for operating, recovery, treatment, and observation room charges. Anesthesia, medical and surgical supplies, pharmaceuticals (except those used in chemotherapy), blood, casts, splints, and donated tissue will also be packaged into the APC. Unbundled, fragmented, or otherwise separated codes will be eliminated from claims prior to payment. APCs were grouped into 346 classes according to ICD-9-CM diagnosis and CPT-4 procedures. There were 134 surgical APCs, 46 significant APCs, 122 medical APCs, and 44 ancillary APCs. Surgical, significant, and ancillary APCs were assigned using only the CPT-4 procedure codes, while medical APCs are based on a combination of ICD-9-CM and E&M CPT-4 codes. Payments are then calculated for each APC by multiplying the facility rate by the APC weight and by a discount factor (if multiple APCs are performed during the same visit). Total payment is the sum of the payments for all APCs. However, no adjustment provisions are made for outliers or teaching facilities, rural hospitals, and disproportionate share or specialty hospitals or facilities. Facilities affected by Medicare's OPPS include those designated by the Secretary of Health and Human Services, such as hospital outpatient surgical centers, hospital outpatient departments not part of the consolidated billing for Skilled Nursing Facility (SNF) residents, certain preventative services and supplies, covered Medicare Part B inpatient services if Part A coverage is exhausted, and partial hospitalization services in Community Mental Health Centers (CMHCs). Exempted facilities include clinical laboratories, ambulance services, end stage renal disease (ESR) centers, occupational and speech therapy services, mammography centers, and durable medical equipment (DME) suppliers. The remaining facilities may experience a slight payment increase if they convert their management information systems (MIS) to APC compliant hardware and software. Compliance measures include electronic interconnectivity, data storage, retrieval, and the security features mandated by the Health Insurance Portability and Accountability Act of 1996 (HIPPA).

AMBULATORY UTILIZATION REVIEW: Clinical or economic health care evaluation of outpatient facilities.

AMERICAN ASSOCIATION OF INDIVIDUAL INVESTORS (AAII): Chicago-based nonprofit organization designed to educate all investors about securities and financial investments.

AMERICAN DEPOSITORY RECEIPT (ADR): A receipt evidencing shares of a foreign corporation held on deposit or under the control of a U.S. banking institution. It is used to facilitate transactions and expedite transfer of beneficial ownership for a foreign security in the United States. Everything is done in U.S. dollars and the ADR holder doesn't have voting rights. An ADR is essentially the same as an American Depository Share (ADS).

AMERICAN DEPOSITORY SHARE (ADS): Similar to an American Depository Receipt (ADR), but an ADS is an instrument that is traded, while an ADR certificate represents a number of ADSs.

AMERICAN INSTITUTE OF CERTIFIED PUBLIC ACCOUNTANTS (AICPA): U.S. professional membership organization that represents practicing CPAs. It establishes ethical and auditing standards and service performance standards, provides guidance for specialized industries, and participates with the Financial Accounting Standards Board (FASB) and the Government Accounting Standards Board (GASB).

AMERICAN SOCIETY OF HEALTH ECONOMICS (ASHE): Domestic association formed to increase communication among health economists, foster a higher standard of debate in the application of economics to health and health care systems, and assist young researchers at the start of their careers. Headquartered in Philadelphia, Pennsylvania.

AMERICAN STOCK EXCHANGE (AMEX): Auction market where sellers and buyers gather in open competition for securities in a central location.

AMERICAN STOCK EXCHANGE PRICE CHANGE INDEX: An unweighted market index for all common stocks listed on the AMEX, prepared hourly.

AMERICAN-STYLE EXERCISE: Option can be exercised at any point prior to expiration.

AMERICAN-STYLE OPTION: An option that can be exercised at any time prior to expiration.

AMORTIZE: To pay off or liquidate a debt on an installment basis.

AMORTIZATION: The allocation of the cost of an intangible asset, such as a CT scanner, over a statutory period. Regular payments are made over a period of time to repay principal and interest on a loan.

AMORTIZATION OF DEBT (LOAN): The process of paying the principal amount of a hospital or other debt security by periodic payments either directly to security holders or to a sinking fund for the benefit of security holders.

AMORTIZATION OF PREMIUM: An accounting process by which the book value of a security purchased at a premium above par is decreased during the security's holding period. The amortization reflects the decrease in the security's holding value as it approaches the redemption date. Under a "straight line" amortization method, the amount of the yearly amortization is the same for all years and is equal to the product of the total amount of the premium divided by the number of years to redemption.

AMOUNT BILLED: Value of health care services or goods rendered by a facility or provider on a bill, invoice, or insurance claim.

AMOUNT, DURATION, AND SCOPE: State Medicaid benefits definition of provided health care services.

AMT BOND: *See* Alternative Minimum Tax (AMT) Bond.

ANALYST: One who studies public companies and makes sell or buy recommendations to individuals or corporations.

ANALYTICAL PROCEDURES: Rigorous tests of financial information that examine relationships among economic data as a means of obtaining evidence. Such procedures include: (1) comparison of financial information with information of comparable prior periods; (2) comparison of financial information with anticipated results; (3) study of relationships between elements of financial information that should conform to predictable patterns based on the entity's experience; and (4) benchmarking of financial information with industry norms (ratio analysis).

ANCILLARY BENEFITS: Secondary benefits provided in a health insurance contract providing coverage, such as benefits provided for miscellaneous hospital charges in a basic room and board hospitalization policy.

ANCILLARY CHARGE: Separated charges for additional health care services such as radiology, anesthesia, or pathology that may exceed a health plan's maximal allowable charges.

ANCILLARY/EXTRAS: These are benefits for health-related services that are not covered by Medicare. Health funds vary considerably in services that they offer as benefits; however, most include services, such as dental, optical, physiotherapy, chiropractic, and naturopathy.

"AND INTEREST": A hospital or other bond transaction in which the buyer pays the seller a contract price plus interest accrued since the issuer's last interest payment. Virtually all interest bearing bonds always trade *"and interest."*

ANDERSON, GERARD: Professor of public health and medicine at Johns Hopkins University in Baltimore, Maryland.

ANDERSON, RON, MD: President and CEO of Parkland Health and Hospital System in Dallas, Texas.

ANGEL: A wealthy private investor.

ANKLE BITER: A high-risk and smaller capitalized company. This is a slang term.

ANNUAL ADJUSTMENT: Bilateral health care contract economic provision that allows each party the opportunity to review the terms and conditions of an existing insurance contract for possible financial modifications.

ANNUAL BASIS: Statistical method annualized financial figures of less than 12 months coverage.

ANNUAL DEDUCTIBLE: Yearly minimal threshold payment for most health insurance plans, including Medicare, Medicaid, and others.

ANNUAL EXCLUSION: IRS regulation that allows one to exclude certain types and amounts of income from taxation. The annual exclusion for gifts made in 2006 is $12,000, indexed.

ANNUAL FEES: Predetermined pricing in concierge medicine based on the desired number of patients in a practice. The number of patients in such a model can range from 100 individuals to more than 1,000 patients.

ANNUAL LIMIT: The maximum amount for a health benefit that will be paid in a continuous 12 month period, either calendar year or membership year. If transferred from another health fund, the calculation may or may not include claims paid by the previous fund.

ANNUAL PERCENT RATE (APR): Annual cost to borrow money funds, with full disclosure under the Truth in Lending Act (TLA-Regulation Z).

ANNUAL PREMIUM: The premium amount required on an annual basis under the contractual requirements of a policy to keep a health insurance policy in force.

ANNUAL REPORT: Yearly report sent to a public firm's shareholders. It is a formal statement issued yearly by a hospital, health care firm, or other company to its shareowners. It lists assets, liabilities, equity revenues, expenses, and so on, and is a reflection of the corporation's condition at the close of the business year (balance sheet) and earnings performance (income statement).

ANNUAL REPORT SUMMARY: A summary of assets and liabilities, receipts and disbursements, current value assets, present value of vested benefits, and any other financial information about an insurance plan and company that must be provided annually to participants.

ANNUALIZE: To convert to an annual basis.

ANNUITANT: A person who receives a distribution from an annuity contract.

ANNUITIZE: The progression of an annuity contract from the accumulation or lump sum stage to the payout distribution sage. To distribute funds in a periodic fashion over time.

ANNUITY: A series of equal periodic payments. An insurance investment product in which an investor contributes money into a plan and then elects to receive pay-out in a fixed or variable amount, usually at retirement. Two important features of this product: (1) Tax deferred growth of earnings during the accumulation period. However, it is important to note that when you elect to receive payment you will be taxed at ordinary income rates on everything exceeding the cost basis. (2) The annuity will provide lifetime retirement income for the annuitant through the mortality guarantee. There are two basic forms: fixed and variable. A fixed annuity can make a lump sum payment or periodic lifetime payments to the annuitant. A variable annuity has a separate account attached to the annuity contract. This type of contract is considered a security, because it is dependent on equities, and its total value is subject to fluctuate due to market risk. There are several annuity varieties: Annuity Certain, Annuity Due, Deferred Annuity, Fixed Annuity, Life Annuity, Ordinary Annuity, Perpetuity, Variable Annuity, and others.

ANNUITY CERTAIN: Annuity that pays a predetermined monthly benefit for a specific time period.

ANNUITY DUE: A series of equal periodic payments made at the beginning of the period.

ANNUITY FACTOR: A multiplication factor for the first annuity cash flow amount that represents the Present Value (PV) of the remaining annuity corpus.

ANNUITY UNIT: Unit used to value the separate account of an annuity during the pay-out (annuity) phase. The number of annuity units is a fixed amount designated when electing to annuitize. With a variable annuity, the value of the units will vary according to the performance of the investments in the separate account, while in a fixed annuity the value remains constant.

ANTICIPATED HOLDING PERIOD: The time period an asset is expected to be owned.

ANTICIPATED INFLATION: The estimated rate of health care inflation based on reasonable economic assumptions and previous history.

ANTICIPATION NOTE: A short-term liability extinguished by specific revenues.

ANTICIPATORY HEDGING: The placement of a hedge prior to placement of the actual position. This sometimes occurs when a firm knows that it will receive investment funds later that day or week and prefers to hedge numerous potential risks at the earlier date.

ANTIDILUTION: Environment that may increase the computation of EPS or decrease loss per share solely because of the inclusion of common stock equivalents, such as options, warrants, convertible debt, or convertible preferred stock, and so forth.

ANTIDILUTIVE: Common stock conversion method that increases, rather than decreases, earnings per share.

ANTIKICKBACK STATUTES: Forbids payer, facility, medical provider, and family member referral payments (kickbacks) for Medicare and Medicaid patients as reviewed by the Office of Inspector General (OIG). *See also* Stark I; Stark II.

ANTIREBATE LAWS: State laws that prohibit an insurance agent or company from giving part of the premium back to the insured as an inducement to buy health or other insurance coverage.

ANTITRUST EXEMPTION: State action immunity providing exclusions from federal antitrust review under certain safe-harbor guidelines for health care joint ventures or mergers and acquisitions.

ANTITRUST LAWS: Legislation, such as the Sherman and Clayton Acts, to promote health care competition and control monopoly.

ANTITRUST STATUTES: Laws that attempt to prevent unfair health care business practices that may give rise to monopoly power.

APPARENT AUTHORITY: An agent's power to bind an organization to third-party contracts.

APPEAL: Reconsideration request for a nonpayment of a medical claim.

APPLEYARD, DIANE: President and CEO of Health Care Research and Development Institute in Pensacola, Florida.

APPLICATION FEE: Fees that are paid upon application.

APPRAISAL: The act or process of determining value, especially for a health care business entity, clinic or medical practice, and so forth. It is synonymous with valuation.

APPRAISAL COSTS: The expenses incurred to detect poor quality product or goods.

APPRAISAL REPORT: Written report by an appraiser containing an opinion as to value and the reasoning leading to that opinion.

APPRAISED VALUE: A business appraiser's or medical practice valuator's conclusion. It is an opinion of value.

APPRECIATION: Asset value increase in response to inflation, and/or through increases in market supply-and-demand factors.

APPROPRIATIONS: Government sponsored fundraising for a specific purpose and time period.

APPROVED AMOUNT: Reasonable fee limits sanctioned by Medicare in a given area of covered service. The fee is approved by payment by private health plans, and the items are likely reimbursed by the insurance company. It may or may not be the same as the approved charge.

APPROVED CHARGE: Limits of expenses paid by Medicare in a given area of covered service. The charges may be wholly or proportionally approved for payment by private health plans, and the items may or may not be reimbursed by a health insurance company.

APPROVED SERVICES: Services and supplies covered under an insurance agreement, contract, or certificate within the benefit period.

APPROXIMATE PERCENT COST: Estimate of the annualized interest rate incurred by not taking a health care insurance premium or similar other product or service discount.

ARBITRAGE: The simultaneous purchase and sale of the same or equal securities, such as convertible securities, in such a way as to take advantage of price differences prevailing in separate markets. The risk is usually minimal and the profit correspondingly small.

ARBITRAGE PRICE THEORY (APT): A multivariable systematic risks method to estimate the cost of equity capital.

ARBITRATION: A system offered under various Standards Review Organization (SRO) rules for resolving disputes, under which two parties who have a disagreement involving a securities transaction may submit the disagreement to an impartial panel for resolution. Securities dealers may be compelled to arbitrate disputes. Customers cannot be compelled to arbitrate disputes involving securities law claims, although they can be forced to resolve general contractual disputes through arbitration if a valid arbitration agreement had been previously executed. Decisions of an arbitration panel are binding on the parties to the claim.

ARGES, GEORGE: Senior director of the health data management group for the American Hospital Association in Chicago, Illinois.

ARITHMETIC MEAN: The sum of a set of numbers (data points) divided by the number of data numbers (data points) in the set $3 + 5 = 8 \div 2 = 4$.

ARITHMETIC MEAN LENGTH OF STAY (AMLOS): Benchmark average for utilization analysis of hospital inpatient time for a given diagnostic related group (DRG).

ARMS' LENGTH TRANSACTION: Economic dealings void of conflicts-of-interest and conducted as though the parties were unrelated.

ARREARAGE: Overdue payments. These are cumulative preferred stock dividends that have been aggregated but not paid out.

ARREARS: Health care, insurance, or other entity or membership contributions that have not been paid by the due date.

ARREARS AND ADVANCES: Any salary, accounts receivable, accounts payable, and so forth, as the total of amount due up to and including the current week or month. Advances are the total premiums paid in advance of the current week or month.

ARRICK, MARTIN: Senior not-for-profit health care analyst at Standard & Poor's in New York City.

ARROVIAN UNCERTAINTY: Measurable risk or variations in possible outcomes on the basis of knowledge or believed health care economic or financial assumptions a priori.

ARROW, KENNETH J., PhD: Authority who helped formalize the separate and distinct field of health economics and whose many interests have led to significant contributions in areas such as social policy, risk management and asset allocation, portfolio optimization, asymmetric information interchange, and medical insurance. In 1963 he introduced the idea of moral hazard and adverse selection. He revised the way people viewed health and economics by exploring the relationship between insurers who do not observe medical care needs, and insured who overuse care, because physicians must side with them. The subsequent establishment of HMOs attempted to overcome overutilization by allowing the same delivery organization to provide the health insurance. He also has examined insurance annuities and demonstrated that those who buy them for income after a certain age live longer than those who buy regular life insurance. In 1972 he received the Nobel Prize, and in 2004 he was selected as one of eight recipients of the 2004 National Medal of Science. Now 84, Dr. Arrow is the Joan Kenney Professor of Economics and Professor of Operations Research, Emeritus, as well as a senior fellow at the Center for Health Policy at Stanford's Freeman Spogli Institute for International Studies, the Center for Primary Care and Outcomes Research at Stanford School of Medicine, and the Stanford Institute for Economic Policy Research.

ARROW-PRATT MEASURE: Attribute of a health care utility risk aversion or function u(c); defined by: $RA = -u''(c)/u'(c)$. It is invariant to the utility function, because it does not affect the preferences expressed by u( ). If RA( ) is decreasing in c, then u( ) displays *decreasing absolute risk aversion*. If RA( ) is increasing in c, then u( ) displays *increasing absolute risk aversion*. If RA( ) is constant with respect to changes in c, then u( ) displays *constant absolute risk aversion*.

ARTICLES OF INCORPORATION: State documents filed by the founders of a corporation.

AS OF: A financial transaction processed on one date, but actually conducted on a different date.

ASIAN OPTION: Option contract settled on the average value of the underlying asset during the contract period.

ASK PRICE: (1) The price at which a health care security, stocks, bonds, or mutual fund's shares can be purchased. The asking or offering price means the net asset value per share plus sales charge. (2) The offer side of a quote.

ASSEMBLY OF FINANCIAL STATEMENTS: Presentation of accounting or data-processing services, the output of which is in the form of financial statements to be used solely for internal medical management and/or decision-making purposes. It is non-FASP and non-GAAP.

ASSERTION: Representations by medical management that are contained in financial statements and for which an auditor obtains and evaluates evidential matter when forming an opinion.

ASSESSED VALUATION: The appraised worth of hospital or other property set by a taxing authority for purposes of ad-valorem taxation. It is important to note that the method of establishing assessed valuation varies from state to state, with the method generally specified by state law.

ASSESSMENT: The regular collection, analysis, and sharing of information about health conditions, risks, and resources in a community. The assessment function is needed to identify trends in illness, injury, and death; the factors that may cause these events; available health resources and their application; unmet needs; and community perceptions about health issues.

ASSET: Resources (human resources, time, money, equipment, cognitive knowledge, etc.) and other inputs used to produce a health care output, and one of three major balance sheet categories. It is any owned item, real or intangible, of exchange or commercial value, such as the resources owned by a clinic, health care, or other organization. This includes everything of value that a health care company owns or has due: cash, investments, money due, materials, inventories, which are called current assets; buildings and machinery, which are fixed assets; and patents and good will, which are intangible assets.

ASSET ALLOCATION: Apportioning of the investment portfolio among categories of assets, such as money market instruments, stocks, bonds, put and call options, and possibly tangible assets such as precious metals, real estate, and collectibles. The portfolio manager of an asset allocation mutual fund has more latitude than that of any other. *See also* modern portfolio theory.

ASSET BACKED SECURITIES: Loan vouched for by company accounts receivable, insurance, or other assets. Security backed by notes or receivables against assets other than health care entity or medical practice real estate.

ASSET BASED APPROACH: Medical practice valuation method using assets net of liabilities.

ASSET CLASS: Category of assets. The three main asset classes are stocks, bonds, and cash.

ASSET COVERAGE, OVERALL: Percentage of total assets, to the aggregate of all prior obligations, including the liquidation value of specific securities issues under consideration. The ratio of total assets to the sum of all prior obligations, including the liquidation value of the specific issue under consideration.

ASSET DEMAND FOR MONEY: The quantity of money patients hold as a store of value (save), and which varies inversely with interest rates, especially for HSA and MSA accounts.

ASSET FINANCING: The conversion of certain assets to working-cash in exchange for a security or ownership interest in them as collateral.

ASSET LIMIT USE: Assets limited to a specific purpose.

ASSET MERGER MODEL: A legal model for mature and integrated health care delivery systems using a top-down economic management approach.

ASSET MIX: Percentage of assets relative to the total number of assets in a health care or other organization.

ASSET PLAY: Attractive value stock with a currently depressed price.

ASSET PURCHASE: The acquisition of tangible or intangible health care or other resources that are expected to produce income or appreciate over time.

ASSET STRIPPER: The sale of large assets to repay large debts.

ASSET TURNOVER: A financial ratio or proportion of net sales to revenues, divided by average asset value, during a specific sales or revenue generating period.

ASSET VALUE, PER COMMON SHARE: The current net market value of a firm's resources (after netting out preferred stock liquidation value, liabilities, and accrued dividends), divided by the number of current common shares outstanding.

ASSET VALUE, PER PREFERRED SHARE: The current net market value of a firm's resources (after netting out preferred stock liquidation value, liabilities, and accrued dividends), divided by the number of current preferred shares outstanding.

ASSETS, COMPANY: Those assets that include all funds, property, goods, securities, rights, or resources of any kind, less such items as are declared nonadmissible by state laws. Nonadmissible items consist mainly of deferred or overdue insurance premiums.

ASSETS, LIMITED: Funds available for specific functions and not for general use.

ASSETS UNDER MANAGEMENT (AUM): Total assets under a portfolio's manager's control, for which a fee is charged (usually 1%).

ASSETS VALUE: Net market value on a per share basis.

ASSIGN: To transfer ownership.

ASSIGNMENT: The noncourt affiliated liquidation of a health care entity, business, or other firm. The form imprinted on a registered securities certificate which, when completed and signed by the registered owner, authorizes the transfer of the security into the name of a new owner (designated on the form as the "assignee"). The assignment also usually provides for the granting by the registered owner of power of attorney to another person (usually the new owner or someone acting on his or her behalf) to accomplish the transfer. Assignments are often executed by the registered owner "in-blank," with the name of the assignee and the person granted power of attorney filled in subsequently.

ASSIGNMENT BENEFITS: Payment of medical benefits directly to the provider or health care facility, rather than the patient.

ASSIGNMENT CLAIM: Medical claims reimbursement arrangement where a provider submits a claim for a patient and is paid by the HMO or insurance plan directly, and accepts it as payment-in-full.

ASSIGNMENT NOTIFICATION: By the Options Clearing Corporation (OCC) to the writer (seller) of an option that the holder has exercised the option and the terms of the settlement must now be met. The OCC makes assignments on a random basis.

ASSIMILATION: New stock absorption by the public after all shares are sold by the underwriting syndicate of investment banks.

ASSOCIATED PERSON: Any partner, officer, director, or other employee of a stockbroker or dealer other than persons whose functions are solely clerical or administrative. In the case of a bank dealer, the term refers only to persons who are involved in the bank dealer's activities (or have some control over them). Associated persons are most often (but not always) registered as representatives or principals.

ASSOCIATION FOR INVESTMENT MANAGEMENT AND RESEARCH (AIMR): The nonprofit organization that confers the professional designation of Chartered Financial Analyst (CFA©) on those who pass a three-leveled examination process. Practitioners are also known as securities analysts. The new current name of the organization is the CFA© Institute.

ASSUMED-INTEREST-RATE (AIR): The rate of interest used by a health insurance company to calculate its reserves. Historically, this rate is usually rather low, from 2% to 3% for sake of safety.

ASSUMPTION: The act of taking on the liabilities of another company. Also, the foundation on which health care economic and financial models are built.

ASSUMPTION OF FINANCIAL RISK: The prospective economic risk that a HMO or MCO bears on behalf of its member, according to financial rule CFR-42.

ASYMMETRIC INFORMATION: Differing degrees of relevant economic and financial information in which to make informed health care decisions.

AT PAR: The price of securities at face value.

AT RISK: Contract in which a medical provider and payer receives a certain payment amount for care. Cost overrides are not additionally compensated.

AT RISK LIMITATIONS: The at risk limitations (rules) affect investor basis and are important because investor cost basis establishes an upper limit on deductions. For those investments that are affected by the at risk limitations, the investor is only allowed to include recourse debt in his basis.

AT THE CLOSE ORDER: A securities order executed at a stock market at the close of trading for the day.

AT THE MARKET: A security sold at the next available market price.

AT THE MONEY: An option is at the money if the underlying security is selling for the same price as the exercise price of the option.

AT THE OPENING ORDER: An order to buy or sell at a limit price on the initial transaction of the day for a given security. If unsuccessful, it is automatically canceled.

ATTRIBUTION RULES: Securities tax treatment by affiliates or familial relatives as if owned by the taxpayer.

AUCTION MARKET: A market for securities, typically found on a national securities exchange, in which trading in a particular security is conducted at a specific location with all qualified persons at that post able to bid or offer securities against orders via outcry.

AUDIT: An examination of a health care firm's financial statements and the systems, records, and accounting records and controls that produced them. There are several types of audits that a health care organization might need to perform:

- Baseline audits are preliminary assessments to develop a reference point. Until a health care organization establishes a track record with items such as coding accuracy, billing, or documentation to support medical necessity, it is difficult to determine any performance issues. In the spirit of collegiality the information that is shared should be done in a nonpunitive manner to demonstrate that the intent of the process is to create a positive environment geared toward fixing the problems.
- Periodic audits are performed on an ongoing basis depending on the volume of billing. These may occur weekly for a large multispecialty ambulatory clinic to quarterly for a small medical practice. These periodic audits can be random or scheduled.
- New employee audits are needed until there is confidence in their capabilities. Background checks are often helpful to find out whether there are any potential financial conflicts. In hospitals, health plans, surgery centers, and other regulated facilities, background checks are a normal part of the credentialing process. This process typically includes Medicare violations, which would show up on the National Practitioner Data Bank report. However, independent medical practices do not have access to this type of information and may have to rely on other organizations to obtain the information. The OIG and the General Services Administration both maintain a database of excluded persons and entities that can be accessed through the Internet. As part of the organization's initial and periodic audits, queries of these two databases should be performed for all employees and independent contractors (*locum tenens* physicians). Failure to do so can put the practice at risk of large civil money penalties ($10,000 for each occurrence) and liability for refunds of all claims the excluded individual had part in providing or billing.

- Consumer and beneficiary complaint audits are like HIPAA privacy complaints, and the current Medicare program is heavily geared toward responding to consumer or beneficiary complaints. The Medicare program relies on patients to be the first party to indicate a problem with an individual practitioner billing pattern or health care organization claims submissions in order to initiate the investigation process. The entire system is focused on capturing complaints and evaluating what is true and factual.

AUDIT ADJUSTMENT REPORT: Medicare audit statement of proposed medical provider cost changes.

AUDIT DOCUMENTATION: The basis for an auditor's conclusions that provide the support for audit representations, whether contained in a report or otherwise (i.e., working papers).

AUDIT ENGAGEMENT: Agreement between an auditor or accountant, and clients, to perform an audit.

AUDIT RISK: Chance or uncertainty that an auditor may unknowingly fail to appropriately modify opinions on financial statements that are materially misstated.

AUDIT SAMPLING: Application of procedures to less than 100% of the items within an account balance or cohort of transactions for the purpose of evaluating some characteristic of the balance or class.

AUDIT TRIAL: A sequential accounting record tracing source documents, papers, electronic transactions, and financial transactions.

AUDITING STANDARDS: Professional AICPA guidelines (GAAP) to which an auditor adheres, as well as heuristic judgments in performance and report preparation (FASB).

AUDITOR: One who evaluates a medical provider's utilization, cost, delivery quality, quantity, and level of medical care for reimbursement purposes. One who audits financial accounts and records, both private and public accounting firms registered with the Public Company Accounting Oversight Board.

AUDITOR'S REPORT: The certification and written report of an auditor's findings, including adjustments, if needed.

AUNT MILLIE: A disparaging slang term for an unsophisticated investor, especially a doctor or medical professional.

AUTHORITY: A unit or agency of government established to perform specialized functions, usually financed by service charges, fees, or tolls, although it may also have taxing powers. In many cases, authorities have the power to issue debt that is secured by the lease rental payments made by a governmental unit using the facilities constructed with bond proceeds. An authority may function independently of other governmental units, or it may depend upon other units for its creation, funding, or administrative oversight. Examples of authorities include hospital and health facilities authorities, industrial development authorities, and housing authorities.

AUTHORIZATION APPROACH: A top-down authoritarian approach to financial, health care, or business management with little rank-and-file input.

AUTHORIZED STOCK SHARES: The maximum number of shares permitted by a State Secretary and issued by a newly chartered hospital, health care, or other corporation.

AUTOCORRELATION: The statistical dependency of financial items within a time series.

AUTOMATED TELLER MACHINE (ATM): Machine that allows a customer to perform common teller transactions, such as cash withdrawals and transfers. It is generally accessible 24 hours a day, 7 days a week.

AUTOMATIC CLEARING HOUSE (ACH): Electronic check processing between banks and financial institutions, and customers, hospitals, and clinical and medical practices.

AUTOMATIC EXERCISE: Occurs after an option expires. Each exchange and its clearing house have rules that govern this exercise. There are minimum in-the-money requirements. A holder of an option must inform the clearing house not to automatically exercise an option. These instructions not to exercise may be due to relatively high transaction costs, increases in position limits, or unacceptable alterations in position profiles.

AUTOMATIC INVESTMENT PLAN: A service that allows investors to invest automatically, by transferring money from bank or brokerage accounts at regular intervals.

AUTOMATIC REINVESTMENT: The option available to security or mutual fund shareholders whereby fund income dividends and capital gains distributions are automatically put back into the fund to buy new shares and thereby build up holdings.

AUTOMATIC STABILIZERS: Federal expenditures or receipts that solidify the economy without Congressional intervention.

AUTOMATIC STAY: A bankruptcy court petition to prevent creditor prepetition debt collection.

AUTONOMOUS HEALTH CARE CONSUMPTION: The portion of annual consumer health care purchases that is not affected, or is independent of, current disposable income.

AUTONOMOUS HEALTH CARE PURCHASES: Health care purchases or autonomous consumption that induce a shift in aggregate purchases.

AVERAGE: The arithmetic and mathematical mean of a set of data points. The total divided by a proportion.

AVERAGE ANNUAL COMPOUND RETURN: The simple rate of return at the end of a specified calendar period, assuming all dividends and capital gains, stated as the percentage gained or lost per dollar invested.

AVERAGE ANNUAL TOTAL RETURN: The average annual profit or loss realized at the end of a specified calendar period, assuming all dividends and capital gains, stated as the percentage gained or lost per dollar invested.

AVERAGE CHARGE PER DAY: The average charge billed by hospitals for one day of care, which is adjusted total charges (ATC) divided by total days of care. Only patients discharged are included in this calculation.

AVERAGE CHARGE PER STAY (ACS): The average charge billed by hospitals for an inpatient stay (from the day of admission to the day of discharge), which is adjusted total charges (ATC) divided by number of discharges. Only patients discharged are included.

AVERAGE COLLECTION PERIOD (ACP): The number of days needed to collect accounts receivable (ARs).

AVERAGE COST: Total costs divided by the number of output units, produced over time.

AVERAGE COST METHOD: Medical inventory costing method that equates ending inventory using a weighted average unit cost. When prices are rising, cost of goods sold is less than under LIFO, but more than that under FIFO, and hence income manipulation is also possible.

AVERAGE COST PER CLAIM (ACPC): Approved and allowable clinical and administrative health care charges for services provided as listed within admissions, physician, and outpatient categories.

AVERAGE COST PRICING RULE: A marketplace theory that sets health care prices equal to their average total cost.

AVERAGE DAILY BALANCE (ADB): Mean dollar amount in an account over a specific period of time. The formula for calculating the ADB is accomplished by adding the daily balances over a period of time and dividing by the total number of days in that period.

AVERAGE DAILY CENSUS (ADC): The number of patients serviced each day, divided by the number of service days in a given time period. It is also known as the mean daily patient census.

AVERAGE DOWN: Sequential securities or other goods, purchased over time as share prices or costs fall.

AVERAGE EARNINGS CLAUSE: An optional provision in a disability income insurance policy that permits the company to limit the monthly income disability benefits to the amount of his or her average earnings for the 24 months prior to the disability. This is generally found only in guaranteed renewable and noncancelable policies.

AVERAGE EQUITY: A brokerage trading account's average daily balance.

AVERAGE FIXED COST: Total fixed cost per unit of health care output. The total fixed health care costs divided by output produced over a given time.

AVERAGE HOURLY EXPENSE: Salaries and wages paid to all employees in a specific health care cost center or service and in a given classification for hours worked divided by the total hours worked by those employees.

AVERAGE INPUT COST: The cost or price of a health care input.

AVERAGE LENGTH OF STAY (ALOS): The sum of hospital patient days, divided by the number of patients served in a given time period. It is also known as the mean length of patient stay.

AVERAGE MARKET PRICE: Total share price divided by the number of investments.

AVERAGE MATURITY: Mean time to maturity for a portfolio basket of fixed term debt investments. Bond investors can determine a mean for the maturity dates of a portfolio's debt securities to come up with the portfolio's average maturity. Generally, the longer the average maturity, the greater the portfolio's sensitivity to interest rate changes, which means more price fluctuation.

AVERAGE MONTHLY WAGE: Figures per week used to determine a worker's primary insurance amount (PIA) for Social Security benefits or worker's compensation.

AVERAGE PAYMENT PERIOD: Ratio that suggests how long it takes for a medical provider or health care organization to pay its bills.

AVERAGE PAYMENT RATE: The amount of money that the Centers for Medicare and Medicaid Services (formerly HCFA) could conceivably pay an HMO for services to Medicare recipients under an at risk contract.

AVERAGE PRODUCT, INPUT: Total health care product or service input produced over a given time period, divided by the number of units of that input used.

AVERAGE PRODUCT, LABOR: Total health care output per unit of labor.

AVERAGE PROPENSITY TO CONSUME (HEALTH CARE): The fraction of total disposable income spent on health care consumption, equal to personal consumption expenditures, divided by disposable income. Health care consumption divided by disposable income.

AVERAGE PROPENSITY TO SAVE (HEALTH CARE): The fraction of total disposable income saved on health care consumption, equal to personal production, divided by disposable income. Health care savings divided by disposable income.

AVERAGE REVENUE: Total health care or other revenue received per unit of good, product, or service sold.

AVERAGE REVENUE PRODUCT: Total health care revenue divided by the quantity of the health care product or service produced.

AVERAGE TAX RATE: Total taxes paid divided by total taxable income.

AVERAGE TOTAL COST: Total costs of a health care corporation divided by its health care outputs. Average fixed costs plus average variable costs.

AVERAGE UNIT COST: The average unit cost of all lots of securities held in an asset management account. The sum of share prices, multiplied by price, and divided by total units.

AVERAGE VARIABLE COST: Variable cost divided by the number of units of health care or other products, services, or outputs produced over a period of time.

AVERAGE WHOLESALE PRICE (AWP): Commonly used in pharmacy contracting, the AWP is generally determined through reference to a common source of information.

AVERAGES: Various ways of measuring the trend of securities prices, including the most popular Dow Jones Industrial Average of 30 stocks listed on the New York Stock Exchange. The average is computed by totaling the prices of the 30 stocks and then dividing by a divisor that is intended to compensate for past stock splits and stock dividends. As a result, point changes have a transient relationship to dollar price changes in stocks, which are included in the average.

AVERAGING: A system of buying securities at regular intervals with a fixed dollar amount at the dollar's worth rather than by the number of shares. In the long run, more shares end up being purchased when prices are low rather than high. *See also* dollar cost averaging.

AVOIDABLE COST: Variable or incremental cost. *See also* out-of-pocket expense.

AVOIDABLE FIXED COST: A fixed cost that may no longer be needed if the medical product line, or health care service, is discontinued.

AWAIT INSTRUCTIONS: Designation for matching of financial transactions. It also refers to additional handling instructions for a transaction for a specific account. Such instructions supersede the standard or default instructions.

AWAY FROM THE MARKET: A low limit order or higher offer price than current market value of a security.

B

B2B: Business to Business.

B2C: Business to Consumer (Client).

B2P: Business to Patient.

BABY BONDS: Bonds that have denominations of less than $1,000 per bond.

BACK DATING: The predating of a letter of intent to allow an investor to incorporate recent large deposits for the purpose of qualifying for a load discount on a purchase of open-end investment company shares.

BACK END LOAD: A surrender charge deducted in some financial and insurance products. Most have a decreasing back end load that generally disappears completely after a certain number of years.

BACK FLOW: The return of a health care labor force to its country of origin.

BACK LOG: Medical claims not paid or adjudicated.

BACK SPREAD: Holding position that occurs when more options are purchased relative to the number sold. It is a strategy placed in the expectation of a dramatic move.

BACK UP: The reverse of a market trend.

BACK UP LINE: Line of credit if new credit notes cannot be secured to cover maturing older notes.

BACK UP WITHHOLDING: Financial payers of interest, dividends, and other reportable payments must withhold income tax funds at a rate equal to the fourth lowest rate applicable to single filers if they fail to supply a federal ID number or certify that they are not subject to it.

BACKING AWAY: Failure to make good on a bid for a minimum number of securities.

BACKWARD BENDING HEALTH CARE LABOR SUPPLY CURVE: A graphical curve suggesting that the substitution effect on a health care worker's labor services outweighs the income effect only at relatively low wages.

BACKWARD INTEGRATION: Company acquisition of its suppliers and vendors.

BACKWARDATION: A market condition where the deferred or more forward delivery months are at a progressive discount to the spot or nearby month.

BAD DEBT EXPENSE: Amount owed to a health care or other business entity that will not be paid.

BAIL OUT: To sell securities fast regardless of price.

BAKED-IN-THE CAKE: A slang term for some factor already reflected in a securities market price, such as adverse publicity, a charge-back, natural disaster, and so on.

BAKER, ROSS: Chairman for the Association of University Programs in Health Administration in Washington, D.C.

BALANCE: The residual amount of money due a company from its agent after all credits and charges are calculated. It is the sum of debit entries minus the sum of credit entries. If positive, the difference is called a debit balance. If negative, the difference is called a credit balance.

BALANCE AVAILABLE: The amount of money that can be withdrawn from a savings or checking account without any limitation. The available balance does not include funds on hold or interest not yet posted.

BALANCE BILLING: (1) Physician charges in excess of Medicare or contractually allowed amounts, for which Medicare or contractual patients are responsible, subject to a limit. (2) In Medicare and private fee-for-service health insurance, the practice of billing patients in excess of the amount approved by the health plan. In Medicare, a balance bill cannot exceed 15% of the allowed charge for nonparticipating physicians.

BALANCE CURRENT: Amount of money in a savings or checking account, including funds on hold but excluding interest not yet posted.

BALANCE OF PAYMENTS DEFICIT: Situation where the sum of the balance on current health care accounts and the balance on the capital account is negative.

BALANCE OF PAYMENTS SURPLUS: Situation where the sum of the balance on current health care accounts and the balance on the capital account is positive.

BALANCE ON CAPITAL ACCOUNT: Capital inflows less outflows.

BALANCE ON CURRENT ACCOUNTS: Health care exports less imports, plus net investment income and transfers.

BALANCE ON GOODS AND SERVICES: Health care exports less imports.

BALANCE SHEET: One of four major financial statements for a health care organization. It presents a summary of assets, liabilities, and net assets for a specific date. It is a condensed statement showing the nature and amount of assets and liabilities, shown in dollar amounts, including what the company owns, what it owes, and the ownership interest (shareholders' equity).

BALANCE SHEET EQUATION: Assets equal liabilities plus stockholder's (owner's) equity.

BALANCE SHEET RESERVE: Amount expressed as a liability on a company's balance sheet for benefits owed to owners.

BALANCE SHEET RESERVE PLAN: A funding plan that sets up a bookkeeping entry acknowledging some or all of the liability incurred for the payment of benefits and taking this liability into account in determining profits and the stockholders' equity.

BALANCED BUDGET ACT: Title IV, in 1997, that included financial provisions for Medicaid, Medicare, Medicare+Choice, child care, Medical Savings Accounts, Health Savings Accounts, Medigap plans, rural health care, military retirees, and other health care economic initiatives.

BALANCED FUND: Investment portfolio or mutual fund that strives to minimize market risks while at the same time earning reasonable current income with varying percentages of bond, preferred, and common stocks.

BALANCED INVESTMENT: Assets or securities purchased to obtain high returns with a low-risk strategic position.

BALANCED SECURITY: A health care economic concept used in needs analysis to determine the amount of income a family would require should the chief wage earner die or become sick, hospitalized, or disabled. It is based on the accounting concept of income versus expenses.

BALLOON INTEREST: The final large interest payment needed to retire a debt.

BALLOON MATURITY: Maturity within a serial issue of securities that contains a disproportionately large percentage of the principal as the amount of original issue. It is generally distinguished from a term bond by the presence of serial maturities in the years immediately preceding the balloon maturity.

BALLOON PAYMENT: The final large principle payment needed to retire a debt.

BANK CHECK PLAN: A simplified method of monthly health insurance premium payment. With the prearranged consent of the insured, the insurance company automatically deducts the monthly premium due from the insured's checking account.

BANK DRAFT: Check drawn by one bank against funds deposited into its account at another bank, authorizing the second bank to make payment to the individual named in the draft.

BANK GUARANTEE LETTER: Bank certification that a put option writer or grantor has sufficient funds at the bank to cover the write. The funds are equal to the exercised value of the put. This value is equal to the strike price multiplied by the number of shares. It effectively reflects an outright purchase of the underlying security at the strike level.

BANK INSURANCE FUND (BIF): One of the two separate FDIC deposit insurance funds generally covering insured deposits in banks and certain savings institutions.

BANK LINE: Moral, not legal, commitment of a bank to make a loan.

BANK MARKET: The spot and forward markets for currencies with known counterparties to the transactions.

BANK RATE: Minimum interest rate for short term advances made by the U.S. Treasury to charted bank members and deposit institutions. *See also* discount rate.

BANKERS ACCEPTANCE: Low-interest bills of exchange guaranteed (accepted) by a bank or trust company for payment within 1 to 9 months, to provide DME or medical manufacturers and exporters with capital to operate between the time of manufacturing (or exporting) and payment by purchasers. Bids and offers in the secondary marketplace are at prices discounted from the face value.

BANKMAIL: A bank's agreement not to finance another firm's takeover bid.

BANKRUPT: Unable to pay debts.

BANKRUPTCY: A legal proceeding from the Bankruptcy Reform Act (BRA) of 1978, ordering the distribution of an insolvent company or person's property among creditors, thus relieving this individual of all liability to these creditors, even though this payment may be less than the full obligation to them:

- Chapter 7: Business forced asset sale and liquidation.
- Chapter 11: Business debt reorganization.
- Chapter 13: Personal debt reorganization.

BANS: Notes issued by a governmental unit, usually for capital projects, which are paid from the proceeds of the issuance of long-term bonds.

BAR: Colloquial slang term for one million dollars.

BARBAKOW, JEFFREY: Chairman and CEO of Tenet Health Care Corp. in Santa Barbara, California.

BARBELL PORTFOLIO: Bond distribution where most maturity dates either fall at the short-term or long-term end of a given time period, with few intermediate maturity bonds.

BAREFOOT PILGRIM: Colloquial slang term for an unsophisticated investor.

BARELLA, HANS: President and CEO of Philips Medical Systems in Best, Netherlands.

BARGAIN SALE: A sale of property to a charity for less than the property's fair market value. [Regs. §1.1011.2]

BARNETT, LAUREN: Executive director for the Society for Health Care Strategy and Market Development of the American Hospital Association, in Chicago, Illinois.

BAROMETER: Set of financial market place data and economic indicators designed to predict or represent larger industry trends, such as the Dow Jones Industrial Average (DJIA) or the Dow Jones Utility Average (DJUA).

BARRIER: Threshold for an option feature to become active or inactive depending on the specifications.

BARRIER TO ENTRY: A constraint that prevents sellers from entering the marketplace, such as health care entity Certificate of Need (CON) legislation for Ambulatory Surgery Centers (ASCs) or private specialty hospitals. It's also an impediment, such as education, a degree, or licensure protecting a company from competition or business launch, as in a medical practice.

BARRON'S CONFIDENCE INDEX: A measure of investor confidence of the direction and level of securities prices.

BARRY, DENNIS: Chairman-elect for the American Hospital Association in Chicago, Illinois. He is also president and CEO of Moses Cone Health System in Greensboro, North Carolina.

BARTER: The process of exchanging health care or other goods, products, or services for other goods, products, or services. It is a type of reciprocal professional courtesy.

BASE: Supportive price level in technical securities analysis.

BASE CAPITATION: A specific amount per person each month, to cover health care costs usually excluding pharmacy and administrative costs as well as optional coverage, such as mental health/substance abuse services.

BASE CURRENCY: Common currency used in an international portfolio.

BASE MARKET VALUE: Mean market price of a basket or group of securities at any given time.

BASE PERIOD: A reference point for economic and financial comparison.

BASE RATE: Interest rate charged by banks to their best and most creditworthy customers.

BASE YEAR: A 12-month reference point for economic and financial comparison.

BASE YEAR COSTS: Medicare term for the amount of money a hospital actually spent to render care in a specific previous annual time period.

BASIC ACCOUNTING EQUATION: Assets equal liabilities plus stockholder's (owner's) equity.

BASIC DRG PAYMENT RATE: The payment rate a hospital will receive for a Medicare patient in a particular diagnosis-related group. The payment rate is calculated by adjusting the standardized amount to reflect wage rates in the hospital's geographic area (and cost of living differences unrelated to wages) and the costliness of the Diagnostic Related Group (DRG).

BASIC EARNING POWER RATIO (BEPR): EBIT divided by total assets.

BASIS: Property basis is the original cost adjusted by charges (such as deductions for depreciation) or credits (such as capitalized expenditures for improvements). It sets the base for calculating depreciation and assists in establishing the gain or loss on sale of the property. An investor's basis establishes the gain or loss on sale of the investor's unit(s) and sets an upper limit on his ability to take any losses generated by a property.

BASIS BOOK: A book of mathematical tables used to convert yields to equivalent dollar prices and vice versa. The factors contained in the book are time redemption, interest rate, yield (or basis), and dollar price. It is used to find the dollar price when yield is known for a given interest rate and time, or to find the yield for a given dollar price when interest rate and time are known.

BASIS POINT: One-tenth of 1% of yield. If a yield increases from 8.35% to 8.50%, the difference is referred to as a 15 basis point increase. The exchange rate where one percentage point equals 100 basis points (bps).

BASIS PRICE: A price of a security expressed in terms of the yield to maturity to be realized by the purchaser.

BASIS RISK: The risk in the basis time series, influenced by many variables, although the total impact is less than the exposure for a naked position. For example, when a hedge is placed, price risk is transformed into basis risk. Basis risk is substantially less than price or inventory risk in terms of dollars.

BASKET: Unit of stocks used in program trading activities.

BATCH: A group of health care or medical claims.

BEAR: A pessimistic stock market outlook.

BEAR HUG: Corporate takeover bid on very attractive terms for stockholders, but not necessarily management.

BEAR MARKET: A declining securities market in terms of prices.

BEAR RAID: The short sale of a large number of securities.

BEAR SPREAD: The purchase of a combination of puts and calls on the same security at different strike prices in order to profit as prices fall.

BEAR TRAP: A bear market reversal confronting short sellers of securities.

BEARER BONDS: Bonds that do not have the owner's name registered on the books of the issuing corporation and that are payable to the bearer, frequently called coupon bonds. None have been issued since 1984.

BEARISH: An adjective describing the belief that a stock (or the market in general) will decline in price.

BEARISH APPROACH: The strategy an investor employs when it is thought that a securities price will decline.

BEFORE-TAX EARNINGS: One's gross income from salary, commissions, fees, and so forth, before deductions for federal, state, or other income taxes.

BEGINNING INVENTORY: The quantity or amount of durable medical equipment or other inventory available at the start of an accounting period.

BEHAVIORAL ASSUMPTION: Theory that suggests motivations for understanding health care cause-and-effect relationships among economic and financial cost variables.

BEHAVIORAL COST FUNCTION: Patterns and analysis from actual cost data across a medical facility, hospital, or health care system.

BEHAVIORAL FINANCE: Field of psychological study of human financial and investment behavior challenging traditional models suggesting that investors will always behave rationally.

BEIGE BOOK: Federal Reserve Board report summarizing domestic economic conditions that is published eight times per year.

BELL: Alarm sound that signals the opening and closing of a major stock exchange.

BELLWETHER: Security seen as an indicator of market direction or general trends.

BENCHMARK: The comparison of a health care entity or its financial statements to a recognized standard.

BENEFICIAL OWNER: The owner of securities who receives all the benefits, even though they are registered in the "street name" of a brokerage firm or nominee name of a bank handling his account.

BENEFICIARY: One who receives assets, usually as a bequest, or health care benefits as an insurance contract.

BENEFICIARY INCENTIVE PROGRAM: Under this program, Medicare beneficiaries are encouraged to report any suspicious billing activities. When a claim results in collection of funds of at least $100, the beneficiary may be paid a portion of the collections, up to $1,000 for each occurrence. Because this process does not require the same amount of time and resources associated with whistle blowing actions, there has been activity generated by senior groups leading to various enforcement actions. This program has allowed the Medicare carriers to send notices to patients that encourage them to call, report, and possibly be rewarded if the report results in action.

BENEFIT: Amount payable by a managed care or insurance company for health care services delivered to plan members.

BENEFIT COST ANALYSIS: The decision methodology to deploy health care resources and the quantity and costs of those resources, in relation to their marginal benefits and marginal costs.

BENEFIT COST RATIO: Present value of future returns divided by the present value of an investment outlay.

BENEFIT STABILIZATION FUND: A Medicare economic risk per capita withhold pool, established by HCFA (now CMS), to reduce benefit payment fluctuations.

BENJAMIN-YOUNG, SALLY: Vice president of communications for Baxter International in Deerfield, Illinois. She is also the board chair for the Society for Health Care Strategy and Market Development in Chicago, Illinois.

BEQUEST: The money or assets given to a beneficiary using provisions in a will.

BERNANKE, BENJAMIN: Economist and U.S. Federal Reserve Board Chairman.

BERTRAND COMPETITION: Price bidding war in which the bidders result in a zero profit.

BERWICK, DONALD, MD: President and CEO of the Institute for Health Care Improvement in Boston, Massachusetts. He is also a clinical professor of pediatrics and health care policy at Harvard Medical School in Cambridge, Massachusetts.

BEST BID: Highest price at which an asset or security is purchased or offered.

BEST EFFORTS OFFERING: An offering of newly issued securities in which the investment banker acts merely as an agent of the corporation, promising only "best efforts" in making the issue a success, but not guaranteeing the corporation its money for an unsold portion.

BEST'S RATING: Insurance company creditworthy rating score issued by the AM Best Company.

BET: Slang for a financial markets position.

BETA: Systemic risk measurement benchmark correlating with a change in a specific index. The measure of a stock's volatility relative to the market, where a beta lower than 1 means the stock is less sensitive than the market as a whole, and a beta higher than 1 indicates the stock is more volatile than the market. The health care industry is considered to be increasingly volatile and hence possesses a higher beta. For example, a health care beta of 1.35 would indicate that the security moves 1.35 times the movement in the S&P or 35% greater variability. The S&P 500 is considered to have a beta of 1.00.

BID AND ASK (QUOTATION OR QUOTE): The *bid* is the highest price anyone has declared that he wants to pay for a security at a given time, and the *ask* is the lowest price anyone will accept at the same time.

BID ASK SPREAD: Difference between the bid and ask price of securities.

BID FORM: A document submitted by an underwriter for a competitive municipal security bid.

BID PRICE: The price at which a buyer is willing to buy an option or stock.

BID WANTED: Announcement that an owner is desirous of selling securities.

BIDDER: One ready to buy securities at a specific price.

BIDDING UP: The sequential movement upward of securities price bids to disallow unexecuted orders.

BIG BOARD: Slang term for the New York Stock Exchange (NYSE).

BIG FOUR (FEW): Top four U.S. accounting firms as measured by business revenues.

BIG UGLIES: Slang term for out of favor securities.

BILATERAL MONOPOLY: A situation where only one buyer and one seller trade health care or other products, goods, or services in a marketplace.

BILL: Slang term for "bill-of-exchange" involving a third party, or "bill-of-sale" document directly from a buyer to seller. It is a statement of money funds owed.

BILL FORM: A document generally included with the notice of sale, to be completed by underwriters interested in submitting a bid on a new issue of municipal securities to be sold at a competitive sale. A bidding underwriter will state on the bid form its proposed interest rate(s) on the issue and the price it would be willing to pay for the new issue (subject to any conditions stated by the issuer in the notice of sale), and may be asked to propose a structure for the issue.

BILL REDEMPTION PRICE: The price at which a mutual fund's shares are redeemed (bought back) by the fund. The bid or redemption price usually means the net asset value per share.

BILLED CHARGES: The submitted charges billed for health care services provided to a covered person that have been submitted by a health care provider or facility to a payer. Maximum payment ceilings exist.

BILLED CHARGES MAXIMUM: The submitted charges by a health care provider or facility to a payer, but with a payment ceiling or cap.

BILLED CLAIMS: The fees or billed fees for health care services provided to a covered person that have been submitted by a health care provider or facility, to a payer. Maximum payment ceilings exist. *See also* submitted charge.

BILLING CODE OF 1992 (UB-92): A Federal code billing form that requires hospitals to follow specific billing procedures. It is similar to the Centers for Medicare and Medicaid (HCFA) 1500 form, but reserved for the inpatient component of health services.

BILLING COLLECTIONS AND DISBURSEMENT POLICY: Tools that health and managed care organizations use to increase the amount of cash available by increasing cash premium receipts and slowing cash disbursements for benefits.

BILLING CYCLE: The exact date for which certain medical services are billed.

BILLING FLOAT: Time delayed between medical services provision and invoicing the third party or patient.

BINARY OPTION: An option that has two outcomes. Generally, it is structured to pay a predetermined fixed amount when in the money or pay nothing when out of the money.

BINDER: Good faith money used as evidence until a transaction is finalized.

BLACK BOX: A software program used for proprietary trading or analytical purposes. The key rules, codes, and core algorithms are not revealed to the end user.

BLACK MARKET: A marketplace where health care or other purchasers buy from health care or other sellers for above market rates.

BLACK-SCHOLES MODEL: A sophisticated options pricing method published by Fischer Black, PhD, and Myron Scholes, PhD, in the May–June 1973 edition of *The Journal of Political Economy*. It laid the foundation for the quantitative analysis and practical calculation of puts and calls. The model indicated that options would eliminate risk from stock portfolios subject to some assumptions. The lognormal model stated that option values could be determined by using the current stock price, time left to expiration, the strike or exercise price, the variance of the stock's rate of return (standard deviation applied) and the risk-free rate of interest.

BLAKENEY, BARBARA: President of the American Nurses Association in Washington, D.C.

BLANKET MEDICAL EXPENSES: A health insured's ability to collect up to maximum policy expenses incurred without limit, and without limits on individual medical expenses, subject to policy constraints.

BLENDED CAPITATION: A hybrid of traditional-indemnity and fixed-rate medical reimbursement models.

BLENDED FUND: A mutual fund holding stocks, bonds, and cash with other financial products, negotiable instruments and/or derivatives.

BLENDED PER DIEM: Hybrid charge per hospital day, combining fee-for-service with a fixed reimbursement element.

BLENDED TRADE: The combination of two or more bonds executed as a single position. Often this is done to offset the individual, lopsided risks in two very different instruments. By doing such a trade, a medical investor or health care portfolio manager is trying to create a more stable investment.

BLIND POOL: An investment fund in which the investors are unaware of the specific properties that will be purchased by the partnership at the time they make their partnership contributions.

BLIND TRUST: A portfolio where a third party is given fiduciary discretion on behalf of its beneficiaries.

BLITZKREIG TENDOR OFFER: Slang term for an attractively priced tendor offer.

BLOCK: A very large quantity of securities.

BLOCK GRANT: Federal monies supplied to a state in order to support Medicare beneficiaries.

BLOCKAGE DISCOUNT: Discount for a public security due to trading size and market incongruities.

BLOTTER: A trading record prepared each business day as the primary data entry for a securities dealer or proprietary stock trader. Orders are recorded in a chronological sequence. When customer orders are involved, the price, quantity, instrument, and customer identification are recorded with time stamping.

BLOWOUT: A fast sale of all shares of a new securities offering.

BLUE CHIP: The common stock of a large, well-known corporation with a relatively stable record of earnings and dividend payments over a period of many years (i.e., Microsoft Corporation or Johnson & Johnson).

BLUE LIST, THE: The daily publication *(The Blue List of Current Municipal Offerings)* listing municipal bonds and notes being offered by dealers in the interdealer market. The par value, issuer, interest rate, maturity date, price or yield, and offering dealer are indicated for each security offered. Many municipal offerings are for health care related entities.

BLUE LIST, TOTAL: The total of the par values of all municipal securities (except zero coupon bonds) offered for sale in *The Blue List. The Blue List Total,* as a measure of the supply of municipal securities available for purchase, is considered to be an indicator of the status of the secondary market for municipal securities. Many municipal offerings on *The Blue List* are for health care related business entities.

BLUE-SKY: Slang term meaning to register securities in a specific state.

BLUE-SKY LAW: Protection of investors against securities fraud.

BLUE-SKYING THE ISSUE: The efforts of the underwriters' lawyers to analyze and investigate state laws regulating the distribution of securities and to register particular issues under these laws.

BLUMENTHAL, DAVID, MD: Director of the Institute for Health Policy at Harvard University in Cambridge, Massachusetts.

BOARD OF DIRECTORS (BOD): Those individuals responsible for overseeing the affairs of an entity, including the election of its officers. The board of a company that issues stock is elected by stockholders.

BOARD OF GOVERNORS: The governing body of the National Association of Securities Dealers (NASD) comprised of persons elected by the general membership.

BOGEY: Achieving some securities exchange buy or sell target objective.

BOILER ROOM: High pressure and fast telephone solicitors attempting to sell speculative or fraudulent securities.

BOLSA: The Spanish stock exchange.

BOND: A certificate representing creditorship in an issuer and issued to raise long-term funds. The issuer pays interest, usually semiannually, plus principal when due. It is a long-term corporate financial liability, as for a municipal hospital.

BOND ANTICIPATION NOTE (BAN): Municipal short-term debt instrument paid off with the proceeds of an impending bond issue.

BOND ARBITRAGE HEDGE FUND: Attempts to capture interest rate differentials or spreads due to bond mispricing or better financing than general market participants can attain.

BOND BUYER, THE: A trade paper of the municipal securities industry, published each business day, that contains advertisements for offerings of new issues of municipal securities, notices of bond redemptions, statistical analyses of market activity, results of previous bond sales, and articles relating to financial markets and public finance. A second publication, *Credit Markets,* provides similar information on a weekly basis. It also contains new issue worksheets for computing bids.

BOND BUYER INDEXES: Indicators published on a periodic basis by *The Bond Buyer* showing the price levels for various groups of municipal securities. Three of the indexes represent weekly averages, based upon estimates from municipal securities underwriters, of the yields which would be offered to investors if an issuer were to bring certain types of securities to market at par on a given day. These indexes are named after the number of issuers in each index (the same issuers are used each week).

BOND COUNSEL: An attorney retained by the issuer to give a legal opinion that the issuer is authorized to issue proposed securities, the issuer has met all legal requirements necessary for issuance, and interest on the proposed securities will be exempt from federal income taxation and, where applicable, from state and local taxation. Typically, bond counsel may prepare, or review and advise the issuer regarding authorizing resolutions or ordinances, trust indentures, official statements, validation proceedings, and litigation.

BOND CROWD: Stock exchange members who execute bond trades on its floor.

BOND EQUIVALENT YIELD: The return on a discounted security figured on a basis that permits comparison with interest-bearing securities. On a short-term (under 6 months) discounted security, the bond equivalent yield is an annualized rate of return. On a longer-term discounted security, the bond equivalent yield is determined by a computation that adjusts for the absence of periodic payments over the life of the security.

BOND FOURTH INDEX: The Bond Buyer Municipal Bond Index represents an average of the prices, adjusted to an 8.00 yield of 40 recently issued securities, based on quotations obtained from five municipal securities broker's brokers. The 40 component issues are selected according to defined criteria and are replaced by newer issues on a periodic basis. This index is published daily and serves as the basis of a commodities futures contract.

BOND FUND: A mutual fund consisting of bonds whose objective is to provide income and minimize capital risk.

BOND INDENTURE: Terms, conditions, restrictions, and covenants of a loan, bond, or debt.

BOND RATING: The risk and likelihood of loan default.

BOND RATING AGENCY: Firms that assess the credit worthiness of companies, health care providers, clinics, hospitals insurers, and facilities or managed care plans (e.g., Duff and Phelps, Fitch, Moody's, and Standard & Poor's).

BOND SWAP: The simultaneous sales and purchase of like amount bonds.

BOND YEAR: $1,000 of debt outstanding for 1 year. The number of "bond years" in an issue is equal to the product of the number of bonds (1 bond equals $1,000 regardless of actual certificate denomination) and the number of years from the dated date (or other stated date) to the stated maturity. The total number of bond years is used in calculating the average life of an issue and its net interest cost. Computations are often made of bond years for each maturity, or for each coupon rate, as well as total bond years for an entire issue.

BOND YIELD: The annual rate of investment return on a debt or bond:

- 2 BOND INDEX: An estimation of the yield which would be offered on 20-year general obligation bonds with a composite rating of approximately Aa or AA. The 11 issuers which comprise this index are also included in the 20 Bond Index.
- 20 BOND INDEX: An estimation of the yield which would be offered on 20-year general obligation bonds with a composite rating of approximately "A."

- 25 BOND INDEX: An estimation of the yield that would be offered on 30-year revenue bonds. The 25 issuers used for this index cover a broad range of types of issues (transportation, housing, hospitals, water and sewer, pollution control, etc.) and vary in ratings from Moody's Baa to Aaa and Standard Poor's A to AAA, for a composite rating of Moody's AI or Standard Poor's A+.

BONDING: An insurance guarantee of payment for financial loss due to the adverse actions of an employee, or by a contingency in which an employer has no control.

BONFERRONI CRITERION: A test of statistical significance on enough randomly selected subsets of a patient base, to find some subsets in which statistically significant differences are distinguished by the treatment. It is a redefinition of the statistical significance testing of many subgroups.

BONUS PAYMENT: An additional amount paid by Medicare for services provided by physicians in health professional shortage areas. Payment varies with Medicare's share of allowed charges. Also, physician or medical provider contingency reserve funds.

BONUS POOL: Financial contingency reserve for medical providers.

BOOK: A broker's client list. Also, the size and variety of a trader's or trading desk's positions, or the process of recording a trade or financial transaction.

BOOK BUSINESS: A list of patients/clients and/or payer names.

BOOK ENTRY: A system for the transfer of ownership of securities through entries on the records of a centralized agency. The centralized agency holds securities on behalf of their owners. When the securities are sold, ownership is transferred by bookkeeping entry from the seller to the purchaser. In the case of U.S. Government securities, securities certificates are not issued, and ownership of the securities is evidence in computer records maintained by the Federal Reserve System. For other types of securities, book-entry clearance is made available through linked or interfaced systems maintained by four securities depositories, which hold securities and act on behalf of their participants.

BOOK TRANSFER: Change in securities ownership without a physical delivery.

BOOK VALUE: Cost of capital assets minus accumulated depreciation for a health care or other organization. The net asset value of a health care company's common stock. This is calculated by dividing the net tangible assets of the company (minus the par value of any preferred stock the company has) by the number of common shares outstanding.

BOOK VALUE OF ASSET (BVA): Acquisition cost minus accumulated depreciation.

BOOK VALUE PER SHARE (BVPS): Common stock equity divided by the number of shares outstanding.

BOOKS: The accounting records or the Official Books and Records of a health care or other organization, person, or financial institution.

BOOT: Cash, property, or other assets added to a financial transaction in order to equalize value. It is a slang term to describe any cash or other property that is received in exchange of property that would be otherwise nontaxable.

BOOT STRAP: To start a corporation from scratch.

BOPP, KENNETH, PhD: Health care economist who first examined the physician-patient relationship in terms of medical malpractice and professional liability insurance costs.

BOT: Slang term for bought.

BOTTOM: A support level for securities.

BOTTOM FISHER: One who purchases low priced securities before they increase in value.

BOTTOM LINE: Net profitability (profits or losses) of a health care business entity.

BOTTOM UP INVESTING: Investment strategy that relies on the assessment of individual health care or other companies' potential based on factors that may include financial condition, management strength, and earnings potential, as opposed to factors such as general industry, economic or market trends. It is the opposite of top-down investing.

BOUNCE: Nonpayable check returned by the bank. Also, a sharp upward movement in the price of a security.

BOUTIQUE FINANCIAL PRACTICE: A small specialized brokerage firm. Also, a financial investment advisory practice that provides concierge services for a niche segment, such as physicians or the health care industry.

BOUTIQUE MEDICAL PRACTICE: Noncovered, nonparticipating, fee-for-service private medical practice that is electively reimbursed by an annual fee or retainer. It is a non-Medicare participating provider, such as concierge medicine.

BOVENDER, JACK: Chairman and CEO of HCA in Nashville, Tennessee.

BOWIE BONDS: A slang term indicating debt first floated against the assets of musician David Bowie or similar other rockstars.

BRADY BONDS: U.S. denominated public bonds of Latin America or other developing countries.

BRAILER, DAVID, MD: First ever national coordinator for Health Care Information Technology (HCIT) for the Department of Health and Human Services in Washington, D.C., who resigned in April, 2006. Now, current Vice President of the American Health Information Community (AHIC).

BRAIN DRAIN: The emigration or loss of highly educated physicians, nurses, and medical workers from the U.S. health care work force. Also, a dearth of bright students entering the field.

BRAND NAME: The distinctive modifier of a health care entity, doctor, hospital, clinic, device, drug, or medical procedure. It is a nongeneric, or trade name.

BREADTH: The percentage of securities participating in a particular movement or direction.

BREAK: Volume pricing purchasing discounts.

BREAK-EVEN ANALYSIS: Approach to analyze health care or other revenue, costs, and volume. It is based on production or medical service costs between those which are variable (change when output changes) and those that are fixed (not directly related to volume).

BREAK-EVEN POINT: The HMO membership level at which total revenues and total costs are equal and therefore produces neither a net gain nor loss from operations. It is the point at which investment gains equal losses.

BREAK OUT: Sharp rise or fall in securities price relative to some pre-existing resistance level. It is a departure from a trading range.

BREAK POINT: The dollar level of investment necessary to qualify a purchaser for a discounted sales charge on a quantity purchase of open-end management company shares. It is the health care output at which total revenue equals total cost and at which profit is zero.

BREAK POINT SALES: The soliciting of mutual fund orders in dollar amounts just below the breakpoint level. This practice is considered contrary to equitable principles of trade.

BREAUX, JOHN: U.S. senator (D-La.) and chairman for the Special Committee on Aging.

BRENT METHOD: Economics algorithm for selecting the step lengths when numerically calculating maximum likelihood financial estimates.

BRETTON WOODS SYSTEM: International monetary framework of fixed exchange rates drawn up after World War II by the United States and Britain in 1944. J. M. Keynes was one of the architects. The system ended on August 15, 1971, when President Richard Nixon terminated gold trading at the fixed price of $35/ounce, thereby ending formal links between the major world currencies and real commodities.

BRIA, WILLIAM, MD: President of the Association of Medical Directors of Information Systems in Keene, New Hampshire.

BRICKS AND MORTAR: A tangible and physical business such as a hospital, clinic, or medical practice.

BRIDGE LOAN: A short-term or swing loan.

BROAD TAPE: Projected Dow Jones or other ticker tape onto a large viewing screen.

BROKER: A registered representative (stockbroker), agent, or intermediary who sells and buys securities for an investor or investor corporation. It is someone licensed by the state to place health care insurance business with several different insurers.

BROKER CHANNELING: Steering business to a specific company for increased commissions, kickbacks, or profits or, the opposite is done by health care providers and facilities when a patient has little or no insurance or expensive catastrophic injuries or conditions. *See also* buffing.

BROKERED CD: A large certificate of deposit purchased by a broker from a bank and then distributed and sold in smaller portions or *tranches* to investors.

BROKER/DEALER (BD): A general term for a securities firm that is engaged in both buying and selling securities on behalf of customers and also buying and selling on behalf of its own account.

BROKER'S BROKER (MUNICIPAL SECURITIES BROKER'S BROKER): A stockbroker who deals exclusively with other municipal security brokers and dealers, and not with public investors. The services of a broker's broker are available, generally at a standard fee established by each broker's broker, only to certain municipal securities professionals that are selected by the broker's broker. Broker's brokers do not take inventory positions in municipal or hospital municipal issues.

BROUGHT-OVER-THE-WALL: Slang term meaning to migrate from the research department to the underwriting department of an investment bank (Chinese wall).

BUBBLE: Highly inflated securities priced well beyond intrinsic value.

BUCEK, CHARLES LYNN, CPA, CVA, CMP©: Medical practice valuation expert in Houston Texas and member of the National CPA Health Advisory Association (NCPAHAA).

BUCK: A slang term for one U.S. dollar.

BUCKET: Securities or derivative categories.

BUCKET SHOP: Illegal brokerage firm that is slow to execute client order to augment profits.

BUCKETING: Illegal stockbroker practice of executing a client's order for his or her own account hoping for a later profit.

BUDGET: Document of the financial planning control cycle using the cash conversion cycle for a health care or other organization.

BUDGET CONSTRAINT: The suggestion that health care product or services income must equal health care expenditures.

BUDGET DEFICIT: The amount by which a health care corporation or other expenditures exceed health care or other revenues.

BUDGET EQUATION: Methodology that suggest the limits to health care consumption for a given income level and at given prices.

BUDGET LINE: A graph that demonstrates the different combinations of two health care products, goods, or services that a patient may purchase with a given money supply. It is a limit to health care consumption choices.

BUDGET NEUTRAL: For the Medicare program, adjustment of payment rates when policies change so that total spending under the new rules is expected to be the same as it would have been under the previous payment rules.

BUDGET PLAN: A plan whereby large policies of health insurance are divided into smaller policies to expire and be renewed on consecutive years, with the policies being written at pro rata of the long-term rates so that the premium payment is spread over several years.

BUDGET SURPLUS: The amount by which health care revenues exceed health care expenditures.

BUDGET VARIANCES: Differences between budgets plans and that which was achieved.

BUFFING: A slang term for the transference of a high-cost patient to another medical provider or facility, within a cost constrained environment. *See also* channeling.

BULGE: A fast but temporary price rise in the value of securities.

BULL: A belief that the market is rising.

BULL MARKET: A rising securities market in terms of price.

BULL SPREAD: Put or call option strategy that pays off when the underlying stock price increases.

BULLET: Credit security that repays the total principal on its maturity date.

BULLET BOND: Noncallable debt whose face value is paid off at maturity.

BULLET LOAN: A balloon debt paid off in one payment at maturity.

BULLISH: An adjective describing the belief that a stock (or the market in general) will rise in price.

BULLISH APPROACH: The strategy an investor employs when it is thought that a security's price will increase.

BUNCHING: Combing several odd or round lot orders on the floor of a stock exchange.

BUNDLED BILLING: All-inclusive global fee or packaged price for medical services for a specific procedure, treatment, or intervention.

BUNDLED CASE RATE: A single professional fee or facility charge for all medical services rendered.

BUNDLED PAYMENT: A single, comprehensive payment for professional fees or facility charges for all medical services rendered.

BUNDLED SERVICE: Combines related medical specialty and ancillary services for an enrolled group or insured population by a group of associated health care providers.

BUNDLING: A single payment for a group of related medical services.

BURDEN: Overhead costs or indirect, nonassignable costs and expenses.

BURN RATE: Speed of cash use in venture capital financing before cash flows from business operations is achieved.

BUSINESS APPRAISER: One qualified to appraise a medical practice or other business, its goodwill, and its tangible and intangible assets.

BUSINESS COMBINATIONS: Union of two entities. Under the accounting Purchase Method one entity is deemed to acquire another, and there is a new basis of accounting for the assets and liabilities of the acquired company. In the Pooling of Interests method, two entities merge through an exchange of common stock, and there is no change in the carrying value of the assets or liabilities.

BUSINESS CYCLE: Fluctuations in aggregate health care production as measured by the waxing and waning of real Gross National Product, or in a specific sector such as the health care space.

BUSINESS ENTERPRISE FIRM: Health care operations or other investment entity pursuing an economic and financial activity.

BUSINESS RISK: Degree of uncertainty regarding the future life, returns, management, and profit of a business.

BUSINESS SEGMENT: Any smaller subunit or matrix division of an organization authorized to operate, within prescribed or otherwise established limitations, under substantial control by its own management (e.g., radiology department within a hospital that is responsible for its own profits and losses).

BUSINESS UNIT: An organizational or corporate *matrix unit* responsible for its own profit and loss (net income statement) within a larger enterprise.

BUSINESS VALUATION: Art of potential sale price determination at fair market value.

BUST UP TAKEOVER: Asset sales of a target company in a leveraged buy out used to pay for the debt that financed the takeover attempt.

BUSTED CONVERTIBLE: Valueless conversion feature of a convertible bond due to a low underlying common stock price.

BUTTERFLY OPTION SPREAD: Strategy using three strike prices for the same instrument and same expiration date. It can consist of the sale of two at-the-money options (puts or calls), the purchase of one (put or call) at a higher strike price, and the purchase of one (put or call) at a lower strike price.

BUY: To purchase assets or securities for money.

BUY BACK: To buy a long (owned) contract to cover a short (nonowned) position in a commodity.

BUY HOLD: To purchase securities for the long-term in order to profit through appreciated prices and reduced capital gains taxes.

BUY MINUS: An order to purchase securities at a lower than current market value price.

BUY ORDER: Order to a stockbroker to purchase securities at the current market price.

BUY OUT: To purchase a controlling amount of company stock.

BUY STOP ORDER: A stop order to buy at the market only when someone else executes an order at or above the stop price. It is frequently used as a protective device for a short position.

BUY WRITE: The purchase of stocks and the writing of covered call options on them for potential profit.

BUYER OF AN OPTION: One who purchases a call or put option.

BUYER'S MARKET: An oversupply of securities and the dearth of cash to purchase them at low prices. It allows purchaser flexibility.

BUYER'S OPTION CONTRACT: A securities contract in which the seller's delivery of the certificate is due at the purchaser's office on the date specified at the time of the transaction.

BUYER'S RESERVATION PRICE: The highest price that a patient or health care purchaser is willing to pay for medical services, products, or goods.

BUYING POWER: The amount of marginable securities an investor may purchase in a margin securities account.

BYLAWS: The legal documents outlining the relationship between shareholders and a health care or other corporation or business entity. Bylaws are approved by a corporation's stockholders in a stock corporation, or other owners in a nonstock corporation.

C

C2C: Client to Client.

C CORPORATION: The most common (double) taxable corporate entity, with limited stockholder liability, under the current IRS Code.

CAFETERIA PLAN: An employee benefits system that allows the selection of health care or other fringe benefits applied on a taxable or nontaxable basis and under which each employee has the opportunity to select the benefits they desire. Certain minimum choices and nondiscriminatory rules apply.

CALENDAR: List of securities about to be offered for sale.

CALENDAR EFFECT: Historic propensity of equities to perform better during certain days or months of the year than others.

CALIBRATION: Economic educated guess for some parameters of a financial model, using the assumption that the model is correct.

CALL: Option contract granting the right to buy a specific amount of underlying securities at a specific price and within a specific time frame.

CALL AWAY: A bond or debt issue redeemed prior to full maturity.

CALL DATE: The date after which a securities issuer has the redemption option at par, or at par plus a premium.

CALL FEATURE: (1) A feature of preferred stock through which it may be retired at the corporation's option by paying a price equal to or slightly higher than either the par or market value. (2) A bond feature, by which all or part of an issue may be redeemed by the corporation before maturity and under certain specified conditions. The call price is usually a premium (never below par) that declines reaching par shortly before maturity.

CALL LOAN: A broker's loan from a commercial bank using margin account customer's securities as the bank's protection. (Usually the securities are worth about one-third more than the amount of the loan.) It is sometimes referred to as a "demand" loan because either party can terminate it on 24 hours' notice.

CALL MONEY RATE: Percentage of interest a broker/dealer pays on a broker's collateral loan, usually a bit lower than prime.

CALL OPTION: The right to buy a stated number of shares or other units of an underlying security at the exercise price, within a stated period of time.

CALL PENALTY: Call feature exercise premium cost.

CALL PREMIUM: The amount in excess of par paid when a security is called.

CALL PRICE: The price, as established in the bond contract, at which securities will be redeemed, if called. The call price is generally at or above par (although it may be at or above the "compound accreted value" on certain types of securities) and is stated as a percentage of the principal amount called.

CALL PRIVILEGE: Right of a corporation or issuer of debt to pay off the loan at an agreed upon price prior to scheduled maturity.

CALL PROTECTION: The aspects of the redemption provisions of an issue of callable securities that partially protect an investor against an issuer's call of the securities or act as a disincentive to the issuer's exercise of its call privileges. These features include restrictions on an issuer's right to call securities for a period of time after issuance (for example, an issue that cannot be called for 10 years after its issuance is said to have "10 years call protection"), or requirements that an issuer pay a premium redemption price for securities called within a certain period of time after issuance. The term may also be used to refer to market factors that would discourage an issuer from calling the securities (for example, a security callable at par which has a current trading market value of 70 is said to have "30 points of call protection").

CALL RISK: The potential for a bond to be called or redeemed prior to maturity, and without its current income.

CALL WRITER: The receipt of a premium and temporary obligation to sell an underlying security at a specific price at the call buyer's discretion.

CALLABLE BONDS: Loans that may be redeemed prior to maturity.

CALLABLE INSTRUMENT: Bond, note, debt, or loan that accords an issuer the right to redemption before it is due.

CALLABLE PREFERRED (STOCK/BOND): Stocks or bonds that may be redeemed by the issuing corporation before their stated maturity at a prestated "call price" that is higher than the original issue price.

CALLING: The act of exercising a call and redeeming securities prior to maturity.

CALPERS: California Public Employee Retirement System of 1 million employees who negotiate reduced health insurance premium and payment rates.

CANNIBALIZATION: Purging or decreasing revenue or cash flows from an existing service or product because of a new one.

CAP: A limit placed on the number of dollars that a health plan will pay in a specified period of time.

CAP RATE: Medical reimbursement fee per person/per month, regardless of quantity or intensity of service. *See also* capitation rate.

CAPACITY: The number of health care goods, products, or services that can be delivered during a specific time period. It is the output at which the average total cost for health care output is at a minimum.

CAPITAL: The source of funds to finance noncurrent assets of a health care or other organization (instruments, machines, material, etc.). The total worth of an individual, partnership, and/or all the shares of company stock. It includes the assets, intellectual skills, and principal as contrasted with income (which may or may not result from ownership and/or use of those assets or that principal).

CAPITAL ACCOUNT: The recorded capital inflows and outflows of a hospital, clinic, medical practice, health care, or other company.

CAPITAL ACCOUNT DEFICIT: A negative balance on the capital account of a health care or other business entity.

CAPITAL ACCOUNT SURPLUS: A positive balance on the capital account of a health care or other business entity.

CAPITAL ACCUMULATION: The growth of health care capital resources.

CAPITAL APPRECIATION: The increase in value of an investment over time.

CAPITAL ASSET: An item not ordinarily bought and sold in the course of business, but having monetary value, and often the source of income or used in the production thereof. It includes trade accounts, notes receivable, depreciable property, and real estate used in a trade or health care or other business.

CAPITAL ASSET PRICING MODEL (CAPM): An economic model that uses beta and market return to help investors evaluate risk return trade-offs in investment decisions. The model defines a security's expected return as risk-free rate of return (for a short-term Treasury bill, for example) plus a risk premium.

CAPITAL BUDGET: A method used to forecast and justify capital expenses.

CAPITAL CASH FLOW: The disbursements and receipts between health care or other organizations and its capital suppliers, and sources of funding (bankers, investors, venture capitalists, etc.).

CAPITAL CHARGES: The funds necessary to cover interest upon and amortization of monies invested in an enterprise. It covers the cost of borrowed money.

CAPITAL CLAIM: A capital (money supplier) vendor's claim on a health care or other organization, as evidenced by securities, equity, partnerships, and so forth.

CAPITAL COSTS: Depreciation, interest, leases and rentals, taxes, and insurance on tangible medical or health care assets such as physical plant and equipment.

CAPITAL EXPENDITURES: Outlays of cash or other property or the creation of liability in exchange for property to remain permanently in the business. These usually include land, buildings, machinery, and equipment.

CAPITAL FINANCING: Financing of noncurrent assets.

CAPITAL FLIGHT: The flow of discretionary savings from traditional health insurance premium paying products to higher deductibles by lowering premium payments. HSAs or MSAs where money flows to so-called high-deductible health plans.

CAPITAL FORMATION: The investment in health care plant, facilities, and equipment.

CAPITAL GAIN (OR LOSS): Profit (or loss), or increase/decrease in value, from the sale of a capital asset. Capital gains may be short term (12 months or less) or long term (more than 12 months). Capital losses are used to offset capital gains to establish a net position for tax purposes.

CAPITAL GAINS DISTRIBUTIONS: Payments to mutual fund shareholders of gains realized on the sale of the fund's portfolio securities. These amounts, if any, are paid once a year.

CAPITAL GAINS TAX: A provision in the federal income tax law that previously subjected profits from the sale of capital assets to less tax than would be required for ordinary income.

CAPITAL GOODS: Health care products, goods, or services added to capital resources.

CAPITAL GROSS WORKING: Current assets.

CAPITAL GROWTH: Asset or security value increase over time.

CAPITAL INFUSION: To add new sources of money (capital) or financing to a health care or other entity.

CAPITAL INTENSIVE: Medial specialty, health care, or other business that requires large outlays of capital, often with low expenses or high margins, for example, GI doctors versus internists and doers versus thinkers.

CAPITAL LEASE: Renting an asset for its entire economic life span, such as renting of a health care or other asset for almost all of its economic life.

CAPITAL LOSS CARRYOVER: Allows taxpayers to carry over unused capital losses indefinitely. Capital loss carryovers can be deducted in subsequent years, first from capital gain for that year, then from ordinary income to the extent of $3,000. Any unused loss is then carried over.

CAPITAL MARKET: The market for equity securities (stocks) and debt obligations with maturities in excess of one year. Also, the market for long-term investments involving banks, insurance companies, pension funds, and trust companies.

CAPITAL MARKET LINE: Represents a spectrum of two-asset portfolios, moving from a portfolio invested in 100% of the least risky asset to a portfolio invested in 100% of the most risky one. The Capital Market Line is plotted on a graph with percent of return plotted on the Y-axis and risk (standard deviation) plotted on the X-axis.

CAPITAL NET WORTH: A business's total assets, less its liabilities.

CAPITAL PROJECTS FUNDS: Funds used by a not-for-profit hospital, clinic, or other organization to account for all resources used for the development of a land improvement or building addition or renovation.

CAPITAL RATIONING: Limitation or constraint on the total size of a capital investment.

CAPITAL RISK: The potential for monetary loss unrelated to an issuer's financial strength.

CAPITAL STOCK: A firm's outstanding preferred and common stock, listed at par value.

CAPITAL STOCK AUTHORIZED: The stock authorized but not yet issued by a company.

CAPITAL STOCK ISSUED: The stock issued and authorized by a company's charter.

CAPITAL STOCK OUTSTANDING: The stock issued and still outstanding by a company's charter.

CAPITAL STRUCTURE: The permanent and long term financing structure of a health care or other organization including long-term debt, preferred stock, and net worth, but not including short term debt or reserve accountants.

CAPITAL STRUCTURE RATIOS: The relationship and structure of a health care or other organization's assets, and whether the company can assume new debt.

CAPITAL SUM: The amount provided in life or health insurance for the loss of life, of two bodily members (such as arms or legs), the sight of both eyes, or of any two members and eyes. Indemnities for loss of one member or the sight of one eye are usually percentages of the capital sum. It is often used interchangeably with principal sum or accidental death benefit.

CAPITAL SURPLUS: Corporate money in excess of stated stock value at the time of first sale. It includes paid-in capital plus paid-in surplus.

CAPITAL TURNOVER: Services, products, or sales revenues divided by average stockholder equity (net worth).

CAPITAL UTILIZATION METHOD: A method of determining the amount of money needed to satisfy future income needs based on the projection that both the earnings and principal will be spent at the end of the period during which the income will be needed.

CAPITALISM: The economic system characterized by private ownership, freedom of choice, competition, and reliance on free markets.

CAPITALIZATION: The monetary total of the securities (bonds, preferred stocks, and common stocks) issued or authorized by a corporation. Total capitalization also includes retained earnings, the process of converting (obtaining the present worth of) future incomes into current equivalent capital value.

CAPITALIZATION EARNINGS: Income approach valuation method used to convert earnings for a single period into value using a capitalization factor or rate.

CAPITALIZATION FACTOR (RATE): A divisor or multiplier to estimate financial activity of a single period into a value estimate.

CAPITALIZATION INTEREST: The process of automatically adding the unpaid interest to the principal of a policy loan.

CAPITALIZATION RATE: The ratio of net operating income divided by the value (or purchase price) of a property. Also known as rate of return.

CAPITALIZATION RATIOS: Analysis of the components of a health care or other company's capital structure, including debt (bonds), stock, and surplus, which show the relative importance of the sources of financing.

CAPITALIZED COST: To record a cost as part of an asset rather than an expense. It is an expenditure identified with medical goods or health care services acquired and measured by the amount of cash paid or the market value of other property, capital stock, or services surrendered, or written off during two or more accounting periods.

CAPITALIZED INTEREST: Money cost incurred during the time necessary to bring an asset to the condition and location for its intended use and included as part of the historical cost of acquisition.

CAPITALIZED LEASE: Leasehold recorded as an asset acquisition accompanied by a corresponding liability by the lessee.

CAPITALIZED VALUE: The money valuation of a business arrived at by dividing the annual profits by an assumed rate of earning, which is usually the current capitalization rate for similar risks.

CAPITATED PAYMENT: A per member/per month (PM/PM) medical capitation model requires the payment of a fixed sum of money to a medical care provider to cover a defined set of health care services for an individual enrollee over a defined period of time. Under PM/PM capitation, the doctor assumes the risk for (1) the incidence (utilization rate) of medical conditions requiring procedures specified in the medical care organization

(MCO) contract, (2) actuarial accuracy, (3) cost of delivering medical care, and (4) adverse patient selection. The characteristics of capitation payments are:

- Discounted payment from HMOs and MCOs,
- Proactive prevention of illnesses,
- Population cohorts are treated collectively, not individually,
- Chronic diseases are treated before acute disease exacerbates,
- Care is rendered in the home or other subacute care facility, and
- Outcomes are evaluated on the basis of results, not specialty care.

CAPITATION: (1) Method of payment for health services in which a physician or hospital is paid a fixed amount for each person served regardless of the actual number or nature of services provided. (2) A method of paying health care providers or insurers in which a fixed amount is paid per enrollee to cover a defined set of services over a specified period, regardless of actual services provided. (3) A health insurance payment mechanism that pays a fixed amount per person to cover services. Capitation may be used by purchasers to pay health plans, or by plans to pay providers.

CAPITATION ARBITRAGE: Medical care payment bid discrepancies in managed care fixed reimbursement contracts prior to marketplace competition and increased cost compressions. Premiums or discounts are achieved for volume providers or early entrants.

CAPITATION CONTRACT: Health insurance contract that pays a fixed fee per each patient it covers.

CAPITATION LIST: Members or subscribers to a managed care capitation contract including any retroactive deletions or plan member additions.

CAPITATION PAYMENT: The periodic fixed payment to medical providers or health care facilities to care for a group of patients or subscribers, regardless of services delivered.

CAPITATION RATE: The amount of money paid to health care providers or facilities, per patient head *(capitus)* on a contracted monthly or annual basis, for medical services (i.e., 25–185 cents, per patient, per month), and usually multiplied by the number of patients contracted, regardless of medical care services or quantity delivered, in the aggregate. Capitation rates may include lower payment for partial-care risk, or high payments for full-care risk by the providers and/or facilities.

CAPLAN, ARTHUR: Director of the Center for Bioethics at the University of Pennsylvania School of Medicine in Philadelphia, Pennsylvania.

CAPPED INDEX OPTIONS: Limit the gain/loss potential from trades in index options. For example, the holder of an *i*MBA, Inc., 330 call with a 30-point cap would only realize a 30-point maximum gain even if the index closed at 390. Likewise, the writer has a maximum loss of the cap minus premium.

CAPPING: Form of market manipulation in which a broker/dealer with an established short position in calls sells large blocks of the underlying security in an attempt to force the price down and lower the loss potential on the naked calls.

CAPTIVE ENROLLMENT BROKER: A health care insurance company or managed care plan broker.

CAPTIVE PATIENT BROKER: A patient broker for a health insurance or managed care plan.

CAPTURE THEORY: The suggestion that rules and regulations exist to maximize health care provider surpluses.

CARDINAL UTILITY: The quantitative value of a health care good or service benchmarked in some unit of measure.

CARMONA, RICHARD, MD: U.S. Surgeon General in Washington, D.C.

CARRY BACK/FORWARD: Losses that are carried back or forward to reduce federal income taxes.

CARRYING COST: The interest expense on money borrowed to finance a stock or option position. It represents the cost of maintaining inventory in a clinic, office, or storage facility and includes rent, utilities, insurance, taxes, employee costs (e.g., labor and human resource costs, salary, fringe benefits, holidays, vacations, etc.), and also the opportunity cost of having space or capital tied up.

CARRYING VALUE: Amount, net, or contra-account balance that an asset or liability shows on the balance sheet of a company. *See also* book value.

CARRYOVER: Provision of tax law that allows current losses or certain tax credits to be utilized in the tax returns of future periods.

CARRYOVER DEDUCTIBLE: Allows any amount applied toward the deductible during the last quarter of the calendar year to apply also toward the next year's deductible. For example, expenses incurred during November or December will apply toward the next year's deductible amount.

CARTEL: A group of health care or other business entities that attempt to control prices and coordinate product output and service decisions as if it were a single unit.

CARVE OUT: Excluded health care coverage by contract.

CASE MIX: Percentage of diagnostic related group relative weights per number of Medicare cases.

CASE MIX INDEX: Numerical assortment of patient cases usually treated in a hospital and based on medical acuity and degree of care.

CASE-RATE: Flat fee paid for a patient's treatment based on medical diagnosis or presenting problem. For this fee the provider covers all of the services the client requires for a specific period of time. It is also known as a bundled rate or flat fee-per-case, and is often used as an intervening step prior to capitation. In this case, the provider is accepting some significant risk, but does have considerable flexibility in how it meets the patient's needs. Keys to success in this mode: (1) properly pricing case rate, if provider has control over it, and (2) securing a large volume of eligible patients.

CASH: Coins, currency, or other liquid marketable securities used to finance a health insurance, managed care, or other organization's daily operations.

CASH ACCOUNT: A customer account, required by Securities Exchange Commission Regulation T to be paid in full for securities purchased, within 1 day of the standard NASD payment period.

CASH ASSETS: Assets such as cash or cash equivalents that can be quickly converted into cash.

CASH BASIS OF ACCOUNTING: Accounting system that recognizes revenues when cash received and expenses when paid.

CASH BUDGET: A projection of cash inflows and outflows for a health care entity, or business, over a scheduled period of time.

CASH COLLATERAL: The use of cash or cash equivalents as collateral for a debt, loan, or bond.

CASH CONVERSION CYCLE (CCC): Inventory conversion period, plus receivables collection period, minus payables deferral period. It is the length of time between the delivery of health care products and/or services, and ultimate payment. The hospital industry average is about 45–48 days, non-electronic, and outlined below:

- Hospital Admission to Patient Discharge
- Patient Discharge to Hospital Bill Completion
- Hospital Bill Completion to Insurance (TPA) Payer Receipt
- Third Party Payer Receipt to Mailing of Hospital Payment
- Payment Mailed to Receipt by Hospital
- Payment Receipt by Hospital to Bank Deposit

CASH COW: A security, investment, or health care project that generates an abundance of free funds. It may be due to private pay patients, a monopolistic market position, or special advantage afforded by patents, licenses, medical providers, reputation, or other economic properties. It is the basic franchise of a health care business entity.

CASH CYCLE: The length of time between the delivery of health care products and/or services and their ultimate reimbursement. *See also* cash conversion cycle.

CASH DISBURSEMENT JOURNAL: Ledger used to record cash payments by check.

CASH DISCOUNT: Cost reduction received for upfront cash payments.

CASH DIVIDEND: Stock dividends paid in cash, rather than more stock.

CASH EQUIVALENTS: Assets that can be readily converted into cash.

CASH FLOW: Reported net income of a corporation plus amounts charged off for depreciation, depletion, amortization, and extraordinary charges to reserve accounts for the particular year under consideration. All of these additional items are bookkeeping deductions and are not paid out in actual dollars and cents. The cash flow may be from operations, financing, or investing activities. It includes the net of cash receipts and cash disbursements relating to a particular activity during a specified accounting period.

CASH FLOW ANALYSIS (CFA): Business methodology to determine the effects of past strategic business decisions in quantitative form, as well as to answer important questions such as:

- How much cash was generated by the health care entity?
- How can a cash account be overdrawn when the accounting department said the clinic or hospital service segment was profitable?
- How much was spent for new equipment and supplies, and where was the cash for the expenditures acquired?

CASH FLOW EQUIVALENT: Barter, or the exchange of noncash or non–near-money assets for products or services rendered (i.e., vendor financing).

CASH FLOW FINANCING: Cash-out and inflows from business or health care entity financing activities, as opposed to operating activities.

CASH FLOW INVESTING: Cash-out and inflows from business or health care entity investing activities, as opposed to operating activities.

CASH FLOW OPERATIONS: Cash-out and inflows from business or health care entity operations, as opposed to financing and investing activities.

CASH FLOW PER SHARE: Earnings after taxes plus depreciation, on a per share basis, to measure financial strength.

CASH FLOW STATEMENT: A nonaccounting financial statement of prior or forecasted (pro forma) cash or cash flow equivalents for a health care or other organization.

CASH INDEMNITY BENEFITS: Monetary sums paid to a patient for health insurance incurred services and/or covered claims.

CASH LESS EXERCISE AND SELL PROGRAM: Arrangement that allows employees to exercise stock options and sell the acquired employer stock without being required to pay cash for exercising the options.

CASH MANAGEMENT ANALYSIS: Business methodology used to determine how:

- Health care entities self insure professional liability risks to offset the current medical malpractice insurance crisis.
- Nonprofit health care entities must replace plants and equipment with cash or debt, not by issuing investor owned equity funds.
- Hospital bonds and pension plans must be funded.
- Hospital donations, gifts, and endowment funds must be managed.

CASH OUT: Money back when refinancing a present debt. The cash a borrower receives upon refinancing all existing loans against a property with a new loan or loans that is greater than the amount needed to pay off the existing loans.

CASH RECEIPTS JOURNAL: Ledger used to record cash receipts.

CASH RESERVE: The assets that are quickly convertible into cash for the purpose of meeting unforeseen health care entity operating expenditures or reductions in income.

CASH RETURN: The rate of return on an investment measured by the cash returned to the investor compared to the cash invested without regard to any tax savings.

CASH SETTLEMENT: The process by which the terms of an options, or other, contract are fulfilled through the payment or receipt in dollars of the amount at which the option is in-the-money, as opposed to delivering or receiving the underlying stock.

CASHIER CHECK: A check drawn on a bank or similar institution's own account.

CASHIER DEPARTMENT: A department of a broker/dealer or other organization responsible for the physical handling of securities and money, delivery and receipt, collateral loans, borrowing, lending, transfer of securities, and other financial transactions.

CATASTROPHE CALL: The redemption of a bond by an issuer because of a catastrophic event.

CATEGORY BASED PRICING: Hospital care that provides fixed pricing for selected or diagnostic related group services. It is global pricing or global per diem fee.

CATS (CERTIFICATES OF ACCRUAL ON TREASURY SECURITIES): A slice of interest payments or coupons called strips or zeroes for which the discounted bond principal is referred to as the *Corpus*.

CATS AND DOGS: Slang term for speculative equities with short operating histories.

CAUSATION: A direct relationship indicating cause and effect (increased smoking leads to increased lung cancer rates).

CEILING: Term referring to the limit that certain itemized deductions may not exceed. For example, charitable contributions may not exceed 50% of AGI. Also, the inflation-indexed wage base, upon which Social Security is computed for the self-employment tax, represents a ceiling. It is a legally established maximum price for goods or services.

CENSUS: The number (quantity) of patients in, or serviced by, a health care entity at any given time period.

CENTERS FOR MEDICARE AND MEDICAID SERVICES (CMS): U.S. federal agency that administers Medicare, Medicaid, and the State Children's Health Insurance Program. The Medicare and Medicaid programs were signed into law on July 30, 1965 by President Lyndon B. Johnson, in Independence, Missouri. Since then the most significant legislative change to Medicare (Medicare Modernization Act) was signed into law by President George W. Bush, on December 8, 2003. This historic legislation added an outpatient prescription drug benefit to Medicare. The mission of CMS is to assure health care security for beneficiaries and its vision is to open all programs to full partnership with the entire health community to improve quality and efficiency in an evolving health care system. The goals and objectives of CMS are to:

- Protect and improve beneficiary health and satisfaction.
- Foster appropriate and predictable payments and high quality care.
- Promote understanding among beneficiaries, healthcare community and public.
- Promote the fiscal integrity and be a steward of public funds.
- Foster excellence in the design and administration of all programs.
- Provide leadership in the broader health care marketplace to improve health.
- To expand health care choice and strengthen programs and services.
- Improve quality of care and health outcomes for beneficiaries.
- Improve access to services for underserved and vulnerable beneficiary populations, including eliminating health disparities.
- Protect beneficiaries from substandard or unnecessary care.

CENTRAL BANK: A bank of the U.S. Federal Reserve System.

CERTAINTY: The absence of economic, business, accounting, security, financial, physical, or other risk.

CERTIFICATE: The actual piece of paper that is evidence of ownership or creditor ship in a corporation. Watermarked certificates are finely engraved with delicate etchings to discourage forgery. Misplacement of a certificate by its holder will cause at least great inconvenience and at worst financial loss.

CERTIFICATE OF DEPOSIT (CD): Negotiable securities issued by commercial banks against money deposited with them for a specified period of time. They vary in size according to amount of deposit and maturity period and may be redeemed before maturity only by sale in a secondary market. With "Jumbo" CDs, the usual minimum size may vary. They are unsecured by any specific bank asset.

CERTIFICATE OF INCORPORATION (CHARTER): A state-validated certificate recognizing a business organized as a legal corporate entity.

CERTIFICATE OF LIMITED PARTNERSHIP: The legal document used to form the limited partnership, usually filed with the appropriate state government. Two or more persons must sign the certificate, although as a practical matter, the limited partners often execute a power of attorney authorizing the general partner to act on their behalf in filing the certificate.

CERTIFICATE OF NEED (CON): The formal justification of capital expenditures from a governmental health care agency, especially for a new specialty hospital, outpatient center, medical clinic, and so forth.

CERTIFICATE OF TITLE: Statement provided by an abstract company, title company, or attorney stating that the title of an asset is legally held by the current owner.

CERTIFIED CHECK: A check guaranteed by the bank upon which it is drawn.

CERTIFIED FINANCIAL PLANNER© (CFP©): A designation awarded by the Certified Financial Planning Board of Standards to those who have passed courses in insurance, investing and securities, taxes, retirement, estate planning, and other economic areas.

CERTIFIED INTERNAL AUDITOR (CIA): One who has satisfied the examination requirements of the Institute of Internal Auditors (IIA).

CERTIFIED MANAGEMENT ACCOUNTANT (CMA): A licensed accountant who possesses specific managerial knowledge and usually works for a single company. It is also the accreditation conferred by the Institute of Management Accountants (IMA) that indicates the designee has passed an examination and attained certain levels of education and experience in the practice of accounting in the private sector.

CERTIFIED MEDICAL PLANNER© (CMP©): Professional designation first charted in 2003 that integrates the personal financial planning process (taxation, insurance, investing, retirement, and estate planning) for physicians, with specific knowledge of contemporaneous managed care principles such as: the Health Insurance Portability and Accountability Act (HIPAA); Sarbanes-Oxley (SARBOX); Occupational and Safety Health Administration (OSHA); human resource management and employee outsourcing; medical information technology; fixed rate capitation and traditional medical reimbursement; Medicare, Medigap, Medicaid, and private health care econometrics; activity based medical costing, medical practice valuations and appraisals, office sales and contracting; medical unions, medical compliance matters, physician HMO, IPA, MCO, and PPO contracting; marketing, advertising, sales, and cost volume profit analysis; succession planning and a host of other health care business concepts as accredited by the Institute of Medical Business Advisors, Inc. in Atlanta, Georgia (www.MedicalBusinessAdvisors.com); a CMP© charterholder, CMP© professional, or CMP© certificant.

CERTIFIED PUBLIC ACCOUNTANT (CPA): A licensed accountant who serves the general public rather than a company. CPAs must meet numerous requirements and pass examinations of accounting knowledge.

CES PRODUCTION FUNCTION: Constant elasticity of substitution that describes health care production, usually at a microeconomic level, with two inputs which are usually financial capital and human labor (medical providers).

CETERIS PARIBUS: Latin phrase for: "all things being equal," which acknowledges noncontrollable possibilities in a controlled testing hypothesis situation.

CHANGE IN AGGREGATE HEALTH CARE DEMAND: Change in the amount of final health care goods or service products to be purchased induced by something other than a change in price levels.

CHANGE IN AGGREGATE HEALTH CARE SUPPLY: Change in the amount of final health care goods or product services supplied and induced by something other than a change in price levels.

CHANGE IN AMOUNT CONSUMED: An increase or decrease in health care consumption.

CHANGE IN AMOUNT SAVED: An increase or decrease in health care savings due to increased efficiencies or health improvement.

CHANGE IN CONSUMPTION SCHEDULE: An increase or decrease of health care consumption at various levels of disposable income.

CHANGE IN DEMAND: Alteration of the relationship between health care or other prices and quantity demanded induced by a change in something other than price.

CHANGE IN INPUT DEMAND: A relationship change between price of a health care or other input and quantity demanded, induced by a change in one of the determinants of input demand other than price.

CHANGE IN QUANTITY DEMANDED: An alteration in the amount of health care or other goods and services patients and purchasers are willing and able to purchase in response to a change in prices.

CHANGE IN QUANTITY SUPPLIED: An alteration in the amount of health care goods and services medical professionals and health care entities are willing to sell in response to a change in prices.

CHANGE IN RELATIVE PRICE: An increase or decrease in the price of a health care good or service, relative to the average price of all other goods or services.

CHANGE IN SAVINGS SCHEDULE: An increase or decrease in health care monetary savings at various levels of disposable income.

CHANGE IN SUPPLY: A change in the relationship of the price of a health care unit of output, and the quantity supplied, in response to a change in a supply determinant other than price.

CHANNELING: Directing, presenting, offering, cajoling, or giving patients incentives to use particular medical providers or health care entities.

CHANNELING INCENTIVE: The money, gifts, token, bonus, or perks for giving patients or doctors an economic reason to use a particular medical provider or health care entity. Also known as turfing, it is the act of cherry picking the most financially sound patients.

CHAPTER 7: Bankruptcy form that requires asset liquidation due to insolvency.

CHAPTER 11: Bankruptcy form that requires court reorganization of outstanding debt while the health care business entity continues its operations. *See also* solvency.

CHAPTER 13: Personal debt reorganization.

CHARGE: The posted prices, expense, or cost of medical provider services, products, or goods.

CHARGE BACK: The amount of money reimbursed to an HMO. It is usually the difference between the average discount price and the price bid to the pharmaceutical manufacturer.

CHARGE BASED SYSTEM: A system in which medical providers set the rates for health care services.

CHARGE DOCUMENT: A bill or invoice for health services.

CHARGE MASTER: A comprehensive review of a physician, clinic, facility, medical provider, or hospital's charges to ensure Medicare billing compliance through complete and accurate HCPCS/CPT and UB-92 revenue code assignments for all items including supplies and pharmaceuticals.

CHARGE OFF: Bad debt expense.

CHARITABLE GIFT ANNUITY: An arrangement under which a donor makes a gift to a charity, such as a health care organization, in exchange for systematic payments of income for a period of time. [Regs. §1.170A-1(d)]

CHARITABLE INCOME TRUST: A trust created by a donor that provides for income payments to a charity for a period of time, after which the remainder is paid to a noncharitable beneficiary. Payments to the charity are limited to the amount of income earned by the trust. [Rev. Rul. 79–223]

CHARITABLE LEAD TRUST: A trust created by a donor that provides for payments to a charity for a period of time, after which the remainder is paid to a noncharitable beneficiary. Payments to the charity are either a fixed amount annually or a fixed percentage of the value of assets in the trust at the beginning of each year. Payments are not limited to the amount of income earned by the trust. [IRC §664(a)]

CHARITABLE REMAINDER ANNUITY TRUST (CRAT): An annuity trust created by a donor that provides for payments to a noncharitable beneficiary for a period of time, after which the remainder is paid to a charity. Payments to the noncharitable beneficiary are a fixed amount annually. Payments are not limited to the amount of income earned by the trust. [IRC §664(d)(1)]

CHARITABLE REMAINDER TRUST: A trust created by a donor that provides for payments to a noncharitable beneficiary for a period of time, after which the remainder is paid to a charity. Payments to the noncharitable beneficiary are a fixed amount annually. Payments are not limited to the amount of income earned by the trust. [IRC §664(a)]

CHARITABLE REMAINDER UNITRUST (CRUT): A trust created by a donor that provides for payments to a noncharitable beneficiary for a period of time, after which the remainder is paid to a charity. Payments to the noncharitable beneficiary are a fixed percentage of the value of assets in the trust at either the beginning or the end of each year, depending on the trust agreement. Payments are not limited to the amount of income earned by the trust. [IRC §664(d)(2)]

CHARITY CARE: Free health care rendered on an indigent or pro bono basis.

CHART OF ACCOUNTS: A ledger list of all business or patient accounts and their numbers.

CHARTER: The relationship between a company and the state of incorporation.

CHARTERED FINANCIAL ANALYST© (CFA©): Designation awarded by the Association for Investment Management and Research (AIMR), now known as the CFA© Institute, in Charlottesville, Virginia.

CHARTERED FINANCIAL CONSULTANT (ChFC): An insurance designation given by the American College in Bryn Mar, Pennsylvania, to insurance agents who complete financial planning courses.

CHARTERED LIFE UNDERWRITER (CLU): A designation given by the American College in Bryn Mar, Pennsylvania, to insurance agents. Recipients must pass examinations in business courses and have professional experience in life insurance planning.

CHARTING: Another term for technical securities analysis. *See also* chartist.

CHARTIST: A type of financial analyst, known as a technician, who predicts securities patterns and trends based on past performance.

CHASTITY BONDS: Debt redeemable at par, when and if a corporate takeover occurs.

CHEAP: A slang term used in value analysis. The cash flow characteristics, when analyzed against a benchmark or comparison bond, suggest an undervalued security or other asset.

CHECK: A bill-of-exchange or bank draft drawn on the writer's account.

CHECK SAFEKEEPING: Process of digitizing paid checks. A digital image becomes the official record of the transaction and is kept by the financial institution. Canceled checks are stored electronically rather than being returned to the customer.

CHECKING ACCOUNT: An account that allows the account owner to write checks against the account on deposited funds.

CHENOWETH, JEAN: Executive Director for Solucient in Evanston, Illinois.

CHICAGO SCHOOL: Economic perspectives from the University of Chicago circa 1970. These include a preference for financial models in which information is perfect, and an associated search for empirical evidence that choices, not health care institutional limitations, result in outcomes for patients (i.e., smoking represents an informed tradeoff between health risk and gratification).

CHINESE WALL: Slang term for the artificial and imaginary separation between investments, research, and financial departments of a brokerage house.

CHOKE PRICE: Fee at which it no longer pays to use a health care input resource because it lacks economic feasibility.

CHRONIC CARE CAPITATION: Capitation care carve-outs and fixed payments for long standing conditions, rather than acute medical problems, on a PM/PM basis.

CHU, BENJAMIN, MD: President for Kaiser Permanente/Southern California Region in Oakland, California.

CHURNING: The practice of a provider seeing a patient more often than is medically necessary, primarily to increase revenue through an increased number of visits in a fee-for-service environment. It is a practice in violation of Securities Exchange Commission rules, where a salesperson affects a series of transactions in a customer's account which are excessive in size and/or frequency in relation to the size and investment objectives of the account. An insurance agent who is churning an account is normally seeking to maximize the income (in commissions, sales credits, or markups) derived from the account.

CIMASI, ROBERT JAMES, MHA CMP©: Health care entity valuation and financial expert and founder and president of Health Capital Consultants, LLC in St. Louis, Missouri.

CIPHER: To calculate, as in mathematics; encryption.

CIRCUIT BREAKERS: Exchange methods to temporarily stop trading following prespecified market drops.

CIRCULAR FLOW OF INCOME: The flow of money from patients, to third party payers, to health care providers in the health care industrial complex.

CIVIL MONETARY PENALTY: Health care professional prohibition from submitting medical claims for services that the individual or entity "knows or should have known" were not actually provided. This provision applies to persons or entities that know or should know that the claims are false or fraudulent. It also prohibits anyone from providing false or misleading information on coverage that could reasonably be expected to influence a decision regarding when to discharge a person from inpatient hospital services. Violation may result in civil monetary penalties of up to $11,000 per claim, and is applicable for any individual who is responsible for providing false or misleading information, and assessment payments (with part going for restitution) of up to three times the amount claimed. Physicians who certify the need for home services and who know that all of the requirements for this care are not met, are subject to civil monetary penalties of not more than the greater of $5,000 or three times the amount of payments for services that are made pursuant to certification.

CLAIM: Request for payment made to the insurance company by medical facilities, members or practitioners for health services provided to plan members. A claim may be approved (cleared for payment), rejected (not approved for payment), or pended or suspended (put aside for further investigation).

CLAIM AGENT: An individual authorized by an insurance company to pay a loss.

CLAIM LAG: The time lapse between an incurred medical claim, its submission, or payment.

CLAIM MANUAL: Administrative guidelines for medical claim submissions and adjudication.

CLAIM FOR REFUND: Refund not automatically mailed, even if due.

CLAIMANT: One who submits a claim for payment of benefits for a suffered loss, according to the provisions of a health or other insurance policy.

CLAIMS CLEARINGHOUSE: Organizations that examine and format claims for adherence to insurer requirements before the claim is actually submitted to the health or insurance company for payment.

CLAIMS EXPENSE: Cost incurred to adjust a health or insurance claim.

CLAIMS LIMIT: Time limit on health care claims that usually must be made within 2 years of the service or they will not be reimbursed.

CLAIMS MANAGER: One who oversees those who process medical claim submissions.

CLAIMS RESERVE: Those amounts set aside to cover future insurance payments or medical claims already incurred.

CLAIMS REVIEW: Bill evaluation for necessary medical care in an appropriate setting and for a reasonable price.

CLAIMS REVIEWER: The person or method by which an enrollee's health care service claims are reviewed prior to reimbursement. The purpose is to validate the medical necessity of the provided services and to be sure the cost of the service is not excessive. *See also* utilization review (UR).

CLAIMS SETTLED: Amount of provider bill that is discharged when a claim is processed.

CLAIMS STATUS: Current classification of a health care claim awaiting disposition.

CLARKE, RICHARD: President and CEO for Health Care Financial Management Association in Westchester, Illinois.

CLASS OF OPTIONS: Options of the same type (call or put) covering the same underlying security.

CLASS OF SHARES: Securities shares or classes (*tranches*) with varying rights, terms and conditions.

CLASSIFIED STOCK: Equity separated into several types, such as Class A, B, C, and so forth, and distinguished by charter, indentures, terms, and conditions.

CLAYTON ACT: 15-USC, 13–19 establishes safeguards that reduce the potential for health care entity monopolies or lessening market competition. *See also* antitrust laws; Sherman Act.

CLEAN: Free of, wholly owned, or without leverage or debt.

CLEAN CLAIM: A claim that meets all insurer requirements and is submitted before the filing limit.

CLEAN OPINION: Audit opinion not qualified for any material scope restrictions or departures from GAAP. It is an unqualified opinion.

CLEAR TITLE: Title that is free of liens or legal questions as to ownership of assets.

CLEARING CORPORATION: An organization registered as a clearing agency with the Securities and Exchange Commission which provides specialized comparison, clearance, and settlement services for its members, but which does not safe keep securities on their behalf. Clearing corporations typically offer services such as envelope delivery systems, automated comparison systems, and transaction netting systems. The four registered clearing corporations are the Midwest Clearing Corporation (Chicago), the National Securities Clearing Corporation (New York), the Pacific Clearing Corporation (Los Angeles/San Francisco), and the Stock Clearing Corporation (Philadelphia).

CLEARING HOUSE FUNDS: Funds drawn on one commercial bank that are deposited in another commercial bank. It may take one or more days after the date of deposit for payments presented in this form to be credited and available to the recipient.

CLEARS: Market occurrence when the quantity demanded of every health care good or medical service at those prices is met.

CLIOMETRICS: The study of economic history with the use of statistics, equations, mathematics, probability, and distribution theorems.

CLONE FUND: A mutual fund that mimics or attempts to match another, with reduced fees and expenses.

CLOSE: The last price of a security on a particular day.

CLOSE CORPORATION: A private corporation such as a medical practice, whose stock is held by a small number of stockholders or investors. It is a privately held, nonpublic company.

CLOSE DOWN CASE: Occurs when a hospital, health care entity, or other business experiences an economic loss greater than its total fixed costs if it were to produce any output greater than zero.

CLOSE MARKET: A market with a narrow spread between the bid and asked price.

CLOSE OUT PROCEDURE: The procedure taken by either party, to a financial transaction, when the contrabroker defaults. The disappointed purchaser may "buy in" and the rejected seller, may "sell out," or liquidate.

CLOSED CLAIM: A medical claim for which benefits have been fully paid.

CLOSED ECONOMY: An economy or industry economic sector that neither imports nor exports health care goods, products, or services.

CLOSED END (INVESTMENT) MANAGEMENT COMPANY (FUND): An investment company whose equity capitalization remains constant. A fixed number of shares outstanding that are traded based on supply and demand and are not redeemable.

CLOSED END PROVISION: A mortgage bond provision in the indenture that, in the event of default or liquidation, entitles the first bondholders to a claim upon assets senior to second and subsequent bondholders, whenever the same real assets are used as collateral for more than one issue of debt.

CLOSED POSITION: To sell or eliminate a security from a portfolio.

CLOSELY HELD CORPORATION: A medical practice, clinic, or private health care entity with shares of stock that are not required to be registered under the Securities and Exchange Act and that generally are owned by a relatively limited number of stockholders. Often, the entire stock issue is held by one family or individual, resulting in little, if any, trading of the shares. Therefore, there is no established market for the stock and such sales as occur at irregular intervals seldom reflect all of the elements of a representative transaction as defined by the term fair market value [Revenue Ruling 50–60, 1959–1, CB 237]. This type of business is also referred to as a "close corporation."

CLOSING: The time and place at which all documents for debt or loan assumption or asset transfer are signed, dated, and notarized.

CLOSING ACCOUNTS: Posting and journalizing closing account entries to set the balance of revenues, expenses, and equity to zero.

CLOSING COSTS: Fees paid by borrowers or sellers during the closing of a debt assumption or asset transfer or purchase.

CLOSING ENTRY: Drawing individual accounts into the general account.

CLOSING PRICE: The final price at which a transaction was made, but not necessarily the settlement price.

CLOSING PROCESS: The process of posting and journalizing closing account entries to set the balance of revenues, expenses, and equity to zero.

CLOSING PURCHASE ORDER: A transaction in which an investor wishes to buy an option having exactly the same terms as an option that he had previously sold, and terminating the obligation.

CLOSING SALE: A transaction in which an investor wishes to liquidate an open position as an option holder by selling an option having the same terms as the option originally purchased.

CLOSING TRANSACTION: A reduction or an elimination of an open position by the appropriate offsetting purchase or sale. An existing long option position is closed out by a selling transaction. An existing short option position is closed out by a purchase transaction.

COALITION: A group-purchasing alliance that bargains for reduced medical service rates because of economies of scale.

COASE THEOREM: Suggestion that in the presence of complete competitive health care markets and the absence of transactions costs, an efficient set of inputs to services production and outputs from services production will be chosen by patients regardless of how control over the inputs is assigned.

COAT-TAIL: Mimicking, or following a successful investor.

COB RECOVERY: Recoupment of unnecessary medical care payments after a coordination of benefits review.

COBB-DOUGLAS PRODUCTION FUNCTION: Standard relationship to describe how much health care output two medical inputs used for health care production may serve.

COBLE, YANK JR., MD: President of the American Medical Association in Chicago, Illinois.

COBWEB MODEL: A theoretical competitive health care model of adjustments that occurs when a price/quantity or supply/demand graph exhibits a spiral toward equilibrium.

COBURN, THOMAS: U.S. Senator for Oklahoma in Washington, D.C.

COD TRANSACTION: A purchase of securities on behalf of a customer promising full payment immediately upon delivery of the certificates to an agent bank or broker/dealer, to be settled no later than the 35th calendar day; cash on delivery.

CODE OF ARBITRATION: Rules established and maintained by the NASD Board of Governors to regulate arbitration of intramember and customer/member disputes involving securities transactions.

CODE OF FEDERAL REGULATIONS (CFR): Public health regulatory document (CFR-42) that outlines requirements for federally qualified HMOs and CMPs, under CMS and HHS.

CODE OF PROCEDURE: Rules established and maintained by the NASD Board of Governors for the administration of disciplinary proceedings stemming from infractions of the Rules of Fair Practice (RFP).

CODER: One who converts a written diagnosis or medical treatment into a number-letter code for payment.

CODING: The transference of disease, injury, and medical treatment descriptions and narratives into designated and approved alphanumeric form.

CODING CREEP: A slang term for elevated (increased acuity) coding, in order to increase medical payments and reimbursement.

CODING CONVENTION: The typeface, font, indentation, and punctuation mark used to determine how *ICD-9-CM Codes* are interpreted.

COEFFICIENT OF VARIATION: The standard deviation divided by the mean average.

COINCIDENCE OF WANTS: Occurs when a health care or other item that one wishes to obtain is the identical item another desires to relinquish.

COINCIDENT: An economic benchmark that varies directly with the business cycle and may be used as a surrogate for the economy or an individual sector.

COLD CALL: Unsolicited and/or unwanted calls or contacts enticing one into a stock, bond, or other securities purchase in order to make a commission.

COLLATERAL: Assets on which a lender can claim in case of default.

COLLATERAL FLOAT: The spread or time period between fund issuance and fund availability for use by a health care or other entity.

COLLATERAL SECURITIES: Assets or cash against which loans are made.

COLLATERAL TRUST BOND: A bond issue that is protected by a portfolio of securities held in trust by a commercial bank. The bond usually requires immediate redemption if the market value of the securities drops below or close to the value of the issue.

COLLATERIZED MORTGAGE OBLIGATION (CMO): Bonds or debt backed by home mortgages and sold by varying maturity classes, slices, or *tranches.*

COLLECTION FLOAT: Time lag between medical bill submission and ultimate payment.

COLLECTION PER THOUSAND: Utilization benchmark for health care resources by determining total collections, divided by covered lives, for a set period and multiplied by 1,000.

COLLECTION POLICIES AND PROCEDURES: Instructions that address when and how to collect health care revenue.

COLLECTIONS: To pursue receipts for the sales of health care services, products, DME, or other products and goods.

COLLUSION: Occurs when firms act in concert to drive up prices.

COLLUSIVE AGREEMENT: Output restriction in order to raise health care product and service prices and profits.

COMBINATION: An option strategy combining a call and a put (either both long or both short).

COMBINATION FINANCIAL STATEMENTS: Formal documents comprising the accounts of two or more entities.

COMFORT LETTER: Missive provided by a company's independent public accountant to an underwriter when the underwriter has a due diligence responsibility under Section 11 of the Securities Act of 1933 regarding financial information included in an offering statement. It is an auditor's statement that no material change has taken place in a prospectus or security offering registration agreement since inception. It is not an indicator of accuracy.

COMMAND HEALTH CARE ECONOMY: An economy where decisions are made using a top-down approach for resource allocation in state or federally sponsored health care programs.

COMMERCIAL BANK: A bank established primarily to accept demand deposits that can be withdrawn at any time, such as checking account deposits, and to make short-term loans to businesses.

COMMERCIAL PAPER: Unsecured, short-term (usually a maximum of 270 days) obligations in denominations from $100,000 to $1 million, issued principally by industrial or the most creditworthy corporations. It is usually traded in the securities market at a price discounted from face value.

COMMINGLING: The ill-advised mixing of client-owned securities with firm-owned securities.

COMMISSION: A broker's fee for handling transactions or executing orders for a client in an agency capacity.

COMMISSION BROKER: A member of the NYSE executing orders in behalf of his own organization and its customers.

COMMITMENT FEE: The unused portion of a line-of-credit. It is also payment to a lender to guarantee a loan, bond, or mortgage.

COMMITTEE ON UNIFORM SECURITY INTIFICATION PROCEDURES (CUSIP): An agency of the NASD responsible for issuing identification numbers for virtually all publicly owned stock and bond issues.

COMMODITIES: Tangible products and goods whose future value is subject to fluctuation. This includes an article, asset, or product used for commerce (meat, poultry or farmland agricultural products, metals, financial instruments, etc.).

COMMODITY FUNDS: Investments in futures and options on futures, which may include the tradition grains, metals, and livestock, as well as stock indices, currencies, and other financials.

COMMODITY MONTH ALPHABETIC CODES: Letters which represent different delivery months for financial futures and options on futures contracts:

- F—January Delivery Month.
- G—February Delivery Month.
- H—March Delivery Month.
- J—April Delivery Month.
- K—May Delivery Month.
- M—June Delivery Month.
- N—July Delivery Month.
- Q—August Delivery Month.
- U—September Delivery Month.
- V—October Delivery Month.
- X—November Delivery Month.
- Z—December Delivery Month.

COMMON COSTS: Cost that is shared by a number of departments or health care services, such as rent, utilities, sales, administrations, and other general expenses.

COMMON SIZE STATEMENTS: Financial statements that present each line item as a percentage of the total, rather than in dollars.

COMMON STOCK: Partial company owners who exercise greater control, and therefore benefit more from dividends and capital appreciation, than owners of preferred stock or bonds. They are paid, however, only after preferred stocks and bondholders, and their interest in the assets in the event of liquidation are junior to all others.

COMMON STOCK FUND: A mutual fund whose portfolio consists primarily of common stocks. The emphasis of such funds is usually on growth.

COMOVEMENT: The degree to which an asset moves with other assets.

COMPANY DOCTOR: A slang term for a corporate turnaround outside specialist from another company.

COMPANY LEVEL CONTROLS: Controls that exist at a corporate level that have an impact on controls at the process, transaction, or application level.

COMPANY RISK: Investment risk attributable to an individual stock and not to the market as a whole. Diversifying among different stocks and industries is a common way to manage company risk.

COMPARABLE WORTH: Similar salary for health care jobs deemed identical or like-kind.

COMPARATIVE ADVANTAGE: A health care entity that produces goods or services at a lower opportunity cost per unit output than a related firm does.

COMPARATIVE COST: Production quantity that one health care product, good, or service must be reduced in order to increase production of another health care product, good, or service.

COMPARATIVE FINANCIAL STATEMENT: Formal presentation in which the current amounts and the corresponding amounts for previous periods or dates also are shown.

COMPARATIVE STATISTICS: Methodology to measure and adjust to new information regarding health care economics and finance.

COMPARISON: A term used to refer to an interdealer confirmation.

COMPENSATING BALANCE: Fund amount required in a banking institution to maintain free checking, a line of credit, or other financial services.

COMPENSATION TO EMPLOYEES: Wages paid to a health care industry labor force.

COMPENSATORY BALANCE: Funds that a borrower must keep on deposit as required by a bank or financial institution.

COMPETITION: An open marketplace occurrence where there are a large number of health care buyers (patients-employers) and sellers (doctors-hospitals), and the freedom they possess to enter or leave the market. It is a contest for command over scarce health care resources and inputs.

COMPETITIVE ALLOWANCE PROGRAM: The reimbursement agreement between a health insurance company and providers of health care services for traditional benefit programs. Providers are paid predetermined maximum allowances for covered health care services and agree to file claims on behalf of members.

COMPETITIVE BIDING: A method of submitting proposals for the purchase of a new issue of municipal securities by which the securities are awarded to the underwriting syndicate presenting the best bid according to stipulated criteria set forth in the notice of sale. The underwriting of securities in this manner is also referred to as a competitive or public sale.

COMPETITIVE HEALTH CARE FIRM: The sale of health care products, goods, or services in a perfectly competitive marketplace in which there is a price taker (patient, third party insurance intermediary, or corporate employer).

COMPETITIVE INPUT MARKET: A marketplace where neither individual patients or purchasers, nor individual health care suppliers or vendors, can influence the prices of health care services.

COMPETITIVE LABOR MARKET: A marketplace occurrence where a large number of health care entities require a large number of health care workers.

COMPILATION: Presentation of financial statement data without formal accounting assurance as to conformity with GAAP.

COMPILATION ENGAGEMENT: Agreement between an accounting firm and client to issue a financial report.

COMPILATION REPORT: An accounting report.

COMPLEX TRUST: A trust that permits accumulation or distribution of current income during the tax year and provides for charitable contributions.

COMPLIANCE AUDIT: Formal review of financial and economic records to determine whether a health care or other entity is complying with specific procedures or rules.

COMPLICATION: An adverse or aberrant health condition that increases a hospital stay by at least 1 day in 75% of all cases.

COMPLIMENT: A health care product, good, or service used in conjunction with another health care product, good, or service, such as orthopedic surgery and radiology services.

COMPLIMENTARY GOODS/SERVICES: Health care products, goods, or services for which there is an inverse relationship between the price of one and the demand of another (private medical office visit fees drop when managed care providers enter a marketplace).

COMPONENT CODE: Post-comprehensive code nomenclature that cannot be charged to Medicare when a comprehensive code is also charged.

COMPONENT CODING: Standardized medical report code regardless of physician specialty.

COMPONENT COST OF DEBT (CCD): Kd (1-T).

COMPOSITE: Average financial statement and accounts of a number of companies to signify a same industry trend. It is a surrogate.

COMPOSITE RATE: A group billing rate that applies to all subscribers within a specified group, regardless of whether they are controlled for single or family coverage.

COMPOSITION: An informal method of reorganization and debt reduction.

COMPOUND ANNUITY FACTOR: A multiplication factor for the first annuity cash flow amount that represents the Present Value (PV) of a remaining annuity corpus.

COMPOUND INTEREST: Interest earned on interest. It is interest earned on principal over a given period that is then added to the original principal to become the new principal upon which interest is earned during the new period, and so on, from period to period.

COMPOUND OPTION: An option related to another option.

COMPOUNDING: Interest paid on interest previously earned.

COMPOUNDING INTEREST: The process of reinvesting interest to earn additional interest.

COMPOUNDING INVESTMENT EARNINGS: Earnings on an investment's earnings, over time. Compounding can produce significant growth in the value of an investment.

COMPREHENSIVE CODE: The code following a component code.

COMPREHENSIVE INCOME: Change in equity of a medical or business enterprise during a period from transactions and other events and circumstances from sources not shown in the income statement. The period includes all changes in equity except those resulting from investments by owners and distributions to owners.

CONCENTRATION RATIO: The percentage of total sales by a specific sector of the health care industrial complex made by the top X number of providers in the industry. It is a way of measuring the concentration of market share held by particular medical suppliers in a market, or the percentage of total revenues accounted for by a given number of leading medical practices.

CONCESSION: (1) In the sale of a new issue of municipal securities, the amount of reduction from the public offering price a syndicate grants to a dealer, not a member of the syndicate, expressed as a percentage of par value. (2) In the secondary market, bonds are usually offered to other dealers "less a concession" that is, at a price expressed in terms of a net offering price (in basis or dollar price terms) minus a differential (in points or dollars per security) granted between professionals. This differential is called the "concession."

CONDITIONAL ORDER: Unlike a market order, this securities order has specific conditions that must be met prior to a purchase or sale.

CONDUIT IRA: An Individual Retirement Account established to accept assets from a qualified plan. As long as the assets aren't mixed with other contributions, they may later be moved into another qualified plan. It is a rollover IRA.

CONFIDENCE LEVEL: The statistical or emotional certainty of a financial or economic forecast.

CONFIRM: The written acknowledgment and details of a business transaction.

CONFIRMATION: Accounting or auditor's receipt of a written or oral response from an independent third party verifying the accuracy of financial information requested.

CONFIRMATION (COMPARISON): A written summary of a transaction involving the purchase or sale of securities, which a broker or dealer provides to the contraparty. The confirmation must contain certain information describing the date, securities, and the parties to the transaction.

CONGLOMERATE: A health care or other corporation that produces many different medical goods, products, and services.

CONSENSUS FORECAST: Average collective opinion of a group of securities analysts regarding earnings-per-share estimations.

CONSERVATISM: Concept aimed at long-term capital appreciation with low risk. It is the act of being economically cautious, and showing possible losses but waiting for actual profits. This theory directs the least favorable effect on net income.

CONSERVATIVE STRATEGY: The investment strategy that includes the avoidance of risk and the maximization of financial liquidity and cash equivalents.

CONSERVATOR: Court approved person who manages property or assets for one lacking mental capacity for same.

CONSIDERATION: The exchange of value, for a promise, upon which an insurance contract is based. Consideration is an essential element of a binding contract. In a health insurance contract, the policyowner's consideration is the first premium payment and the application. The health insurance company's consideration is the promise(s) contained in the contract. Future premiums are not consideration but rather a condition precedent to the insurer's obligation.

CONSISTENCY PRINCIPLE: The theory that suggests a health care or other business entity should use the same accounting methods from period to period.

CONSOLIDATED FINANCIAL STATEMENTS: A combination of the financial statements of a large parent company combined with those of its subsidiaries and integrated as one economic unit.

CONSOLIDATED TAX STATEMENTS: An income tax return that combines the income statements of several affiliated health care firms.

CONSOLIDATION: Business combination of two or more health care or other entities that occurs when the entity transfers all net assets to a new company (Nu-Co), created for that purpose.

CONSTANT COST INDUSTRY: An industry where new entrants have no effect on price.

CONSTANT DOLLAR: Inflation-adjusted base-year dollar used to maintain purchasing power.

CONSTANT MATURITY TREASURY (CMT): A calculated value reported by the Federal Reserve Board in Statistical Release H15 to express what the yield would be on U.S. Treasury securities for various specified fixed terms. Data is reported daily for values effective for specific dates and as averages in effect for each week, month, and year.

CONSTANT RETURN TO SCALE: The percentage increase in a health care entity's output is equal to its percentage change in inputs.

CONSTRAINT: Any factors that prohibit the production or sale of a health care or other product, good, or service.

CONSTRUCTIVE RECEIPT: A tax doctrine that can cause deferred compensation benefits to be taxed before they are received if these benefits are made available without restriction in a year before actual payment. It is considered to have received income even though monies are not in hand, as it may have been set aside or otherwise made available.

CONSUMER: The individual, household, or company that purchases health care products and services produced by the health care industrial complex. Also, a patient.

CONSUMER CONFIDENCE INDEX (CCI): Monthly survey that is an indicator of the propensity to shop, buy, or purchase goods or services.

CONSUMER DIRECTED HEALTH PLAN (CDHP): A new benefit option that portends to give employees and patient consumers more choice in the selection and use of health care insurance plans (HSAs and MSAs). Typically included are high deductibles, health reimbursement arrangements, catastrophic coverage, preventive care coverage, and other health care management tools, such as telephonic or online information and call centers.

CONSUMER EQUILIBRIUM: Attained when a patient-consumer-insurer purchases health care services or goods over time, until the marginal utility per dollar spent is the same for all health care goods and services consumed.

CONSUMER GOODS: Goods, products, and services, such as health care, that directly satisfy human wants.

CONSUMER PRICE INDEX (CPI): A measure of the core rate of inflation, according to a diverse market basket of goods and services.

CONSUMER PRICE MEDICAL INDEX (CPMI): A measure of the core rate of medical and health care services inflation, according to a diverse market basket of health care goods and medical services.

CONSUMER SOVEREIGNTY (HEALTH CARE): Responsiveness of the market economy to health care consumer, patient, and insurer demands.

CONSUMER SURPLUS: The difference in patient value between a health care product or service, and its price.

CONSUMPTION: The use of medical services, goods, or services by patients.

CONSUMPTION EQUILIBRIUM: Patient allocation of income to maximize individual health care utility.

CONSUMPTION FUNCTION (HEALTH CARE): Ratio between aggregate health care purchases and disposable income, for a period of time, given all other influences of consumption.

CONSUMPTION GOODS: Health care goods or services that are used as soon as they are delivered or produced.

CONSUMPTION SCHEDULE: Schedule of the amount patients plan to spend on health care at various levels of disposable income (DI).

CONTACT CAPITATION: Capitation scheme for medical specialists or specialty departments, using strong underutilization safeguards for patient protection.

CONTAGION: The dissemination or spread of one economic crisis to another country.

CONTESTABLE MARKET: A marketplace in which seller entry and exit is not costly.

CONTINGENCY: Unexpected change in the financial environment of a health care entity, such as nursing labor shortages, power outage, interest rate hikes, and so forth.

CONTINGENCY FEES: Remuneration based on future occurrences, as when an attorney accepts a medical malpractice case on a contingent basis, to be paid by future settlements, if won.

CONTINGENCY RESERVE: A managed care or health insurance company's assigned fund for future settlements or claims.

CONTINGENT DEFERRED LOAD: A commission due upon sale.

CONTINGENT LIABILITY: A potential liability that may become real if a particular event occurs. It is potential liability arising from a past transaction or a subsequent event.

CONTINUING OPERATIONS: Portion of a business entity expected to remain active, such as a trained and assembled workforce, as in a medical office, hospital, or clinic. These are an ongoing concern.

CONTRA ACCOUNT: A companion-account whose normal balance is the exact opposite of the first account. It is considered to be an offset to another account that is established to reduce the other account to amounts that can be realized or collected.

CONTRA ASSET: The asset value increase that decreases the value of a related asset.

CONTRA PARTY: The securities professional or customer to whom a person has sold securities or from whom a person has purchased securities.

CONTRACT SIZE: Number of units of an underlying security covered by the option contract. The usual size on equity contracts is 100 shares.

CONTRACTION: A downward trend from peak health care or other economic activity in the business cycle in which real GNP (or other benchmark) declines from previous values.

CONTRACTIONARY FISCAL POLICY: Government ideology of reducing spending and raising taxes.

CONTRACTIONARY MONETARY POLICY: Government ideology of raising interest rates charged by the U.S. Central Banks.

CONTRACTUAL ALLOWANCES: The difference between established health care services, goods, or product prices, and those actually paid by the patient or third party because of lower contracted fee schedules or other discounts.

CONTRACTUAL PLAN: A periodic investment plan for a mutual fund by which an investor agrees to invest a fixed sum of money at specified intervals over an extended period.

CONTRARIAN: Following an economic, strategic, financial, or investment strategy against the consensus.

CONTRARIAN INVESTING: Going against conventional wisdom to earn investment returns, for example, buying technology or health care related stocks when most other investors are selling, and vice versa.

CONTRIBUTION: Revenue collections net (minus) variable costs.

CONTRIBUTION MARGIN: What is left after variable costs are removed from revenues and determined on a per-unit or total basis.

CONTRIBUTION MARGIN INCOME STATEMENT: An income statement that groups fixed and variable expenses separately.

CONTRIBUTION MARGIN PER UNIT: The excess of sales revenue per unit over variable expenses per unit.

CONTRIBUTION MARGIN RATIO: Ratio of contribution margin to sales revenue.

CONTRIBUTORY PROGRAM: Insurance payment structure that uses premiums from both employer and employee but does not guarantee medical benefits.

CONTROL: The ability to manage or direct health care or other business entity policy.

CONTROL ACCOUNT: An account whose balance equals the sum of the balance in a group of related accounts in a subsidiary firm's ledger.

CONTROL DEFICIENCY: Exists when the design or operation of an audit or accounting control does not allow medical, executive, or other management or employees to prevent or detect misstatements on a timely basis and in the normal course of business.

CONTROL PERSON: One who owns at least 10% of a public company or a director or officer of an affiliate of a securities issuer.

CONTROL PREMIUM: An economic percentage factor representing control of a business entity.

CONTROL RISK: Measure of uncertainty that errors exceeding a tolerable amount will not be prevented or detected by an entity's internal controls.

CONTROL SECURITY: A security owned by a control person. It is also a policy or procedure to assess its effectiveness in preventing or detecting material misstatements in a financial report.

CONTROL TESTS: Queries directed toward the design or operation of an internal control structure.

CONTROLLABLE COST: A cost or expense that can be directly influenced, positively or negatively, during a specific time period. For example, costs that are controllable over the long run may not be controllable over the short time. In the very long term however, all costs are variable and controllable.

CONTROLLER (COMPTROLLER): The chief accounting officer of a health care or other firm, corporation, or business.

CONVERGENCE: Behavior of cash or the underlying security instrument and its derivative moving toward one another.

CONVERSION: (1) A bond feature by which the owner may exchange his bonds for a specified number of shares of stock. Interest paid on such bonds is lower than the usual interest rate for straight debt issue. (2) A feature of some preferred stock by which the owner is entitled to exchange his preferred for common stock of the same company in accordance with the terms of the issue. (3) A feature of some mutual fund offering's allowing an investor to exchange his shares for comparable value in another fund with different objectives handled by the same management group.

CONVERSION COSTS: The expenses to convert direct materials into finished health care or other products, goods, or services.

CONVERSION FACTOR: Standard dollar value that converts relative value units (RVUs) for each service by the stated economic conversion factor. It is updated and indexed annually.

CONVERSION PARITY: The equal dollar relationship between a convertible security and the underlying stock.

CONVERSION PRICE: Used in convertible bonds to determine the number of shares to be obtained by converting. Divide $1,000 par by the conversion price.

CONVERSION RATIO: The ratio of common stock shares obtained by converting a convertible security.

CONVERSION VALUE AS STOCK: The value of bond debt in terms of the equity stock value into which it may be converted.

CONVERTIBLE BONDS: Although they function like other bonds, convertible bonds have an additional feature. They pay interest and have a maturity date, but they also give the investor an option to "convert" the bond into a specific number of shares of the corporation's common stock. The so-called "equity kicker" occurs when the price of the underlying stock rises. Should it fall, the investor still receives the stated interest and receives principal upon maturity. Some variations of corporate bonds include discount bonds that trade in the secondary market. While the coupon is currently taxed at the client's prevailing rates, the taxable event with respect to principal occurs when the bond matures. By purchasing deep-discount bonds, the investor receives the coupon rate as current income, and the difference between the investor's purchase prices, and either the call price or the face value at maturity, though a gain, is taxed as ordinary income. The effect is to defer the investor's taxes until the bond is called or redeemed. Some of the more actively traded corporate bonds include the following:

- Triple A: Guaranteed Secondary Securities, referred to as TAGSS, are instruments given to bonds with lower ratings, which provide the opportunity to be insured and resold with a top AAA rating. TAGSS are insured by Financial Security Assurance (FSA), Inc., an AAA-rated company formed to guarantee corporate asset-backed and real estate-backed securities.

- Medium-term Notes: Highly rated corporate debt instruments, with maturities ranging from 9 months to 10 years, that can be custom-tailored for an investor in both denomination and maturity. Most are noncallable and interest is paid semiannually.

CONVERTIBLE PREFERRED STOCK: Preferred stock that can be exchanged for common stock.

CONVERTIBLE SECURITIES: Preferred stock or bonds that are exchangeable for a stated number of shares of common stock at a preset price (conversion price). The conversion ratio is determined by dividing the par value of the convertible security by the conversion price. The amount by which the conversion price exceeds the current market price is the conversion premium.

CONVERTIBLES: Bonds or preferred stock with a convertible privilege attached at the time of issuance. The privilege usually gives the holder, for a certain period, the right of exchanging his security for common stock issued by the same company, on a fixed or sliding scale of exchange.

CONWAY-MORANA, PAT, RN, CHE: Vice President and Chief Nurse Executive at Columbus Regional Health Care System in Columbus, Georgia.

COOK THE BOOKS: Slang expression for false, erroneous, or intentionally misleading financial statements.

COOLING OFF PERIOD: The minimum time period between the registration filing date of a security and its effective date. It is part of the 1995 House Ways and Means Subcommittee on Health ruling that allows beneficiaries to change their selection of health care coverage within 120 days.

COORDINATION PERIOD: Occurs when private health insurance is the primary payer, and Medicare is the secondary payer.

CO-PAYMENT (CO-PAY): A cost-sharing arrangement in which the HMO enrollee pays a specified flat amount for a specific service (such as $40.00 for an office visit or $20.00 for each prescription drug). The amount paid must be nominal to avoid becoming a barrier to care. It does not vary with the cost of the service, unlike coinsurance that is based on some percentage of cost.

CORNERING THE MARKET: Volume purchasing of a security or commodity in order to control its price.

CORPORATE ACCOUNTABILITY ACT: Sarbanes-Oxley Act, or the Corporate Responsibility Act (CRA) of 2002, covering financial, accounting, certification, and new protections governing securities fraud. *See also* Sarbanes-Oxley Act.

CORPORATE BONDS: These debt loan bonds issued by large health care or other corporations represent a promise to pay coupon rates quarterly and to repay principal upon maturity. Utilities are generally the largest issuer of corporate bonds in the form of mortgage bonds. These bonds are secured by a lien on the company's property. The issuing corporation has a debt obligation to pay a fixed rate of interest and to repay the principal upon maturity. Maturities on corporate bonds can range from a few months to as long as 40 years. The principal amount is usually $1,000 with the coupon set on issuance. They may be categorized as follows:

- Intermediate Corporate Bonds
- Distressed Securities
- Junk Bonds
- Long Industrials
- Tennessee Valley Authority Bonds
- Utilities

CORPORATION: A separate fictional legal person or business, such as a clinic, medical practice, or hospital, legally incorporated under state laws that grant it a separate identity distinct from its owners, investors, shareholders, stockholders, or stakeholders. It is a form of doing business pursuant to a charter granted by a state or federal government, and is characterized by the issuance of freely transferable capital stock, perpetual life, centralized management, and limitation of owners' liability to the amount they invest in the business.

CORPUS: Latin term for body, or financial principle amount.

CORRECT CODING INITIATIVE: Quarterly guidelines for the appropriateness of CPT codes and combinations for Medicare payment.

CORRECTION: Sharp reverse or downward movement in securities or commodities prices, usually greater than 10%.

CORRECTIVE SUBSIDY: Amount paid to consumers of health care goods or services equal to the marginal external benefit of the goods or services.

CORRELATION: Association between two or more data sets, or variables.

CORRELATION COEFFICIENT: Statistical measurement of the relationship of two variables, usually securities or commodities.

CORRIDOR DEDUCTIBLE: The name for the deductible that lies between the benefits paid by a basic health insurance plan and the beginning of the major medical benefits when a major medical plan is superimposed over the basic health plan.

COSGROVE, DELOS, MD: President and CEO of the Cleveland Clinic Foundation in Cleveland, Ohio.

COSIGNER: One who jointly signs a credit agreement with the principal borrower.

COST: Inputs and/or expenses, both direct and indirect, required to produce an intervention. It is the resources used to produce medical or other products, goods, or services.

COST ACCOUNTING: Accounting field that supplies financial information to internal management for corporate decision-making. It is used for classifying, recording, and allocating current or predicted costs that relate to certain products or services.

COST ALLOCATION: Assignment of funds for various corporate operational or support activities. Also known as budgeting. It is flexible and not objective.

COST ALLOCATION METHODS: There are several types of cost allocation methods:

- Step-down method: is the most common and allocates direct costs, plus allocated costs, to some department based on the ratio of services provided to that department.
- Double distribution method: is a refinement of the step-down method, because after allocating its costs, the original department remains open and receives the costs of other indirect departments. A multiple cost distribution method recognizes that resources flow in multiple directions, and not just from top to bottom. In this modified double distribution cost method, cost centers are not closed on the first pass of responsibility but are reconsidered in an upward direction. The process terminates when all costs are appropriately allocated.
- Simultaneous equation method: is used to more precisely determine the exact cost allocation amounts.
- Reciprocal cost method: recognizes that resources flow in many directions, and requires considerable spreadsheet analysis to solve matrix-like cost allocation problems. Like other costing methods, the goal is to allocate revenues to costs.
- Rate Setting Analysis: a concept related to marginal cost and marginal revenue defined by the equation:

$$\text{Set Rate Price} = \text{Average Cost} + \text{Profit Requirements} + \text{Loss incurred on fixed price patients}$$

- Equipment Payback Method: involves making capital budgeting decisions that do not involve discounting cash flows. The payback period (PP), expressed in years, is the length of time that it takes for the investment to recoup its initial cost out of the cash receipts it generates. The basic premise is that the quicker the cost of an investment can be recovered the better that investment is. This method is most often used when considering equipment whose useful life is short and unpredictable, such as with medical instrumentation.

COST ALLOWANCE: Health care charges recognized by a third party payer.

COST APPROACH: Costing method that adds a marginal charge of the price of an item, such as a laboratory test or drug.

COST AVOIDANCE: Ability of a health care or other organization to obviate the need for costs by operating in new ways.

COST BASED REIMBURSEMENT/PAYMENT (CBR/P): Medical care payment method based on provider costs, or those delivering the services.

COST BASED SYSTEM: A method of medical payments that starts with the provider's costs, as opposed to fees, as the starting point for reimbursement.

COST BASIS: The price paid for an asset including related fees and commissions.

COST BEHAVIOR: The relationship between costs and cost drivers or the study of how costs change in relation to variations in activity, service, or use. Kaizen costing, a Japanese cost behavioral method of cost reduction, is the pursuit of continuous improvement to reduce costs. Its prime purpose is to gather cost data for managerial decision making in health care organizations.

COST BENEFIT ANALYSIS (CBA): Analytical procedure for determining the economic efficiency of a program, expressed as the relationship between costs and outcomes, usually measured in monetary terms.

COST CENTER: A health care or other organizational division, department, or unit performing functional activities within a facility. For each such center, cost accountability is maintained for revenues produced and for controllable expenses incurred.

COST COMPARISON DATA: Methodology to economically benchmark medical providers, health care facilities or other entities that provide medical care, products/DME and/or services for reimbursement, to determine low-cost leaders or high-cost laggards.

COST COMPRESSION: Marketplace forces that drive down health care reimbursement and payments for providers, facilities, DME vendors, drug suppliers, and so forth. It allows for medical cost containment.

COST CONTAINMENT: Actions that control or reduce health care costs. It is the control or reduction of inefficiencies in the consumption, allocation, or production of health care services that contribute to higher than necessary costs. (Inefficiencies in consumption can occur when health services are inappropriately utilized; inefficiencies in allocation exist when health services could be delivered in less costly settings without loss of quality; and, inefficiencies in production exist when the costs of producing health services could be reduced by using a different combination of resources.)

COST CONTRACT: An arrangement between a managed health care plan and HCFA (now Center for Medicare and Medicaid Services) under Section 1876 and 1833 of the Social Security Act, under which the health plan provides health services and is reimbursed its costs. The beneficiary can use providers outside the plan's provider network.

COST DRIVER: Medical or health care events or service activities that cause a cost to be incurred.

COST EFFECTIVENESS: The efficacy of a program in achieving given intervention outcomes in relation to the program costs.

COST EFFECTIVENESS ANALYSIS (CEA): A method that benchmarks the least costly way to achieve a given intervention or medical outcome in relation to the program costs.

COST FUNCTION: Relationship of health care input prices and output quantity. It is the cost of medical output given medical input prices. Form: $c(w_1, w_2, y)$ is the cost of producing output quantity y using inputs that cost w_1 and w_2 per health care unit.

COST HIERARCHY: Expense levels ascribed to a health care organization or other business entity on a prioritized basis. A budget.

COST HMO: A health care maintenance organization structured like a point-of-service plan that is paid by CMS and Medicare with a monthly predetermined fixed amount per member, with annual year end adjustments.

COST MINIMIZATION ANALYSIS: An assessment of the least costly medical interventions among available alternatives that produce equivalent outcomes.

COST MINIMIZING ACTIVITY: Any method used in managed care to reduce health care expenses without jeopardizing patient care, diagnosis, or treatment.

COST OBJECT: Any medical product or service for which a cost is determined (patient exam, visit, test, or intervention).

COST OF CAPITAL: The hurdle rate or required rate of return needed to embark on a capital business project.

COST OF DEBT: The interest rate paid on debt minus any tax savings.

COST OF FUNDS INDEX (COFI): Monthly weighted average cost of mutual or other funds for savings institutions that are members of the Federal Home Loan Bank System Eleventh District (San Francisco). COFI consists of the monthly weighted average cost to Bank members of savings, borrowings, and advances.

COST OF GOODS (MANUFACTURED) AVAILABLE FOR SALE: The cost of finished health care goods, products, or services for sale.

COST OF GOODS SOLD: The cost of inventory that a health care or other entity has sold to patients, customers, or clients.

COST OF GOODS USED: Amount or cost of supplies used to produce a medical service. It may be determined by the product of the numbers of Resource Value Units (RVUs) and RVU service costs.

COST OF ILLNESS ANALYSIS: An assessment of the economic impact of an illness or condition, including treatment costs.

COST OF INSURANCE: The cost or value of the actual net insurance protection in any year (face amount less reserve), according to the yearly renewable term rate used by a company on government published term rates.

COST OF LIVING ADJUSTMENT (COLA): A rider available with some health insurance and managed care policies that provides for an automatic increase in benefits, offsetting the effects of inflation.

COST OF LIVING INDEX: Measures the changing cost of a constant standard of living and is usually a positive number that rises over time to indicate inflation.

COST OF RISK: A measurement of the total costs associated with providing health or managed medical care insurance, for the payer and/or underwriter.

COST OUTLIER: A medical case that is more costly to treat compared with other patients in a particular diagnosis related group. Outliers also refer to any unusual occurrence of cost, cases that skew average costs, or unusual procedures.

COST PER PATIENT PER DAY: The expenses of operating a hospital or health care inpatient facility divided by the number of inpatient days.

COST PLUS APPROACH: Method of determining medical costs with a margin added for profit.

COST PLUS APPROACH CONTRACT: Medical or health care good/service/product price or contract determination that includes a margin for the cost of that medical product, good, or service.

COST POOL: A collection or aggregation of business expenses or costs by like-kind category.

COST PUSH INFLATION: Health care inflation caused by the continual decrease in aggregate supply.

COST RATIO: The decrease in production amount of one health care product or service, when a second health care product or service increases by one unit.

COST RECOVERY: An income tax deduction sometimes called "depreciation." Cost recovery is not dependent on the useful life of the property or its salvage value. The IRS lets the owner of a property, other than land or personal residence, make a tax deduction based on the then-current IRS tax code. It also may be used when the total amount of collections (accounts payable) is highly uncertain, as with health care accounts receivable (ARs).

COST SHARING: Paying a portion of health care or disability costs, such as premiums, deductibles, co-payments, and so forth. It is a payment method where a person is required to pay some health costs in order to receive medical care, either at the time of initiating care, or during the provision of health care services, or both. Cost sharing can also occur when an insured pays a portion of the monthly premium for health care insurance.

COST SHIFTING: Charging one group of patients more in order to make up for underpayment by others. Most commonly, it's the act of charging some privately insured patients more in order to make up for underpayment by Medicaid.

COST TO CHARGE RATIO: The quotient of cost (total operating expenses minus other operating revenue) divided by charges (gross patient revenue) expressed as a decimal.

COST VOLUME PROFIT ANALYSIS: The interrelationships among volume, profits, and costs of goods or health care services.

COSTING: To determine the expense or cost of various health care products, goods, or services.

COUNCIL OF ECONOMIC ADVISORS: A group of economists appointed by the company president to provide insight, wisdom, and counsel on economic policy, including the large health care sector.

COUNTER CYCLICAL STOCKS: Securities that tend to rise in value with a depressed economy and/or decrease in value with a rising economy.

COUPON: The amount of interest to be paid to a debt-holder; the interest rate. (1) A detachable part of a bond which evidences interest due. The coupon specifies the date, place, and dollar amount of interest payable, among other matters. Some older coupons may be redeemed semiannually, by detaching them from bonds and presenting them to the paying agent or bank for collection. (2) The term is also used colloquially to refer to a security's interest rate.

COUPON BOND: A bearer bond or a bond registered as to principal only, carrying coupons as evidence of future interest payments. Prior to June 30, 1983, most bonds were issued in coupon form. However, I.R.C. §103(j) essentially provides that, subsequent to that date, a long-term bond must be issued in registered form.

COUPON RATE: The same as the nominal yield rate. The specified interest rate paid by a bond issuer.

COVARIANCE: Relationship of statistics between two variables (securities) times the standard deviation for each variable. It is the volatility of investments in relation to other investments.

COVENANT: The legal provisions in a life, health, managed care, or other insurance or debt contract.

COVENANTS OR BOND COVENANTS: A debt issuer's enforceable promise to perform or refrain from performing certain actions. With respect to municipal securities, covenants are generally stated in the bond contract. Covenants commonly made in connection with a bond issue include covenants to charge fees sufficient to provide required pledged revenues (called a "rate covenant"); to maintain casualty insurance on the project; to complete, maintain, and operate the project; not to sell or encumber the project; not to issue parity bonds unless certain earnings tests are met (called an "additional bonds covenant"); and, not to take actions that would cause the bonds to be arbitrage bonds.

COVER: To close out an open position. This term is used most frequently to describe the purchase of an option to close out an existing short position for either a profit or a loss.   .

COVERAGE APPROACH: A financial method that settles charges to cover future costs.

COVERAGE DECISION: A health care payer's election to pay, or not to pay, for medical expenses of a plan member based on the terms and conditions of its contract.

COVERED EXPENSES: Health care charges considered for reimbursement under the terms and conditions of a health care insurance, HMO, MCO, or other medical services contract.

COVERAGE GAP: Medicare Part D (2006) basic plan that requires patients to pay all medications costs from \$2,251–\$5,100 resulting in a "hole" (slang). After medication costs exceed \$5,100, patients pay about 5% of the remainder (indexed annually).

COVERAGE RATIOS: The number of times income will meet the fixed charges of bond interest and preferred dividends.

COVERED CALL: An option strategy in which a call option is written against a long stock (stock held in a client's portfolio).

COVERED CALL WRITER: A seller of a call option who owns the underlying security upon which the option is written. A call writer is also considered to be covered if held on a share-for-share basis, a call of the same class as the call written where the exercise price of the call held is equal to or less than the exercise price of the call written.

COVERED CHARGES/EXPENSES: In an insurance contract, those costs for which benefits are payable or which may be applied against a deductible amount. For example, under a medical expense contract, those expenses, such as hospital, medical, and miscellaneous health care, incurred by the insured and for which he or she is entitled to receive benefits.

COVERED LIFE: An insured patient, cohort unit, or company.

COVERED OPTION: An option contract backed by its underlying shares. It's an open short option position that is fully collateralized. If the holder of the option exercises, the writer of the option will not have a problem fulfilling the delivery requirements.

COVERED OPTION WRITING: Selling an owned option.

COVERED PUT: An option strategy in which a put option is written against a sufficient amount of cash (or T-bills) to pay for the stock purchase if the short position is assigned.

COVERED PUT WRITER: A writer of put options is covered only when the writer also holds a long put of the same class, with an equal or higher exercise.

COVERED SERVICES: Reimbursable health care goods, products, or medical services and interventions under the terms and conditions of a health or managed care insurance contract.

COVERED SHORT: The purchase of commodities or securities to cover a short position.

COYE, MOLLY, MD: CEO of the Health Technology Center in San Francisco, California.

CRAM DOWN: Slang term for the forced acceptance by stockholders of unfavorable terms in a corporate merger or acquisition.

CREAMING: A slang term for the act of seeking healthy patients who will utilize medical and health care services less than their premium costs.

CREDIT: Money received in an account from either a deposit or a transaction that results in increasing the account's cash balance. With savings or checking accounts, it is an amount added to a savings or checking account balance, either through deposits or interest earned over time (debit). Also, a loan. In a double entry system, it is the entry on the right side that represents the reduction of an asset or expense, or the addition to a liability or revenue.

CREDIT AGREEMENT: Arrangement in which one party borrows or takes possession of an asset in the present, by promising to pay in the future.

CREDIT BALANCE: Funds remaining after one of a series of bookkeeping entries, which represents a liability or income to the entity. Also, an account balance in a patients' favor.

CREDIT CRUNCH: Restricted credit availability so that financial activity is adversely impacted. It is a more extreme case of credit rationing which has tightened.

CREDIT HISTORY: Record of open and fully repaid debts. A credit history helps a lender to determine whether a potential borrower has a history of repaying debts in a timely manner.

CREDIT INSURANCE: Indemnification policy for unusual losses from unpaid accounts receivable.

CREDIT LIMIT: The maximum one can borrow under a line of credit, home or business equity line of credit plan.

CREDIT RATING SERVICES: Companies that rate public, private, or consumer credit ratings, such as: Duff and Phelps Credit Rating Company, Moody's, and Standard Poor's.

CREDIT RATING SYSTEMS: The classification systems used to indicate the risk associated with a particular bond issue.

CREDIT REPORT: A report of credit history prepared by a credit bureau and used by a lender in determining a loan applicant's creditworthiness.

CREDIT REPOSITORY: An organization that gathers, records, updates, and stores financial and public records information about the payment records of individuals or businesses being considered for credit.

CREDIT RISK: Potential that a bond issuer will default.

CREDIT SPREAD: Option position, the end result of which is a credit. For example, an investor who places a vertical bear call spread receives a credit. Similarly, a trader who places a vertical bull put spread receives a premium credit.

CREDITOR: An entity or person owed money for supplying funds, goods, or health care services on credit.

CREEPING INFLATION: The slow rise in prices of health care or other goods, products, and services that erodes their money value.

CRIMINAL PENALTIES INVOLVING FEDERAL HEALTH CARE: Programs, individuals, and covered entities are prohibited from "knowingly and willfully" making false statements or representations in applying for benefits or payments under all federal and state health care programs. Individuals also are prohibited from fraudulently concealing or failing to disclose knowledge of an event relating to an initial or continued right to benefits or payments. There is also a prohibition against knowingly and willingly soliciting or receiving any remuneration (including any kickbacks, bribes, or rebates) directly or indirectly, in cash or in kind, in exchange for referrals. Violations may result in a felony conviction, with penalties including imprisonment for up to 5 years and a fine of up to $25,000. In addition, there can be civil money penalties assessed of up to $50,000 for each occurrence of illegal remuneration for referrals.

CROSS ELASTICITY OF DEMAND: Used to measure the sensitivity of patient-consumer health care or other purchases to each 1% change in the price of related goods and services.

CROSS PRICE ELASTICITY OF DEMAND: Percentage change in the quantity demanded of one health care good or service, from a 1% change in the price of related goods and services.

CROSS OVER CLAIM: A bill when dual eligibility exists in medical care claims reimbursement, simultaneously, from both Medicare and Medicaid. Medicare pays first.

CROSS SECTIONAL ANALYSIS: Financial analysis of firms in the same industry segment, such as those in the health care space.

CROSS WALK: To cross-reference a CPT code with an ICD-9 dental, anesthesia, or HCPCS codes.

CROWDING OUT: Heavy patient, consumer, business, and federal borrowing during the same time period.

CUM: A Latin phrase meaning "with," "included," or "attached."

CUM DIVIDEND: With dividends.

CUM RIGHTS: With rights.

CUMULATIVE AVERAGE RETURN (CAR): A portfolio's abnormal return (AR) at each time is $AR_t = $ Sum from $i = 1$ to N of each ar_{it}/N. Here ar_{it} is the abnormal return at time t of security i. Over a window from $t = 1$ to T, the CAR is the sum of all the ARs.

CUMULATIVE PREFERRED STOCK: Preferred stock issue that allows for the accumulation of any dividends not paid in prior years due to insufficient earnings. Note that these dividends will accrue and be paid in full in any year that the company wishes to pay common stockholders.

CUMULATIVE TOTAL RETURN: A measure of total value increase of an investment over time, assuming dividends and capital gains distributions are reinvested.

CUMULATIVE VOTING: Method of voting ones shares of common stock that allows the minority (small) shareholder to obtain a better representation on the Board of Directors. This representation is achieved by allowing the shareholder to cast his votes in any manner desired. To illustrate this, let's assume ownership of 100 shares of XYZ and an election for 3 directors' positions is being held. We would have a total of 300 votes that could be cast in any manner. Thus, we could cast all 300 votes for one director's position if we desired, or in any other way. This contrasts with the regular (statutory) voting method where we would have to distribute our votes evenly, meaning 100 votes for each of the 3 positions to be filled.

CURB: A slang term for the American Stock Exchange (ASE or AMEX).

CURRENCY: Paper money and coins.

CURRENCY FUTURES: A contract for the anticipated future delivery of foreign exchange.

CURRENT ASSETS: Assets used or consumed within 12 months. Cash plus any other assets that will be sold, converted into cash, or used during a hospital's "cash conversion cycle," or the cycle of cash to medical services, to third party insurance payer, and back to cash, again. Most commonly included with cash are marketable securities, patient accounts receivable and inventory.

CURRENT COSTS: Expenses usually payable and due within 1 year. Current liabilities.

CURRENT COMPENSATION: Compensation that provides an employee with an immediate benefit, the most obvious example of which is his or her current base pay.

CURRENT DEBT: Same as current liabilities.

CURRENT INCOME: Money received from business operations, work effort, employment, or other conscientious industry.

CURRENT INTEREST RATE: General term used to describe the interest rate of earnings credited to variable and universal life or health products (versus the fixed rate of traditional life or health insurance policies).

CURRENT LIABILITIES: Debts or obligations that must be met within a year. On a stock, the annual dividend divided by the current ask price; on a bond, the annual interest dividend by the current market value. Obligation whose liquidation is expected to require the use of existing resources classified as current assets, or the creation of other current liabilities.

CURRENT MARKET VALUE (CMV): The worth of securities on an account on a particular day and time.

CURRENT PRICE: The worth of a security on a particular day and time.

CURRENT PRINCIPAL FACTOR: A statistic multiplied against an initial principal amount to indicate the current outstanding principal amount.

CURRENT PRINCIPAL VALUE: Adjusted outstanding amount of loan or bond indebtedness computed by multiplying the initial principal amount by the Current Principal Factor (CPF). This factor reflects any accretions in part due to negative amortization, any ordinary principal payments, and accelerated principal payments. The greater the divergence between the ordinary expectation for principal and current principal amount is a reflection of the prepayment events.

CURRENT PROCEDURAL TERMINOLOGY **(CPT):** A standardized mechanism of reporting services using numeric codes as established and updated annually. It was first produced, owned, and copyrighted in 1961 by the American Medical Association.

CURRENT PROCEDURAL TERMINOLOGY **(CPT)** *CODE:* Medical diagnosis or procedure descriptor using a five digit CPT code number.

CURRENT PROCEDURAL TERMINOLOGY **(CPT)** *MODIFIER:* Additional code descriptors used after a five digit CPT code number to indicate the medical service was altered or extraordinary compared to the standard CPT code description for payment:

- 21: prolonged EM services
- 22: unusual procedure services
- 23: unusual anesthesia
- 24: unrelated EM same physician services done post-operatively
- 25: significant and separate EM services by same-day physician
- 26: professional component
- 27: multiple same-day, outpatient EM encounters
- 32: mandated services
- 47: anesthesia by surgeon

- 50: bilateral procedure
- 51: multiple procedures
- 52: reduced services
- 53: discontinued procedure
- 54: surgical care only
- 55: post-operative management only
- 56: preoperative management only
- 57: decision for surgery
- 58: staged related procedure, same physician, post-operative period
- 59: distinct procedure service
- 62: two surgeons
- 63: procedures on infants less than 4 kg.
- 66: surgical team
- 73: discontinued ASC procedure prior to anesthesia administration
- 74: discontinued ASC procedure after anesthesia administration
- 76: repeat procedure by same physician
- 77: repeat procedure by another physician
- 78: return to OP by same physician during post-operative period
- 79: unrelated procedure, same physician, post-operative period
- 80: assistant surgeon
- 81: minimum assistant surgeon
- 82: assistant surgeon when qualified resident surgeon absent
- 90: reference laboratory
- 91: repeat clinical diagnostic laboratory test
- 99: multiple modifiers

CURRENT RATIO: A liquidity measure to determine how easily current debt may be paid (current assets/current liabilities).

CURRENT VALUE: (1) Asset value at the present time as compared with historical cost. (2) The amount determined by discounting the future revenue stream of an asset using compound interest calculations.

CURRENT YIELD: The annual dividend of a stock divided by the current ask price. On a bond, it's the annual interest dividend by the current market value.

CUSIP (COMMITTEE ON UNIFORM SECURITIES IDENTIFICATION PROCEDURES) NUMBER: An identification number assigned to each maturity of an issue, which is usually printed on the face of each individual certificate of the issue. The CUSIP numbers are intended to help facilitate the identification and clearance of securities.

CUSTODIAN: A commercial bank, trust company, or individual with certain qualifications that holds in safekeeping monies and securities owned by an investment company or other individual. Often held for the benefit of another, as in a child.

CUSTOMARY CHARGE: One of the screens previously used to determine a physician's payment for a service under Medicare's customary, prevailing, and reasonable payment system. Customary charges are calculated as the physician's median charge for a given service over a prior 12-month period.

CUSTOMARY AND REASONABLE CHARGES: A basic concept used in health insurance to determine the benefit package in a major medical plan: to pay all reasonable and necessary medical costs, but not to pay excessive or unnecessary costs. Insurance companies and government providers may refuse to cover excessive expenses if they determine that charges made were not within customary and reasonable limits.

CUSTOMARY, USUAL, PREVAILING, AND REASONABLE (CUPR): The method of paying physicians under Medicare from 1965 until implementation of the Medicare Fee Schedule in January 1992. Payment for a service was limited to the lowest of (1) the physician's billed charge for the service, (2) the physician's customary charge for the service, or (3) the prevailing charge for that service in the community. Similar to the usual, customary, and reasonable system used by private insurers.

CUT OFF POINT: The minimum rate of return in capital budgeting acceptable as an investment opportunity.

CUT OFF RATE: Hurdle rate.

CUT RATE: A health, life, or other insurance premium charge that is below a scheduled rate.

CYCLE BILLING: The time period in which accounts receivable invoices, premiums, or other bills are periodically repeated and sent.

CYCLE, OPTIONS: The expiration dates applicable to the different series of options. Traditionally, there were three cycles:

- January/April/July/October
- February/May/August/November
- March/June/September/December

Equity options expire on a sequential cycle that involves a total of four option series: 2 near-term months and 2 far-term months. For example, on January 1, a stock traditionally in the January cycle will be trading options expiring in January, February, April, and July. Index options, however, expire on a consecutive cycle that involves the 4 near-term months. For example, on January 1, index options will be trading options expiring in January, February, March, and April.

CYCLE TIME: Turnaround time from start to finish of the medical claims cash conversion cycle.

CYCLICAL ANALYSIS: The study of recurring or periodic movements in securities prices or other time series.

CYCLICAL COMPANY: A company whose profits and losses are tied to the macroeconomic activity. Medical practices, clinics, and hospitals have traditionally been considered noncyclical.

CYCLICAL INDUSTRY: A space whose profits and losses are tied to the macroeconomic activity. The health care sector has traditionally been considered noncyclical.

CYCLICAL STOCK: Stocks that tend to rise or fall quickly, corresponding to the same movements in the economic business cycle. Automobiles and housing, for instance, are more in demand when consumers can afford high-ticket durables.

D

DAILY BENEFIT: Maximum payment for room and board expense charges in a hospital.

DAILY CENSUS: Mean census or patient population, per 24 hour period.

DAILY COMPOUNDING: Interest calculation in which interest is added to the principal each day. Interest is then earned on the new balance.

DAILY INTEREST: Interest computed or assessed daily and based on the principal and interest left in the account each day. *See also* compound interest.

DAILY OPERATIONS: The customary and usual business activities of a health care or other business organization.

DAILY SERVICE CHARGE: Per day or Diem, health care bills or claims for reimbursement.

DAISY CHAIN: The trading of securities between stock market manipulators.

DATE OF AUDITOR/ACCOUNTANT REPORT: Last day of performed fieldwork and responsibility relating to significant events subsequent to financial statement dates.

DATE OF ISSUE: Date on which a new stock is publicly issued or a bond is issued and effective.

DATE OF PLAN INSOLVENCY: Either the later date that a health or insurance plan is declared and unable to meet its going-concern financial obligations, or the date on which it ceases operations.

DATE OF RECORD: Date of securities ownership in order to receive dividend payments.

DATE OF SERVICE: Calendar date medical service or treatment was rendered.

DATED DATE: The date of issue printed on a security from which interest usually starts to accrue, even though the issue may actually be delivered at some later date.

DAVIDSON, RICHARD: President of the American Hospital Association in Chicago, Illinois.

DAY ORDER: A transaction order that remains valid only for the remainder of the trading day on which it is entered. Also, an individual in the securities business acting as a principal rather than as an agent. Dealers earn their profits from markup and markdown, never a commission.

DAY TRADE: Sale and purchase of securities on the same day.

DAY TRADER: One who makes repeated day trades.

DAYS IN ACCOUNTS RECEIVABLE (DAR): Net accounts receivable divided by average revenue per day (gross patient revenue divided by days in the reporting period). Indicates the time necessary to convert receivables into cash [net ARs / (net patient revenues / 365 days)]. It is the average AR collection period.

DAYS CASH ON HAND (DCOH): The number of days a health care or other entity can cover using its most liquid assets [cash and marketable securities] / [(operating expenses-depreciation) / 365 days].

DAYS PER THOUSAND: Utilization method determining the number of hospital days per year for each thousand lives covered.

DAYS SALES OUTSTANDING (DSO): ARs / Average sales (revenue) per day

DAYS SALES RECEIVABLES (DSR): The average of net accounts receivable to one day's sales revenues.

DEAD CAT BOUNCE: A sharp rise in a securities price, after a sharp drop.

DEAD WEIGHT LOSS: Measure of health care allocative inefficiency as a reduction in patient surplus resulting from a restriction of outputs below efficient levels.

DEALER: A financial organization that transacts trades on the behalf of its proprietary account, as opposed to a broker who transacts trades for the account of its customer and is compensated by the spread. OTC market makers or principals who sell and buy various securities.

DEALER BANK: A bank that is engaged in the business of buying and selling government securities, municipal securities, and/or certain money market instruments for its own account.

DEALER MARKET: Securities transactions between principals or dealers.

DEALER SPREAD: The difference in the buy-sell price for securities dealers or principals.

DEANGELIS, CATHERINE, MD: Editor for the Journal of the American Medical Association in Chicago, Illinois.

DEATH BACK BOND: Debt backed by a life insurance policy.

DEATH SPIRAL: A slang term for the combination of high health insurance premium rates and the underestimation of claims due to adverse patient selection, which results in fiscal insolvency for the medical provider or insurance payer.

DEATH VALLEY CURVE: The rapid use of capital by a small start-up firm, such as an emerging health care organization (EHO).

DEBENTURES: A type of bond that is issued by hospitals or other corporations. Debentures do not have a special lien on the corporation's property, but the bondholders do have first claim on all assets not already pledged. Next are subordinated debentures, which have a claim on assets after the more senior debt is satisfied.

DEBIT: A combination health or life insurance agent's group of policy owners, from whom premiums are regularly collected. A debit book is the insurance agent's list of active policy owners. The term also applies to the territory in which an agent collects premiums, an amount withdrawn or removed from a checking or savings account balance, and credit.

DEBIT BALANCE: Account balance with money owed by the buyer or patient, to the seller or health care provider. It is that which remains after one or a series of bookkeeping entries. An expense or asset of the entity.

DEBIT CARD: A plastic smart card designed to give a customer access to funds in his/her checking account to obtain cash or purchase goods and services.

DEBT: Money, notes, and bonds owed, or the left side of an account.

DEBT EQUITY RATIO: Total company liabilities divided by total owner (shareholder) equity.

DEBT FINANCING: Borrowing money at an interest rate cost, instead of using equity financing.

DEBT LIMIT: The maximum amount of debt that an issuer of municipal securities is permitted to incur under constitutional, statutory, or charter provisions. The debt limit is usually expressed as a percentage of assessed valuation.

DEBT RATIO: Total debt / total assets.

DEBT RATIOS: Comparative statistics showing the relationship between the issuer's outstanding debt and such factors as its tax base, income, or population. Such ratios are often used in the process of determining credit quality of an issue, primarily on general obligation bonds. Some of the more commonly used ratios are (a) net overall debt to assessed valuation, (b) net overall debt to estimated full valuation, and (c) net overall debt per capital.

DEBT RETIREMENT: To pay off, satisfy, or amortize a loan.

DEBT SECURITY: Evidence document of an obligation or liability.

DEBT SERVICE: The amount of money necessary to pay interest on an outstanding debt, the principal of maturing serial bonds, and the required contributions to a sinking fund for term bonds. Debt service on bonds may be calculated on a calendar year, fiscal year, or bond fiscal year basis. Debt service coverage may be calculated as: [excess of revenues over expenses + interest expenses = depreciation expenses) / (interest expense + principle payment)].

DEBT SERVICE FUND: Fund whose interest and principle is set aside and accumulated to retire debt.

DEBT SERVICE RESERVE FUND: The fund in which monies are placed, which may be used to pay debt service if pledged revenues are insufficient to satisfy the debt service requirements. The debt service reserve fund may be entirely funded with bond proceeds, or it may only be partly funded at the time of issuance and allowed to reach its full funding requirement over time, due to the accumulation of pledged revenues. If the debt service reserve fund is used in whole or part to pay debt service, the issuer usually is required to replenish the funds from the first available funds or revenues. A typical reserve requirement might be the maximum aggregate annual debt service requirement for any year remaining until the bonds reach maturity. The size and investment of the reserve may be subject to arbitrage regulations. Under a typical revenue pledge this fund is the third to be funded out of the revenue fund.

DEBTOR: Company, patient, customer, client, vendor, or individual that owes money or other assets to a creditor.

DEBTS SUPPLIER: A vendor who accepts a debtor's claim in exchange for supplied capital (funds).

DEBTS TO ASSETS: Financial ratio of total liabilities, divided by total assets of a health care or other organization.

DEBTS TO EQUITY RATIO: Total liabilities divided by total stockholder (owner) equity.

DECAPITATION: Slang term for inadequate medical capitation payments.

DECEDENT: Individual or patient who has died.

DECIMAL TRADING: Securities trading in decimal increments, rather than 1/8s.

DECLARATION DATE: The time set for the corporate board of directors' meeting at which a dividend distribution is announced.

DECLINING ECONOMY: Economy or industry sector in which net private investment is less than zero.

DECREASE IN DEMAND: Diminution of the quantity demanded of a health care good or service at every price level.

DECREASING RETURN TO SCALE: Percentage change in a health care entity's output is less than the same percentage change in its scale of inputs. *See also* diseconomies of scale.

DEDUCTIBLE: Provision or clause in an insurance contract that the first given number of dollars, or percentage, or expenses will not be reimbursed or covered. (1) The amount paid by the patient for medical care prior to insurance covering the balance. (2) A type of cost sharing where the insured party pays a specified amount of approved charges for covered medical services before the insurer will assume liability for all or part of the remaining covered services. (3) Cumulative amount a member of a health plan has to pay for services before that person's plan begins to cover the costs of care.

DEDUCTIBLE AGGREGATE: Total annual deductible for a health insurance policy.

DEDUCTIBLE CARRY OVER: A life or health insurance policy feature whereby covered expenses in the last 3 months of the year may carry over to be counted toward the next year's deductible.

DEDUCTIBLE CARRY OVER CREDIT: Last quarter deductible that may be used for the next year.

DEDUCTIBLE COVERAGE: A health insurance policy provision stipulating that only the loss in excess of a minimum figure is covered.

DEDUCTIBLE COVERAGE CLAUSE: A provision in a health insurance policy that states that, in return for a reduced rate, the insured will assume losses below a specified amount. In a health insurance policy, for example, that portion of covered hospital and medical charges that an insured person must pay before the policy's benefits begin.

DEDUCTION: An expenditure subtracted from AGI to reduce taxable income.

DEEP DISCOUNT BOND: Debt or bonds selling usually for a reduction of more than 20 basis points from par value.

DEFALCATION: To misuse or embezzle funds or other assets.

DEFAULT: Breach of some covenant, promise to duty imposed by the bond contract. The most serious default occurs when the issuer fails to pay principal, interest, or both, when due. Other, "technical" defaults result when specifically identified events of default occur, such as failure to perform covenants. Technical defaults may include failing to charge rates sufficient to meet rate covenants or failing to maintain insurance on the project. If the issuer defaults in the payment of principal, interest, or both, or if a technical default is not cured within a specified period of time, the bondholders or trustee may exercise legally available rights and remedies for enforcement of the bond contract.

DEFAULT RISK: Possibility of default.

DEFEASANCE: The nullification of certain financial contracts when specific acts are performed as outlined in the terms and conditions statements. It is the annulment of a contract or deed, or a clause within a contract or deed that provides for annulment.

DEFENSIVE STOCK: A stock that, because of the nature of the business represented, is believed likely to hold up relatively well in declining markets. Examples include public utilities, some health care organizations and hospitals, and basic foodstuffs.

DEFERRED ANNUITY: An annuity in which the annuitant wishes to allow earnings received into a separate account during the accumulation phase to accrue tax deferred until some future time.

DEFERRED CHARGE: Costs or expenses incurred for subsequent periods which are reflected in assets.

DEFERRED COMPENSATION: A nonqualified compensation plan, often tied to an executive bonus plan, allowing for payments in the future, such as retirement.

DEFERRED COMPENSATION ADMINISTRATOR: A company that provides services through retirement planning administration, third-party administration, self-insured plans, compensation planning, salary survey, and workers' compensation claims administration.

DEFERRED EXPENSES: Business expenditures that are planned to occur several years in the future and usually requiring large outlays of cash. ·

DEFERRED INCOME: Income received but not earned and reflected as a liability on the balance sheet.

DEFERRED INCOME TAXES: Assets or liabilities from timing or measurement differences between tax and accounting principles.

DEFERRED INTEREST: Interest delayed when a minimum monthly payment is not large enough to pay all the interest that has accrued on a loan for a specific period. The unpaid interest is added to the outstanding principal balance to be repaid over the remaining life of the loan. To avoid deferred interest, a borrower sometimes has the option of making a larger payment that includes what would otherwise become deferred interest.

DEFICIENCY LETTER: Securities Exchange Commission written notice for the expansion or correction of a securities prospectus.

DEFICIENCY IN DESIGN: Exists when a control necessary to meet audit objectives is missing or not properly designed so that even if the control operates correctly, the control objective may not be met.

DEFICIENCY IN OPERATION: Exists when a properly designed control does not operate as designed, or when the person performing the control does not possess the necessary authority or qualifications to perform the control effectively.

DEFICIT: The debt balance of a retained earnings account. It is a financial shortage that occurs when liabilities exceed assets.

DEFICIT SPENDING: Excess of expenditures over revenue income.

DEFINED BENEFIT PENSION PLAN: A traditional nonportable pension plan where benefit is defined in a formula that is often based on the final years of employment. The benefit is paid as a single life annuity for single clients without dependents. It is a qualified retirement plan that suggests the total amount of money received at retirement.

DEFINED CONTRIBUTION PENSION PLAN: A popular portable retirement benefit for health care workers and employees. The most popular versions of this type of plan are the various IRA and 401(k) plan types. The amount of contribution is defined, not the final benefit. The final benefit depends on how well an employee's investments perform. Another important feature is that the employee must choose the investments to which to allocate his or her contributions (and often the employer's contributions). Plans typically offer three or more selections, and the employee decides on the percentage of money to be invested in each.

DEFLATE: Economic process where monetary and fiscal authorities act to stabilize or reverse an upward trend in general price levels. Monetarists view this activity as decreasing the money supply.

DEFLATION: A sustained period of falling interest rates, prices, and economics.

DEFLATOR: Mathematical factor used to convert current dollar amounts into inflation adjusted dollar amounts.

DEGREE OF LEVERAGE: The amount of profits derived from products, services, and sales, in percentage terms.

DELBANCO, SUZANNE: Executive director for the Leapfrog Group in Washington, D.C.

DELINQUENCY: Failure to make debt/bond payments when due.

DELINQUENT CLAIM: Overdue statement of medical charges, issued when a medical bill is not submitted in a timely fashion.

DELIST: Formal removal of securities that were previously approved for trading on a recognized exchange.

DELIVERY: The process of meeting the terms of a written option when notification of assignment has been received. In the case of a short call, the writer must deliver stock and in return receives cash for the stock sold. In the case of a short put, the writer pays cash and in return receives the stock purchased.

DELIVERY CHARGES: The expenses entailed in making or taking a delivery on the futures or cash markets. Also, it is used to reflect the fact that there may be additional risks associated with holding the nearest month in commodity futures contracts. These risks can be potential squeezes, lack of good delivery storage, transportation problems, and other impediments to a smooth and orderly market.

DELIVERY DATE: Same as the security settlement or delivery date.

DELIVERY NOTICE: A document that expresses the intent of the seller to make good delivery to a long paying or long buyer of a futures contract.

DELIVERY PRICE: Invoiced price for a futures contract.

DELIVERY VERSUS PAYMENT (DVP): A method of settling transactions whereby payment on the transaction is made when the securities involved in the transaction are delivered and accepted. The term is often used to refer specifically to a transaction settled in this manner where a customer (typically an institutional investor) has purchased securities from a dealer. The term is also used generally to refer to all types of transactions settled in this way.

DELTA: Relationship between the price of an option and its underlying futures contract or stock price. It is expressed between the range of -1.0 to $+1.0$.

DELTA EQUIVALENCY: Determines the effective market behavior for combined derivative positions.

DEMAND: Relationship between the price of a health care item or service and the quantity demand.

DEMAND CURVE: Graphical relationship between quantity demanded and health care product or service price.

DEMAND DEPOSITS: Checking accounts and bank deposits subject to demand withdrawal.

DEMAND FUNCTION: Relationship between medical quantity demand and price; micro- (individual patient) or macroeconomic demand of society.

DEMAND LOAN: A debt due on demand without a maturity date.

DEMAND PULL INFLATION: Health care or other product. A good or service price rise caused by the increase in aggregate demand.

DEMAND SCHEDULE: Tabular depiction of how the quantity demanded of health care goods and services would change with price, given all other health care demand determinants.

DEMORO, ROSE-ANN: Executive director for the California Nurses Association in Oakland, California.

DENIED CLAIM: A health care bill rejected for insurance payment. An appeals process/protocol is available.

DENOMINATION: The par value amount represented by a particular securities certificate. Bearer bonds are typically issued in denominations of $1,000 or (more commonly) $5,000 par value per certificate. Registered bonds are typically issued in variable denominations, multiples of $1,000 up to $100,000 or more per certificate (although denominations of larger than $100,000 are not acceptable for delivery purposes between dealers unless specifically identified as such at the time of trade). Notes are typically issued in denominations of $25,000 or more per certificate.

DEPARTMENT CAPITATION: Fixed payment per medical specialty service on a PM/PM basis.

DEPOSIT: Posting money or near-money in the bank for payment of health care products, goods, or services rendered.

DEPOSIT IN TRANSIT: A deposit not yet in the bank, or float.

DEPOSIT PREMIUM: A premium deposit required by an insurance company on those forms of health insurance subject to premium adjustment.

DEPOSIT TICKET: A recorded paper trail for a deposit.

DEPOSITORY: A clearing agency registered with the Securities and Exchange Commission (SEC) that provides mobilization, safekeeping, and book-entry settlement services to its participants. The four registered depositories are The Pacific Securities Depository Trust Company (San Francisco), The

Depository Trust Company (New York), The Midwest Securities Trust Company (Chicago), and The Philadelphia Depository Trust Company.

DEPRECIATION: Decreasing value or wasting away, as in depletion over time. The continuous decline in the value of a health care or other company's buildings, instruments, and equipment in the course of its operations. It is an item of expense through which the money paid for the plant and equipment is shown as having been spent in installments over the productive lifetime of the plant or equipment. It may be considered a noncash expense.

DEPRECIATION AMOUNT: The portion of an asset subject to accounting rules regarding depreciation or asset wasting.

DEPRECIATION LIFE: The time period over which the depreciable cost of an asset is expensed.

DEPRECIATION TAX SHIELD: The inflow of funds that provide tax reduction in the amount of taxes owed.

DEPRESSION: A long period of general economic malaise and decline.

DEPRESSED MARKET: A long period of economic malaise and securities decline.

DEPTH OF MARKET: The number of securities that can be sold without substantially affecting market price.

DERIVATIVE: Derivatives are financial arrangements between two parties whose payments are derived from the performance of an agreed-upon benchmark. They can be issued based on currencies, commodities, government or corporate debt, home mortgages, stocks, interest rates, or any combination of the above. The primary purpose of derivatives is to hedge investment risk. In the case of debt securities, derivatives can swap floating interest rate risk for a fixed interest rate. Because the possibility of a reduced interest rate is the most important risk to the investor's capital, coupled with changes in currency values, derivatives can be an important investment tool. Derivatives can be risky if they involve high leverage: both parties to the transaction are exposed to market moves with little capital changing hands. Remember, when the market moves are favorable, the leverage provides a high return compared with the relatively small amount of investment capital actually at risk. However, when market moves are unfavorable, the reverse is true: enormous losses may be incurred. International health care corporations are major investors in derivatives, because exports can suffer upon currency fluctuations or the corporations want to change a floating rate liability to a fixed-rate obligation. However, even though corporations were originally the main purchasers of derivatives (primarily because of the high minimum transaction size), the opportunity is now available for some individuals to take advantage of the benefits of derivatives. This is done primarily through private partnerships (not generally available to the public.)

DERIVATIVE PRICING MODEL: Theoretical determination regarding options and other derivatives useful in evaluating their market value.

DERIVED DEMAND: Demand for a health care input derived from demand for the product that the input is used to produce or serve.

DESCRIPTIVE HEALTH CARE ECONOMICS: The collection, study and reporting of relevant health care economic data.

DESIGNATED ORDER: An order for securities held in a syndicate that is submitted by an account member on behalf of a buyer on which all or a portion of the takedown is to be credited to certain members of the syndicate. The buyer directs who will receive the designation and what percentage of the total designation each member will receive. Generally, two or more syndicate members will be designated to receive a portion of the credit.

DETECTION RISK: Uncertainty that an auditor will not detect a material misstatement in financial records.

DETECTIVE CONTROLS: Detect errors or fraud that have already occurred which could result in a misstatement of financial statements.

DETERMINANTS OF AGGREGATE DEMAND: Factors such as consumption tastes or government spending that shift the aggregate health care demand curve.

DETERMINANTS OF AGGREGATE SUPPLY: Factors such as price and productivity that shift the aggregate health care supply curve.

DETERMINANTS OF DEMAND: Nonprice factors that determine the quantity demanded of health care products, goods, or services.

DETERMINANTS OF SUPPLY: Nonprice factors that determine the quantity supplied of health care products, goods, or services.

DETERMINISTIC FUNCTIONS AND VARIABLES: Nonrandom, in the context of other variables available.

DEVALUATION: The decline in the value of one currency over another.

DEVIANT BILLING: Deviation in billing can be detected through utilization data that insurance companies produce on all providers that submit a claim for payment of services. Insurance companies track utilization through a variety of parameters, including CPT codes, ICD-9-CM, or number of referrals. Different programs utilize certain benchmarks to trigger a review. For example, a physician who sees patients in the office from 8:00 A.M. until 8:00 P.M., 7 days a week and has the highest billing amounts in the region can be subjected to a review. This doctor's activities would be scrutinized. The utilization review department would probably flag this doctor's provider number and request more information on a sampling of his or her claims, based on the volume. Some utilization review activities may occur due to the type of services that a doctor may offer. For example, if a cardiologist should suddenly start billing for a large number of incisions and drainage of abscesses, this might trigger a review, because that might not be a typical scope of service for this doctor in this locality. Thresholds vary from locale to locale regarding what triggers an audit. There are consultants who have suggested querying the local carrier for provider-specific information regarding utilization activity to compare against community performance. Some Carrier Advisory Committee (CAC) representatives have indicated that this may bring undesirable attention from the Medicare program and trigger an audit.

DIAGNOSIS CREEP: Slang term meaning increased medical acuity coding of an illness, disease, injury, or treatment in order to increase reimbursement in a fee-for-service system. Also known as diagnostic upgrading.

DIAGNOSIS AND STATISTICAL MANUAL OF MENTAL DISORDERS, 4TH ED., REV. (DSM-IV-R): American Psychiatric Association manual of diagnostic criteria and terminology.

DIAGNOSIS RELATED GROUPS (DRGS): (1) System of classifying patients on the basis of diagnoses for purposes of payment to hospitals. (2) A system for determining case mix, used for payment under Medicare's prospective payment system (PPS) and by some other payers. The DRG system classifies patients into groups based on the principal diagnosis, type of surgical procedure, presence or absence of significant comorbidities or complications, and other relevant criteria. DRGs are intended to categorize patients into groups that are clinically meaningful and homogeneous with respect to resource use. Medicare's PPS currently uses almost 500 mutually exclusive DRGs, each of which is assigned a relative weight that compares its costliness to the average for all DRGs.

DIALING AND SMILING: Slang sales expression indicating the emotional tone of a stockbroker when cold calling unsuspecting sales prospects.

DIAMONDS (DIA): Represent ownership in a unit investment trust established to accumulate and hold a portfolio of the equity securities that comprise the Dow Jones Industrial Average. They seek investment results that, before expenses, correspond to the price and yield performance of the entire DJIA. Total returns are calculated monthly and quarterly using the daily 4:00 P.M. net asset value (NAV) method. Distributions, if any, are assumed to be reinvested back into the fund on the pay date at the NAV on that date. Performance data quoted represents past performance and is no guarantee of future results.

DICKEY, NANCY, MD: Past president of the American Medical Association in Chicago, Illinois.

DIFFERENTIAL: Brokerage transaction fee for odd lot stock purchases.

DIFFERENTIAL COST: Any expense charge that is present under one alternative but is absent in whole or part under another alternative.

DIFFERENTIATED PRODUCT/SERVICE: A health care product, good, or service that differs in some positive or enticing way to other similar products or services, and is not a perfect substitute.

DIFFUSION PROCESS: The dissemination of a health care innovation, drug, technique, and so forth, from entity to entity or practitioner to practitioner.

DILUTION: The decrease in earnings per share because of new securities issuance.

DILUTIVE EFFECT: The lowering of the book or market value of the shares of a company's stock as a result of more shares outstanding. A company's initial registration may include more shares than are initially issued when the company goes public for the first time. Later, an issue of more stock by a company (called a primary offering, distinguished from the initial public offering) dilutes the existing shares outstanding. Also, earnings-per-share calculations are said to be "fully diluted" when all common stock equivalents (convertible securities, rights, and warrants) are included. "Fully diluted" numbers are used in analysis when there is a likelihood of conversion or exercise of rights and warrants.

DIMINISHING MARGINAL RATES OF SUBSTITUTION: The marginal rates of substitution of health care service A for B, that will tend to decline as more A is substituted for B, along any patient's indifference curve.

DIMINISHING MARGINAL RETURNS: The mathematical and economic concept that incremental health care value is inversely related to existing quantities prior to the value added increment.

DIMINISHING MARGINAL UTILITY: The decline in marginal health care utility that occurs when more and more of a health care product, good, or service is consumed.

DIRECT CAPITATION: Full advanced provider-risk personal fixed rate reimbursement, per patient head, regardless of the quantity or volume of medical care provided but using rolling averages for primary care physicians. It is full persona capitation.

DIRECT CLAIM PAYMENT: Patient-payer interaction void of employer intervention.

DIRECT CONTRACT METHOD: Health care plan that deals directly with medical providers rather than a third party or other intermediary.

DIRECT COST: The cost of a medical service that can be directly traced to a specific patient or medical service. It is the opposite of an indirect cost.

DIRECT DEBT: The sum of the total bonded debt and any short-term debt of the hospital or other issuer. Direct debt may be incurred in the issuer's own name or assumed through the annexation of territory or consolidation with another governmental unit.

DIRECT DEPOSIT: Funds are placed automatically to checking or savings accounts via a pre-authorized system. Some types of direct deposits are Social Security, SSI, VA benefits, annuities, pension benefits, payroll checks, and dividend checks.

DIRECT FINANCING: Financing, especially as with a loan or debt, arranged without a third party intermediary.

DIRECT INVESTMENT: Investing, especially as with a securities purchase, arranged without a third party intermediary.

DIRECT ISSUE: The sale of commercial corporate paper (debt) arranged without a third party intermediary.

DIRECT LABOR: Compensation of traceable labor employee costs.

DIRECT METHOD: Cash flow format for operating activities that list major categories of cash receipts and disbursements.

DIRECT OVERHEAD: Pro rata overhead expenses, also known as the *burden rate*, built into the *cost of goods sold.*

DIRECT PARTICIPATION PROGRAM (DP PROGRAM; DPP): A group investment structured so that investors are direct recipients of all tax consequences. It is a Tax-Advantaged Investment (TAI).

DIRECT PLACEMENT: Securities sales, between two investors, arranged without a third party intermediary.

DIRECT PURCHASE: Purchase of an open-ended company directly from the mutual fund, without a third-party sales intermediary such as a broker.

DIRECT RELATIONSHIP: Two economic or financial variables that change in the same direction.

DIRECT ROLLOVER: Qualified plan distribution directly to a custodian or other trustee.

DIRECT WRITE-OFF: A credit department-type decision to forfeit an uncollectible account.

DIRECTOR: One elected by stakeholders to determine the policy and procedures of a health care or other corporation.

DIRTY CLAIM: Slang term for a rejected health care bill. A dingy or other claim.

DISBURSEMENT: A monetary payout to discharge or reduce a debt or liability.

DISBURSEMENT FLOAT: The amount of time between medical goods or services provided, and payment in a health care organization or other system.

DISCHARGE OF BANKRUPTCY: A legal or court order terminating a bankruptcy proceeding.

DISCLAIMER OF OPINION: Auditor statement indicating inability to express an opinion on the fairness of financial statements and the reason for the inability. This is required to disclaim depending on the limitation in scope.

DISCLOSURE: Divulging financial, economic, or accounting information so that financial statements may be understood.

DISCLOSURE PRINCIPLE: The suggestion that financial statements should be detailed enough for outsiders to make informed decisions about the firm.

DISCONTINUED OPERATIONS: Segment of a medical clinic or hospital business that is terminated.

DISCOUNT: A reduction in premium payments or medical products, goods, or service costs. The percentage or dollar amount below net asset value at which a closed-end company may sell (opposite of premium). The sale of a bond below its par value.

DISCOUNT BOND: A bond that sells below its face amount, usually because interest rates have risen since issue. A decline in the credit standing of the issuer will frequently cause the bond's price to drop as well. Some bonds are originally offered at a discount.

DISCOUNT BROKER: A stockbroker or brokerage firm that charges lower commissions than a full service equivalent.

DISCOUNT DRUG LIST: Certain drugs that are available for a reduced price from a drug manufacturer.

DISCOUNT FOR LACK OF CONTROL: Amount reduced in the economic interest of a business entity for the inability to steer policy or management.

DISCOUNT FOR LACK OF MARKETABILITY: Amount reduced in the economic interest of a business entity reflected in a lack of promotional or advertising endeavors.

DISCOUNT FOR LACK OF VOTING: Amount reduced in the economic interest of a business entity reflected in a lack or reduction of voting rights.

DISCOUNT FROM NET-ASSET VALUE: The amount a closed-ended fund sells below its net asset value (NAV).

DISCOUNT POINTS: Payment made to a lender at the inception of a loan for the purpose of reducing the interest rate of a loan. Each point is equal to 1% of the loan amount (i.e., three points on a $100,000 mortgage would equal $3,000).

DISCOUNT RATE: The amount of interest that Federal Reserve Banks (FRBs) charge their member banks for overnight loans. The rate of return factor used to convert present money value into the future value of money. It is financial return to compensate for financial risk taking in a business project to mitigate the lost opportunity cost of holding money or investing in another project.

DISCOUNT STOCK OPTION: A right given that allows an employee to purchase shares of employer stock at a price that is substantially below the stock's market value on the date the option is granted.

DISCOUNTED CASH FLOWS: The adjusted cash flow to reflect present-value for the cost-of-capital, over time.

DISCOUNTED FEE FOR SERVICE: Agreement between a provider and payer that is less than the medical provider's full fee. This may be a fixed amount per service or a percentage discount. Providers generally accept such contracts because they represent a means to increase their volume or reduce their chances of losing volume.

DISCOUNTED FUTURE EARNINGS: Income approach valuation method converting the present value of a future economic business entity using a discount rate.

DISCOUNTED PRESENT VALUE: The present value of money to be received in the future.

DISCOUNTING: The treatment of time in valuing costs and benefits, that is, the adjustment of costs and benefits to their present values, requiring a choice of discount rate and time frame. The process of determining present value.

DISCRETE CHOICE ANALYSIS: Economic statistical methodology where only one variable is measured and limited in alternatives to values of 1 or 0.

DISCRETIONARY ACCOUNT: An account in which the customer authorizes in writing a registered representative to use his judgment (completely, or within limits) in buying and selling securities including selection, amount, and price. However, judgment as to time and/or price only is not considered discretion.

DISCRETIONARY INCOME: The extra money available after all bills have been paid.

DISCRETIONARY ORDER: An order that empowers a registered representative (stockbroker) with a discretionary account to use his own judgment on the customer's behalf with respect to choice of security, quantity of security, and whether any such transaction should be a purchase or sale.

DISCRETIONARY TRUST: Arrangement in which a trustee has the authority to make investment or other decisions, and has control within the framework of a trust instrument.

DISECONOMIES OF SCALE: An increase in the average cost of health care entity operations resulting from managerial difficulties in large scale business enterprises.

DISHONORED NOTE: Failure to pay or default on a note. A bounced check.

DISINFLATION: A sharp reduction in the annual rate of health care product or services inflation.

DISINTERMEDIATION: The removal of a third party intermediary in a securities, business, economic, or other transaction.

DISINVESTMENT: The reduction in capital investment through the disposition or sales of goods, equipment, or other assets.

DISMAL SCIENCE: Slang term for the study of economics.

DISPENSE AS WRITTEN (DAW): Instructions for a pharmacist to use an expensive brand name drug, rather than a less expensive generic equivalent.

DISPENSING FEE: A fee charge for filling a drug prescription.

DISPERSION: Mathematical deviation from the norm, average, or mean. Common measures include:

- Coefficient of Variation
- Range
- Standard Deviation
- Variance

DISPOSABLE INCOME (DI): Ability to spend or save after the payment of income taxes.

DISPROPORTIONATE SHARE HOSPITAL (DSH): Hospital expenses allocated for indigent care or low income patients, or those with special needs, according to U.S. Code 42: "Grants to States for Medical Assistance Programs."

DISSOLUTION: The termination of a partnership, corporation, or other agreement.

DISTRESS SALE: The sale of assets under less than ideal conditions, for less than current value.

DISTRESSED SECURITIES: Issues in bankruptcy or other severely impaired securities that have very low credit ratings.

DISTRIBUTION DATE: The date when a dividend is paid to shareholders.

DISTRIBUTION EXPENSE: Expense of selling, advertising, and delivery of medical products, goods, and/or health care services.

DISTRIBUTION STAGE: The period of disbursement for an annuity.

DISTRIBUTIONS: Payments by a health care business entity to its owners of items such as cash assets, stocks, or retained earnings.

DISTRIBUTOR: A person or company that purchases open-end investment company shares directly from the issuer for resale to others.

DIVERSIFICATION: Investment in a number of different security issues for the purpose of spreading and reducing the risks inherent in all investing.

DIVERSIFIED COMMON STOCK FUND: A diversified management company that invests substantially all of its assets in a portfolio of common stocks in a wide variety of industries.

DIVERSIFIED MANAGEMENT COMPANY: A management company that has at least 75% of its assets arranged so as to not own securities of one issuer having a value greater than 5% of the management company's total assets and to not own more than 10% of the voting securities of any corporation. There are no restrictions placed upon the other 25% of the company's assets. Up to 30% of assets could be in one stock.

DIVESTITURE: The outright sale of assets, or inventory.

DIVIDED ACCOUNT (WESTERN ACCOUNT): A method for determining liability stated in the agreement among underwriters in which each member of an underwriting syndicate is liable only for the amount of its participation in the issue, and not for any unsold portion of the participation amounts allocated to the other underwriters.

DIVIDEND: Partial premium return when insurance earnings exceed costs. Or, a portion of corporate profit paid back to stockholders.

DIVIDEND ARREARS: Accumulated dividends owed to current stockholders.

DIVIDEND DATE: Entitlement to security dividends or the actual payment date.

DIVIDEND DISCOUNT MODEL: Statistical model to estimate stock value based on the discounted value of future income, dividends, or business cash streams.

DIVIDEND GROWTH VALUATION MODEL: A valuation method that uses dividends and discounted growth back to present values.

DIVIDEND PAYOUT RATIO (DPR): Corporate common stock dividends divided by the net income available for common stockholders. It is the compliment of retained earnings ratio.

DIVIDEND REINVESTMENT PLAN: The reinvestment of cash dividends into stocks.

DIVIDEND YIELD: Ratio of current dividend to the current price of a stock share. For example, if hospital company ABC trades at $90 per share, its $2 dividend provides a dividend yield of $2/$90 or 2.22%.

DIVIDENDS: Distributions in cash to stockholders earned and declared by a corporate health care or hospital board of directors, computed by dividing cash by price per share at purchase. For example, if a health care stock were trading at $100, and the dividends equaled $2.80, then the yield would be 2.80%. Stock dividends are also possible.

DIVISION OF LABOR: The separation of larger health care service projects, into smaller individual tasks, by workers who specialize in those tasks.

DIVISOR: A mathematic factor to adjust stock splits that would otherwise distort comparisons.

DOCUMENTATION COMPLETION DATE: A final set of audit documentation is assembled for retention as of a date not more than 45 days after the report release date.

DOG: Slang for an underperforming asset.

DOGS OF DOW: The 10 best yielding equities of the DJIA, and usually purchased over rolling annual periods. It is a slang term and unproven investing model.

DOING-BUSINESS-AS (DBA): Fictitious nonlegal name of a person or business actually conducting business transactions.

DOLAN, THOMAS: President of the American College of Health Care Executives in Chicago, Illinois.

DOLLAR BEARS: One who believes the U.S. dollar will decrease in value against foreign currencies.

DOLLAR BOND: A colloquial term for a bond that is usually quoted and traded in terms of dollar price rather than yield. Dollar bonds are generally more actively traded securities from larger, term issues rather than securities from serial issues.

DOLLAR COST AVERAGING: Investing equal amounts of money at regular intervals regardless of whether the stock market is moving upward or downward. This reduces average share costs by automatically acquiring more shares in periods of lower securities prices and fewer shares in periods of higher prices. DCA does not assure a profit or protect against depreciation in declining markets. Total dollars invested / number of shares bought.

DOLLAR RATE: One of two factors used to determine prospective diagnostic-related group payment health care rates.

DOMAR AGGREGATION: A principle that suggests the growth rate of a health care aggregate is the weighted average of the growth rates of its individual components, where each component is weighted by the share of the aggregate it makes.

DONATION: Restricted or unrestricted funds provided without the need for repayment.

DONATIVE INTENT: The inclination of a donor to make a gratuitous gift to charity.

DONOR: One who makes a gift to another.

DO NOT REDUCE ORDER (DNRO): A buy limit or a sell stop order that is not to be reduced by the amount of a cash dividend on the ex-dividend date as the customer specifically so requested.

DONSKER'S THEOREM: Synonymous with the Functional Central Limit Theorem.

DOUBLE-BARRELED BOND: A General Obligation bond secured by both a defined source of revenue (other than property taxes) plus the full faith and credit of an issuer that has taxing powers. The term is occasionally, although erroneously, used in reference to hospital bonds secured by any two sources of pledged revenue.

DOUBLE COINCIDENCE OF WANTS: Occurs when patient A desires what provider B is selling, and provider B wants to buy what patient A is selling.

DOUBLE DECLINING BALANCE: A method of accelerated depreciation that multiplies the asset's decreasing book value by a constant percentage that is twofold the straight line depreciation rate.

DOUBLE-ENTRY BOOKKEEPING: Method of recording financial transactions in which each transaction is entered in two or more accounts and involves two-way, self-balancing posting. Total debits must equal total credits.

DOUBLE TAXATION: Health care (Section C) corporate income which is subject to both corporate taxes and individual taxes. Frequently, it is viewed as the case whereby the company's income is taxed and the distribution of that income in the form of a dividend paid to the shareholder is taxed again.

DOUBLE TAX FREE INCOME: Income that is exempt from both federal and state income taxes.

DOUBLE WITCH: The exact date that two related classes of futures and options expire.

DOUGHNUT: Slang term for the coverage gap (hole) in the 2006 Medicare Drug Benefit Plan where patients pay all medication costs from $2,251–$5,100. After medication costs exceed $5,100, patients pay about 5% of the remainder (indexed annually).

DOW JONES INDUSTRIAL AVERAGE (DJIA): A market average indicator consisting (individually) of 30 industrial, 20 transportation, or 15 public utility common stocks [Dow Jones Utility Average, DJUA]. The composite average includes these 65 stocks collectively.

DOW THEORY: A theory predicated on the belief that the rise or fall of stock prices as measured by the Dow Jones Industrial average is both a mirror and a forecaster of business activities.

DOWELL, MARSHA, RN, PhD: Senior editor for the *Journal of the International Society for Research in Healthcare Financial Management,* Towson, Maryland.

DOWN AND IN: Option feature by which a derivative contract becomes active when an indicator, such as price, drops through a trigger point or threshold.

DOWN AND OUT: Option feature by which a derivative contract dies or ceases to exist when an indicator, such as price, drops through a trigger point or threshold.

DOWN GRADE: The lowering of a securities rating by a rating firm, which increases the cost of debt or interest rate.

DOWN PAYMENT: A portion of the upfront payment price to reduce an outstanding purchase balance.

DOWN SIZE: A reduction in health care entity or business size and complexity, but especially a reduction in work force quantity.

DOWN STREAM: Flow of assets, people, money, intellectual capital, or management directives from upper corporate echelons to the rank-and-file.

DOWN STREAM COSTS: Flow of expenses, especially human labor from a primary care provider, and the efficiency improvement methods used to reduce them.

DOWN TICK: The sales of securities at a price lower than the preceding sale.

DOWN TURN: The lowering of a market or economic cycle.

DRAZEN, JEFFREY, MD: Editor-in-Chief for the *New England Journal of Medicine* in Boston, Massachusetts.

DRESSING UP PORTFOLIOS: The purchase or sales of securities by money managers at the end of a time period, usually annually, in order to enhance appearances at the reporting period.

DRG 468–470: Diagnostic related groups which are especially common in medical workload financial analysis:

- 468—extensive operating room procedures unrelated to primary diagnosis
- 469—primary diagnosis invalidated or not matched to discharge summary
- 470—medical records with ungroupable diagnosis
- 477—simple OR procedure not related to primary diagnosis

DRG CREEP: Slang term for diagnostic related group coding creep, or upgrading/up-coding or exaggeration in order to increase reimbursement in a fee-for-service environment.

DRG RATE: Fixed monetary payment (diagnostic related group) amount based on patient averages in a based year for comparison, and adjusted for factors such as inflation, bad debt, specialty, acuity, or other economic factors.

DRG RISK POOL: A hospital's diagnostic related group economic uncertainty.

DRG SPECIFIC PER-CASE PRICE: Fixed diagnostic related group payment rate used by Medicare, with risk limits through the identification of long length of stay (LOS) cases. It is a global fee or category DRG pricing.

DRG WEIGHT: Diagnostic related group assigned index used to reflect relative hospital costs.

DROP DEAD DAY: The absolute final deadline, usually pertaining to payment.

DRUG BENEFIT PLAN: Medicare Part D (2006) basic plan that requires a $250 annual deductible and then 25% of "covered" drug charges between $251–$2,250. Patients pay all medications costs thereafter, from $2,251–$5,100 resulting in a hole or coverage gap. After medication costs exceed $5,100, patients pay about 5% of the remainder (indexed annually).

DUAL DATING: Time sampling of an accountant or auditor report when a subsequent event disclosed in financial statements occurs after completion of field work but before issuance of the report (i.e., "July 20, 2007, except for Note X, as to which the date is January 11, 2008.").

DUE BILL: A legal document that evidences the transfer of title to stock and/or dividends. It must be attached to certificates delivered too late for effective transfer, and will ensure distribution of dividends to the new and rightful owner.

DUE DATE: Government forms scheduled reporting day and payment time stamp. It is the day that one must file and may result in a penalty, fine, and commence interest charges if late.

DUE DILIGENCE: (1) Procedures performed by underwriters in connection with the issuance of a SEC registration statement involving questions concerning the company and its business, products, competitive position, recent financial and other developments, and prospects. Also performed by others in connection with acquisitions and other transactions. (2) Requirement found in ethical codes that the person governed by the ethical rules exercise professional care in conducting his or her activities.

DUE DILIGENCE MEETING: A meeting between corporation officials and the underwriting group to discuss and review detailed information in the registration statement, prepare a final prospectus, and begin negotiation for a formal underwriting agreement. This meeting is held shortly before the anticipated effective date.

DUE ON SALE: A clause in a debt agreement providing that, if the debtor (borrower) sells, transfers, or, in some instances, encumbers the asset, the lender has the right to demand the outstanding balance.

DUMPING: The sales of health care goods and services abroad, at prices below cost, in order to reduce a surplus or gain competitive advantage. OR patient transfer to another medical provider or health care facility because of an inability to pay for care rendered. Slang term.

DUN & BRADSTREET (DB): A for-profit credit information firm.

DU PONT SYSTEM: EI Du Pont de Nemours Company method for determining Return on Assets (ROA) financial performance, by multiplying asset turnover (revenues divided by assets), by return on sales (net income divided by net sales).

DURABLE GOODS: Equipment or instruments with a useful life of 1 year or more, and similar to durable medical equipment (DME).

DURABLE INPUT: Factor of health care production not used up in a single period.

DURATION: The average time to collect a bond's principal and interest payment. A measure of volatility, expressed in years, taking into consideration all of the cash flows produced over the life of a bond. For example, if the duration of a bond is 5 years, then the price of the bond changes 5% for every 1% change in interest rates. Duration is additive in that assets, liabilities, swaps, and other credit instruments can be added to arrive at a portfolio's duration. Some guidelines are:

- Duration of a zero coupon is its maturity.
- Duration of a coupon security is less than its maturity.
- Duration extends with maturity.
- Duration is inversely related to market rate.
- Duration is inversely related to coupon rate.

DUTCH AUCTION: Auction market where price is reduced until sold (U.S. T-bill system).

DUTY: A tariff, import, export, or consumption tax.

DUTY TO ACCOUNT: Obligation to keep factual and accurate financial records and return funds to owners.

DYNAMIC PROGRESS: The development over time of less costly and more efficient health care delivery. It is health care economic progress.

E

E-CODE: *International Classification of Diseases, Ninth Edition, Clinical Modification* code that describes an injury or adverse medicine reaction, rather than disease or illness for medical reimbursement purposes.

EACH WAY: Stockbroker commission made on both the buy and sell side of a securities transaction.

EAFE INDEX: Morgan Stanley Capital International Europe, Australasia, Far East Index of over 1,000 foreign stock prices. The index is translated into U.S. dollars.

EARLY EXERCISE: A feature of American-style securities options that allows the holder to exercise an option at any time prior to the expiration date.

EARN-OUT: Payments not part of the initial acquisition cost of a firm and based on future earnings.

EARNED INCOME: Income derived from the active participation in a trade or business, such as a medical practice, clinic, or health care entity. This includes wages, salaries, professional fees, and other amounts received as compensation for services rendered.

EARNED SURPLUS: Income kept in a health care or other business and not distributed to owners or shareholders, referred to as retained income or as earnings retained in the business.

EARNEST MONEY: A good-faith deposit for a specific transaction.

EARNING ASSET: Any income-producing asset.

EARNINGS: Profit or income from a health care business or other enterprise.

EARNINGS BEFORE TAXES (EBT): Business or corporate profit before taxes, but after bond and debt-holder interest payments have been paid.

EARNINGS LIMITATION: The limitation on the amount of income a patient who is receiving Social Security benefits can earn before those benefits are reduced. Both the earnings limitation amount and the benefit reduction are subject to escalation and are annually indexed.

EARNINGS MOMENTUM: A trend of increasing earnings per share of common stock.

EARNINGS MOMENTUM INVESTING: A style of investing that looks for emerging health care organizations (EHOs) or other companies that are on growth trends similar to a growth style. Two nuances differentiate these two styles: (1) the earnings momentum style focuses mainly on the growth of the earnings of the company, and (2) the earnings momentum style looks for an accelerating increase in the growth of earnings.

EARNINGS MULTIPLIER: The Price / Earnings ratio.

EARNINGS PER PREFERRED SHARE (EPPS): Total earnings divided by total preferred shares outstanding.

EARNINGS PER SHARE (EPS): The amount of company profit available to each share of common stock. EPS = Net income (after taxes and preferred dividends) divided by Number of outstanding shares.

EARNINGS PRICE RATIO: The ratio relationship of earnings per share (EPS) to current stock price.

EARNINGS REPORT: Earnings per share report of a public company for the latest accounting period.

EARNINGS SURPRISE: An earnings report that is either better or worse than expected by analysts.

EARNINGS YIELD: Earnings per share (EPS) for the most recent 12 fiscal months, divided by current market price, per share.

EASTERN ACCOUNT: An undivided brokerage account.

EASY MONEY POLICY: An expanding money supply.

EATING STOCK: An underwriter unable to find buyers for securities and who must purchase them for its own account.

ECONOMETRICS/ECONOMETRICIAN: The study of economics, or one who studies economics, especially health care economics.

ECONOMIC ACTIVITY: What patients do to cope with scarce health care products, goods, or services.

ECONOMIC BENEFITS: Inflows from a health care or business entity, such as cash, insurance payments, accounts receivable, Medicare/Medicaid, and so forth.

ECONOMIC COST: The money value of all inputs in a health care activity or business enterprise over a period of time.

ECONOMIC CREDENTIALING: Evaluating a physician's economic and professional financial behavior (i.e., tests ordered, hospital bed days, outcomes, etc.) in deciding upon medical staff appointment or re-appointment.

ECONOMIC DEPRECIATION: The change in market price of a durable health care good (DME) or service input, over time.

ECONOMIC EFFICIENCY: The state in which the cost of producing a specific health care product, service, or output good is as low as possible. It is the relationship between scarce health care resource inputs and the resulting output of health care goods, products, or services, with a given dollar value and with the smallest expenditures for inputs while obtaining the largest total production of outputs.

ECONOMIC EXCHANGE: Transaction in which two or more parties exchange something of value, such as insurance premiums for health care services.

ECONOMIC GROWTH: Expansion in the general economy or health care services sector production as measured by the annual percentage increase in GNP, currently about 15% for the health care industrial complex.

ECONOMIC INDICATORS: Key statistics that estimate the direction of the economy or a specific sector, such as health care.

ECONOMIC LIFE: The period of time in which a health care or other organization may generate financial benefits.

ECONOMIC MEDICAL VALUE ADDED© (EMVA)©: Concept that combines finance and accounting income to determine medical practice, clinic, hospital, or other health care business-enterprise entity operations value as an ongoing concern. The term was coined by the *Institute* of Medical Business Advisors, Inc., (*i*MBA, Inc.) of Atlanta, Georgia.

ECONOMIC ORDER QUANTITY (EOQ): The optimal or least costly quantity of inventory or Durable Medical Equipment (DME) that should be purchased, and on what schedule. This assumes:

- Constant demand rate
- Constant lead time
- Entire quantity received at once
- Constant unit costs
- No limits on size of inventory

The mathematical formula for EOQ is the square root of 2SO/C: where inputs: S = annual usage or purchases in units; O is the cost per order; and C is the annual carrying cost per unit:

$$EOQ = \sqrt{\frac{2(\text{Annual usage in units})(\text{Order cost})}{(\text{Annual carrying cost per unit})}}$$

ECONOMIC PERSPECTIVE: The viewpoint that rational decisions based on costs-benefit analysis be included in the deeds of the health care industrial complex.

ECONOMIC PROFIT: The difference between total health care or other business revenue, and the cost of all related inputs used by an entity over time. *See also* net present value (NPV).

ECONOMIC RENTS: Health care product, goods, or service earnings that exceed the opportunity costs of the business enterprise.

ECONOMIC RESOURCES: Health care inputs used in the process of delivering health care services or products.

ECONOMIC RISK: Securities losses trigged by domestic or international events.

ECONOMIC VALUE ADDED (EVA): Concept that combines finance and accounting income to determine corporate operations value. The term was coined by the Stern Stewart & Co. of New York.

ECONOMICS, HEALTH CARE: The formal research science and study of resource generation, use, and allocation in the health care industrial complex.

ECONOMIES OF SCALE: Reduction in health care production unit-costs from an increased size in business operations.

ECONOMIES OF SCOPE: The decrease in average total cost made possible by increasing the number of different health care products, goods, or services.

ECONOMIZING: Making the best and highest use of scarce health care resources and inputs.

ECONOMIZING PROBLEM: The discrepancy between wants and needs and the costs and scarce inputs available to produce health care services. It involves the impossibility of unlimited health care.

ECONOMY, HEALTH CARE: The mechanism through which the use of doctors, nurses, labor, land, vehicles, equipment, instruments, buildings, drugs, and other physical and cognitive resources are organized to meet the health care demands of patients in a society.

EDGEWORTH BOX: A schematic diagram that demonstrates visually all fixed allocations of health care goods and services between two economic parties.

EFFECTIVE DATE: The date on which a security can be ordered publicly if no deficiency letter is submitted to the issuer by the Securities Exchange Commission (SEC).

EFFECTIVE INTEREST RATE: The cost of credit on a yearly basis expressed as a percentage. Includes up-front costs paid to obtain the debt, and is, therefore, usually a higher amount than the interest rate stipulated in the debt.

EFFECTIVE TAX RATE: Total income taxes expressed as a percentage of net income before taxes.

EFFICIENCY: The measurement and maximization of health care economic inputs versus health care outputs.

EFFICIENCY WAGE: A salary that minimizes the cost of a unit of health care product or service output.

EFFICIENT ALLOCATION OF RESOURCES: The distribution of scarce health care services inputs, among a production curve of different health care products and services that maximize patient satisfaction, that is, achieve the point of maximum efficiency (PME).

EFFICIENT CAPITAL MARKETS: An exchange that fully reflects all public information.

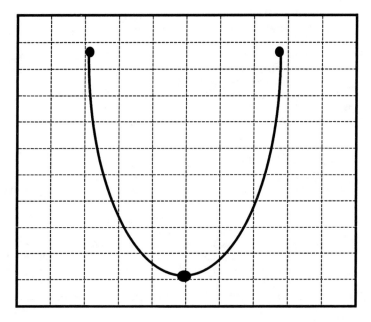

Figure 1: Point of Maximum Efficiency.

EFFICIENT FRONTIER: A graphical leading line that represents the highest rate of return for each particular mix of assets in a portfolio.

EFFICIENT MARKET HYPOTHESIS (THEORY): Belief that all market prices and movements reflect all that can be known about an investment. If all the information available is already reflected in stock prices, research aimed at finding undervalued assets or special situations should be useless.

EFFICIENT PORTFOLIO: The highest investment return possible for a given level of risk.

EITHER/OR ORDER: An order consisting of a limit and a stop for the same security at different prices. The execution of one order will cancel the other.

ELASTIC DEMAND: Occurs when the price of elasticity of demand for health care or other goods, products, or services is greater than one (1) unit.

ELASTIC SUPPLY: Occurs when the price of elasticity of supply for health care or other goods, products, or services is greater than one (1) unit.

ELASTICITY: Responsiveness of patients and health care providers to a change in price or fee schedule.

ELASTICITY COEFFICIENT: The value obtained when the percentage change in health care output quantity-demanded exceeds the percentage change in its price.

ELASTICITY DEMAND: Greater than one unit (1) indicates the quantity demanded of a health care product or service decreases by a larger percentage than a corresponding price increase.

ELASTICITY FORMULA: The medical fee schedule price elasticity of demand, or supply, is equal to:

Percentage change in health care quantity demanded or supplied/ percentage change in price; which is equal to:

Change in quantity demanded or supplied/original quantity demanded or supplied; divided by change in price/original price.

ELASTICITY SUPPLY: The percentage change in the quantity supplied of a health care product or service, divided by the percentage change in its price.

ELASTICITY SUBSTITUTION: Percentage change in capital health care labor from a 1% change in related factor prices.

ELECTION §83(B): An income tax election that allows a health care or other employee who receives employer stock under a tax-deferred arrangement to report income that results from the receipt of such stock in the year the stock is received.

ELECTRONIC BILLING: Medical, DME, and related health insurance bills or premiums submitted though Electronic Data Interchange EDI (nonpaper claims) systems.

ELECTRONIC CLAIM: The digital representation of a medical bill or invoice.

ELECTRONIC FUNDS TRANSFER (EFT): The nonpaper based transfer of funds by electronic means.

ELECTRONIC MEDICAL CLAIMS (EMC): Usually refers to a flat file format used to transmit or transport medical claims, such as the 192-byte UB-92 Institutional EMC format and the 320-byte Professional EMC-NSF.

ELECTRONIC REMITTANCE ADVICE: Any of several electronic formats for explaining the payments of health care claims.

ELEPHANTS: Slang term for large institutional securities investors.

ELIGIBLE EXPENSES: Reasonable and customary charges for health care services incurred while insurance coverage is in effect.

ELLIOT, RALPH NELSON; WAVE: Economic theorist who suggested the concept of technical (nonfundamental) securities analysis and the idea that financial markets and other human endeavors run in cycles with a ratio of 5:3; advancements to declines.

ELLWOOD, PAUL JR., MD: The father of modern managed care who coined the term *Health Maintenance Organization,* along with Stanford University economist Alain Enthoven, PhD, in the Nixon Administration. He is the creator of the managed care competitive concept who has since recanted some of its draconian cost cutting initiatives as counter-productive. He is currently president of Health Outcomes Institute, a nonprofit health policy research organization, and President of the Jackson Hole Group in Teton Village, Wyoming, a health care reform policy think tank. He has been called one of the most important figures in American health care in the last half century, that whose 35 years of health care reform experience confirmed that the American system may be dysfunctional and deteriorating. He is also the founder of InterStudy in Minneapolis, Minnesota.

ELVES: Slang term for an unofficial group of technical analysts and financial forecasters.

ELZINGA-HOGARTY CRITERION: Health care competitive market approach consistent with the economic theory of corporate mergers and acquisitions, which suggests that the outflow of medical goods and services to adjacent areas is relatively small, at the same time that inputs from neighboring markets are also small.

EMANCIPATION: The ability and freedom to assume certain legal responsibilities associated with adulthood.

EMBEDDED OPTION: An option whose characteristics are not formally specified, but are informally implied.

EMERGENCY MEDICAL TREATMENT AND ACTIVE LABOR ACT (EMTALA): A statute intended to ensure that all patients who come to the emergency department of a hospital receive care, regardless of their insurance or ability to pay. Both hospitals and physicians need to work together to ensure compliance with the provisions of this law. The statute imposes three fundamental requirements on hospitals that participate in the Medicare program with regard to patients requesting emergency care. First, the hospital must conduct an appropriate medical screening examination to determine if an emergency medical condition exists. Second, if the hospital determines that an emergency medical condition exists, it must either provide the treatment necessary to stabilize the emergency medical condition or comply with the statute's requirements to affect a proper transfer of a patient whose condition has not been stabilized. A hospital is considered to have met this second requirement if an individual refuses the hospital's offer of additional examination or treatment, or refuses to consent to a transfer, after having been informed of the risks and benefits of treatment. Third, the statute's requirement is activated if an individual's emergency medical condition has not been stabilized. A hospital may not transfer an individual with an unstable emergency medical condition unless: (1) the individual or his or her representative makes a written request for transfer to another medical facility after being informed of the risk of transfer and the transferring hospital's obligation under the statute to provide additional examination or treatment; (2) a physician has signed a certification summarizing the medical risks and benefits of a transfer and certifying that, based upon the information available at the time of transfer, the medical benefits reasonably expected from the transfer outweigh the increased risks; or (3) a qualified medical person signs the certification after the physician, in consultation with the qualified medical person, has made the determination that the benefits of transfer outweigh the increased risks, if a physician is not physically present when the transfer decision is made. The physician must later countersign the certification. Physician and/or hospital misconduct may result in violations of the statute. One area of particular concern is physician on-call responsibilities. Physician practices whose members serve as on-call hospital emergency room physicians are advised to familiarize themselves with the hospital's policies regarding on-call physicians. This can be done by reviewing the medical staff bylaws or policies and procedures of the hospital that must define the responsibility of on-call physicians to respond to, examine, and treat patients with emergency medical conditions. Physicians should also be aware of the requirement that, when medically indicated, on-call physicians must generally come to the hospital to examine the patient. Patients may be sent to see the on-call physician at a hospital-owned contiguous or on-campus facility to conduct or complete the medical screening examination due to the following reasons:

- all persons with the same medical condition are moved to this location;
- there is a bona fide medical reason to move the patient;
- qualified medical personnel accompany the patient; and
- teaching physicians may participate.

EMERGING GROWTH STOCKS: Shares of early health care or other companies participating in new markets or niches with greater future expectations than those in established industries or services. Emerging Health Care Organizations (EHOs), Health Care eBusiness Networks (HeBNs), or other companies are usually smaller and do not yet have steady earnings streams or pay dividends, and they may be more highly priced relative to the rest of the market.

EMERGING HEALTHCARE ORGANIZATION (EHO): Medical providers, hospitals, clinics, health care systems, and payers who are innovating, integrating, or merging because of constant competitive financial influx from the health care industrial complex, and in response to managed care economic compression. The term was promoted by Health Capital Consultants, LLC, St. Louis, Missouri.

EMERGING MARKETS: Developing foreign countries and their associated economies and securities markets.

EMPLOYEE BENEFITS: Corporate expenses incurred for vacation pay, sick leave pay, holiday pay, Federal Insurance Contributions Act (FICA), state unemployment insurance, federal unemployment insurance, workers' compensation insurance, group health insurance, group life insurance, pension, retirement costs, and so forth.

EMPLOYEE BENEFITS PLAN: Compensation arrangement used by employers such as clinics and hospitals in addition to salary or wages. Some plans such as group term life insurance, medical insurance, and qualified retirement plans are treated favorably under the tax law. Most common qualified retirement plans are: (1) defined benefit plans or a traditional fixed promise to pay participants specified benefits that are determinable and based on such factors as age, years of service, and compensation; or (2) defined contribution plans to provide a portable individual account for each participant and benefits based on items such as amounts contributed to the account by the employer and employee and investment experience.

EMPLOYEE RETIREMENT INCOME SECURITY ACT OF 1974 (ERISA): Federal law governing most private pension and benefit plans. ERISA sets standards for funding, administration, and investing.

EMPLOYEE STOCK OWNERSHIP PLAN (ESOP): Employee program that encourages stock purchases in company equities to allow a collective voice in managerial matters. A health care entity or other corporate benefit plan that offers company stock as an investment. Other available plans are leveraged ESOPs, which are highly complex financial arrangements, usually in the form of profit-sharing.

EMPLOYEE STOCK PURCHASE PLAN: A plan that allows a broad spectrum of hospital, health care, or other employees to purchase employer securities at a discount of up to 10–15% of the stock's fair market value.

EMPLOYER COST INDEX: Department of Labor (DOL) quarterly report of domestic wages and benefits adjusted for inflation.

EMPLOYER SECURITIES: Generally, common stock of a health care or other company that is also the employer of the stockholder.

ENCODER: Software that helps assign a diagnostic related group for payment.

ENCOUNTER: Patient contact suitable for payment.

ENCUMBERED: Subject to the terms and conditions of a valid claim by another.

ENCUMBRANCE: A claim against an asset by another party which usually affects the ability to transfer ownership of the asset.

ENDING INVENTORY: The amount of durable medical equipment and/or other health care related inventory-on-hand, at the end of an accounting period.

ENDING PERIOD MARKET VALUE: The total value of a managed investment portfolio as of the prior business day.

ENDORSE: To impart or transfer credibility to another. An imprimatur of respect.

ENDORSEMENT: A signature on the back of a check or security by the person named by the check, stock, or bond as owner.

ENDOWMENT: Principal financial corpus with interest payments usually only available for disbursements, gifts, scholarships, research, and so forth.

ENGAGEMENT COMPLETION DOCUMENT: A statement from an auditor or accountant where all significant findings or issues are noted. The statement should be as specific as necessary in the circumstances for a reviewer to gain a thorough understanding of the findings or issues.

ENGEL'S EFFECT: Changes downward in health care commodity demands by patients because their incomes are rising.

ENGEL'S LAW: Occurrence observed that when a familial income rises, the percentage of money spent on food consumption decreases. Established by Ernst Engel (1857), a Russian statistician.

ENROLLMENT BROKER: A patient's health insurance broker.

ENTERPRISE: A small but growing business, such as an emerging health care organization (EHO).

ENTHOVEN, ALAIN C., PhD: The father of modern managed care and economics professor from Stanford University who helped coin the term *Health Maintenance Organization,* along with Paul Ellwood, Jr., MD, in the Nixon Administration. Currently, Marriner S. Eccles Professor of Public and Private Management, Emeritus, and CHP/PCOR Core Faculty Member.

ENTITLEMENT: Program (federal, state, or local) in which medical care, health services, or other benefits (housing and food) are provided to those who qualify.

ENTITY: A health care, medical, or other organization that produces medical goods or services for sale in an attempt to make a profit. It is also the act of setting up a company in the health care industry.

ENTRY-LIMIT PRICE: Price set by health care businesses or other enterprises that is low enough to prevent new entrants from entering the marketplace.

EOM DATING: Wholesale drug industry practice where purchases made by the 25th of one month are payable within 30 days of the following end-of-month.

EQUAL CREDIT OPPORTUNITY ACT (ECOA): Federal law that requires lenders and creditors to make credit equally available without discrimination based on race, color, religion, national origin, age, sex, marital status, or receipt of income from public assistance programs.

EQUATION OF EXCHANGE: $MV = PQ$; where M is the money supply, V is income velocity, P is price, and Q is volume.

EQUILIBRIUM: The stabilization point where health care or other economic variables neither increase, nor decrease.

EQUILIBRIUM PRICE: The health care product or service price that equilibrates to supply and demand. It is neither a surplus nor a shortage.

EQUILIBRIUM PRICE LEVEL: The intersection of the aggregate health care demand and aggregate supply curves.

EQUILIBRIUM QUANTITY: The quantity of health care products and services bought at similar prices.

EQUILIBRIUM REAL DOMESTIC HEALTH CARE OUTPUT: Actual domestic health care output determined by the intersection of aggregate health care demand and aggregate health care supply.

EQUIMARGINAL PRINCIPLE: The suggestion that to maximize utility, a patient, health care, or other consumer must equalize the marginal utility per dollar, spent on each health care good or service.

EQUIPMENT TRUST BOND: A longer-term bond collateralized by machinery and/or equipment of the issuing health care corporation. It was used historically many times by railroads to finance the purchase of their rolling stock.

EQUIPMENT TRUST CERTIFICATE: A shorter-term paper certification collateralized by machinery and/or equipment of the issuing health care corporation. It was used historically many times by railroads to finance the purchase of their rolling stock.

EQUITIZED MARGIN CALL: The transference of debt for equity, as in an unsatisfied margin call, to eliminate debt and transfer ownership.

EQUITY: The ownership interest of common and preferred stockholders in a health care or other company. The term also refers to the excess of value of securities over the debit balance in a margin (general) account. The money-value of property or interest in property after all claims have been deducted. In connection with cash values and policy loan indebtedness, the policy owner's equity is the portion of cash value remaining to the policy owner after deduction of all indebtedness on account of loans or liens secured by the policy.

EQUITY ACCOUNT: Balance sheet entry that includes capital stock, additional paid-in capital, and retained earning.

EQUITY FINANCING: The purchase of an asset with internally generated funds, such as cash, or stock. An equity supplier.

EQUITY FUND: An investment portfolio that invests primarily in stocks.

EQUITY FUNDING: Combination of a mutual fund (investment) with a life insurance policy, also known as a hybrid.

EQUITY KICKER: Ownership position potential in a loan (debt) deal.

EQUITY LINE OF CREDIT (ELOC): Generic term that allows conversion of home or business equity to cash.

EQUITY METHOD OF ACCOUNTING: Cost basis that is adjusted up or down (in proportion to the percentage of stock ownership) as retained earnings fluctuation. It is used for long-term investments in equity securities of affiliate where the holder can exert significant influence. Ownership of 20% or greater is arbitrarily presumed to have significant influence over the investee/trustee, and so forth.

EQUITY NET CASH FLOWS: The cash available for owners after funding health care or other business operations.

EQUITY OPTION: An option on a common stock.

EQUITY RISK PREMIUM: The risk-free rate-of-return, plus the rate-of-return to reflect the risk of the health care business or other corporate entity over the risk-free rate.

EQUITY RUN: An account statement list of securities, debt, and other holding information.

EQUITY SECURITIES: Capital stock and/or other securities that represent ownership shares, or the legal rights to purchase or acquire it.

EQUIVALENT PRETAX YIELD ON TAXABLE BOND (EPYTB): Municipal bond yield / 1-Tax Rate.

EQUIVALENT TAXABLE YIELD: A comparison of the tax-free municipal bond yield with that of a corporate bond.

EQUIVALENT UNITS: A period of work measure expressed in complete units of service or goods output.

ERGODIC: A stochastic economics process where no sample helps meaningfully to predict values that are very far away in time from a sample.

ERISA SECTION 404(C).: Section 404(c) of the Employee Retirement Income Security Act of 1974 (ERISA) determines whether the third party is an insurance company or an ERISA organization, because state laws through the Freedom of Choice Acts (FCA) preclude discrimination on the part of insurance companies. ERISA programs are covered under federal law and are not subject to the FCA. Generally, patients may sue health plans and employers in federal court, though not in state court, for the cost of a denied benefit, legal fees, and court costs, but not for compensatory or punitive damages. Patients may also sue doctors for malpractice in state court. Federal employees may sue the Office of Personnel Management (OPM) in federal court only for the amount of denied coverage, plus attorney and court costs. If the OPM loses, it can obtain a court order to require the insurer to pay. Thus, ERISA has shielded nongovernmental health plans from punitive and compensatory damages in state courts. This is known as the "ERISA exemption," and it has allowed managed care organizations to flourish. The exemption has been challenged. In 1998, a U.S. district judge upheld a Texas law allowing patients to sue a managed care plan for medical malpractice. The judge's decision did limit lawsuits to cases in which negligence occurs in the actual performance (commission) of medical services, not necessarily the withholding (omission) of services.

ERROR: Financial accounting or economic act that departs from what should be done. It is an imprudent deviation, unintentional mistake, or omission.

ERROR ACCOUNT: Holding pen for temporary but erroneous securities transactions.

ESCALATOR CLAUSE: Terms and conditions in a health insurance or other contract that allows inflation or other cost increases to be passed on.

ESCHEAT: Property of a person returned to the State if abandoned or left by who dies interstate, or without a will.

ESCROW: A third-party intermediary agent.

ESCROW ACCOUNT (IMPOUND ACCOUNT): An account that a borrower pays into and from which the lender makes tax and insurance payments applicable to the borrower.

ESCROW ANALYSIS: Annual review of escrow accounts to determine if current monthly deposits continue to provide the required funds to pay taxes, insurance, or other payments as they come due.

ESTATE: The total assets and liabilities left by a person at death.

ESTATE ASSETS: The property of a deceased person, which may include a functioning medical practice or other businesses, securities, real estate, cash, household and personal effects, the contents of safe deposit boxes, and other items.

ESTATE PLANNING: Planning for the proper disposition of an individual's assets in order to limit gift and estate tax liability.

ESTATE TAX: A tax on the transfer of property at death typically paid from the assets in an estate. The federal government and some states levy estate taxes.

ESTIMATED ANNUAL INCOME: Approximation of the annual amount earned from a security or portfolio, computed as follows:

- Equities: (Last dividend multiplied by 4) multiplied by number of shares
- Fixed Income Securities: Coupon rate multiplied by number of units

ESTIMATED LENGTH OF STAY (ELOS): Average number of hospital days per incident, based on prior utilization history.

ESTIMATED LIABILITIES: Pro forma liabilities, or potential future financial obligations.

ESTIMATED RESIDUAL VALUE: The cash, residual, or salvage value of an asset at the end of its useful life.

ESTIMATED REVENUE OVER EXPENSES: Operating and other health care entity income similar to net income before taxes.

ESTIMATED TAX: Amount of tax one may expect to pay for the current tax period. It is usually paid through quarterly installments.

ESTIMATED THIRD-PARTY SETTLEMENTS: Projected amount due, or from third-party insurance payers, for advances, under-, or overpayments.

ESTIMATED USEFUL LIFE: The length of service expected from an asset.

ESTIMATION TRANSACTIONS: Activities that involve medical management judgments or assumptions in formulating account balances in the absence of a precise means of measurement. Often used as estimated or pro forma financial statements.

EURO: Common currency conversion of the first 11 nations of the European Central Bank (ECB) in Brussels, founded on January 1, 1999.

EURO BONDS: U.S. denominated debt issued abroad.

EURO DOLLAR: U.S. dollars (USD) held in foreign banks.

EUROPEAN OPTION: An option that can be exercised only on the expiration date.

EUROPEAN STYLE EXERCISE: Option can only be exercised the day prior to expiration.

EVALUATION AND MANAGEMENT: Medical provider patient contact code for diagnosis, assessment, and counseling reported with *CPT-4 Codes* for payment.

EVALUATION AND MANAGEMENT SERVICE COMPONENTS: History, examination, and medical decision making for patient medial services and reimbursement. Four additional components include: counseling, coordination of care, nature of problem, and a time factor.

EVANS, MICHAEL K.: Chief economist for the American Economics Group in Washington, D.C., and an advocate of market-driven competitive health care models.

EVANS MODEL: Conceptual framework for describing a profit-maximizing health care entity with a negatively sloping demand curve. It is the concept that physicians do not readily induce health care demand and experience greater incremental displeasure with greater inducements. Supply induced demand (SID).

EVENT RISK: Chance that debt will be downgraded and interest rate costs will rise due to some unexpected negative economic, political, social, business, or financial event.

EVIDENTIAL MATTER: Supporting financial and health care accounting data and other corroborating economic information that supports financial statements.

EX: Latin term for without, or not included.

*EX-***DIVIDEND:** Occurs when dividends are declared by a company's board of directors; they are payable on a certain date ("payable date") to shareholders recorded on the company's books as of a stated earlier date ("record date"). Purchasers of the stock on or after the record date are not entitled to receive the recently declared dividend, so the *ex*-dividend date is the number of days it takes to settle a trade before the record date (currently 3 business days). A stock's price on its *ex*-dividend date appears in the newspaper with an X beside it.

*EX-***DIVIDEND DATE:** A date set on which a given stock will begin trading in the marketplace without the value of a pending dividend included in the contract price. It is normally 2 business days before the record date, except on mutual funds.

EX-GRATIA PAYMENT: Settlement of a claim even though a company does not feel it is legally obligated to pay. Settlement is made in order to prevent an even larger expense to the company as a result of having to defend itself in court, or for goodwill purposes.

_EX_-LEGAL: A term that refers to the absence of a legal opinion. An "_ex_-legal" delivery is a delivery of municipal securities in the secondary market without a copy of the legal opinion being provided.

_EX_-RIGHTS: A term applied to stocks trading in the marketplace for which the value of the subscription privilege has already been deducted and which, therefore, no longer bears such a right. It is literally trading "rights off."

_EX_-WARRANTS: Stocks sold without warrant attached.

EXCESS CAPACITY: The difference between health care outputs corresponding to their minimum possible average cost, and the output produced by a similar monopolistically competitive health care business entity in the long run.

EXCESS EARNINGS: Future estimated economic benefit from a health care concern over the rate of return for a similar business enterprise.

EXCESS EARNINGS METHOD: Health care entity valuation based on the sum value of assets from capitalized earnings excess and the value of selected assets.

EXCHANGE: Any organization that maintains a marketplace for the purchase or sale of securities. It includes the transfer of money, property, or services in exchange for any combination of items.

EXCHANGE LISTED SECURITY: A security listed on a stock exchange for sale or purchase.

EXCHANGE PRIVILEGE: The right to exchange the shares of one open-end fund, or class of funds, for those of another under the same sponsorship, at nominal cost or at a reduced sales charge. For tax purposes, such an exchange is considered a sale and new purchase.

EXCHANGE RATE: The price of a foreign currency relative to another currency.

EXCHANGE RISK: Foreign currency uncertainty regarding value.

EXCHANGE TRADED FUND (ETF): Similar to a mutual fund that represents a basket of stocks that reflect an index such as the DJIA or S&P 500. Unlike a mutual fund that has its NAV calculated at the end of each trading day, an ETF's price changes throughout the day, fluctuating with supply and demand. While ETFs attempt to replicate the return on indexes, they are not guaranteed, such as DIAMONDS, QQQQs, and SPYDRS. A securities index that is traded like stocks, first on the American Stock Exchange (AMEX), and now traded on other exchanges for a commission.

EXCLUSION PRINCIPLE: Economic suggestion that one who does not pay for a health care product or service should not reap the benefits of that product or service.

EXCLUSIONS: (1) Medical services not covered in a health plan because of risk or cost. (2) Income item excluded from a taxpayer's gross income, such as gifts, inheritances, and death proceeds paid under a life insurance contract.

EXECUTION: Signing, delivering, or carrying out a contract or transaction.

EXECUTOR: The person, organization, or combination charged with the responsibility of carrying out the terms of a will.

EXEMPT: Personal income not subject to tax. Individuals, trusts, and estates qualify for an exemption unless they are claimed as a dependent on another individual's tax return.

EXEMPT ORGANIZATION: Firm that does not pay federal income tax, such as certain medical clinics, hospitals, religious organizations, charitable organizations, social clubs, and so forth.

EXEMPT SECURITY: A security exempt from the registration provisions of the Securities Exchange Act of 1933. Among exempt securities would be government and municipal bonds, private placements, and intrastate issues.

EXEMPT TRANSACTION: Any securities transaction that does not trigger state registration and/or advertising requirements under the Uniform Securities Act (USA).

EXERCISE: To place into effect the option rights held by an option buyer. To request the writer to deliver stock at the stated price (call) or to pay the stated price for stock delivered to him (put). To invoke the rights granted to the holder of an option contract. In the case of a call, the option holder buys the underlying stock from the option writer. In the case of a put, the option holder sells the underlying stock to the option writer.

EXERCISE NOTICE: An irrevocable written statement, tendered by a clearing member in whose account an option is held with the Options Clearing Corporation (OCC), that states an option holder's intention to exercise the option.

EXERCISE PRICE: The price at which the holder of an option may purchase (in the case of a call option) or sell (in the case of a put option) the indicated underlying security. Also called the strike price.

EXIT: The act of closing a medical practice, clinic, hospital, or other health care company and leaving the health care industry.

EXPANDING INDUSTRY: Economically profitable industry that will grow its outputs because of supply and demand needs.

EXPANSION: A period of rising or increased business and economic activity. A period of rising health care outputs.

EXPANSION DECISION: Capital investments to increase the operational capacity, and hence profits, of a health care or other organization.

EXPECTATIONS: What patients believe will happen now, or what health care conditions will be like in the future.

EXPECTED CLAIMS: Projection of future health care claims expenses for a member or group of subscribers. It is actuarial projection.

EXPECTED EXPENSE: Expected health insurance related costs, exclusive of managed care claims related costs.

EXPECTED EXPENSE RATIO: Ratio of expected incurred health or disability insurance costs, with written premiums received.

EXPECTED RATE OF RETURN: Mean average possible rate-of-return on an asset or investment.

EXPECTED RETURN: The sum total of anticipated investment returns: capital gains, plus dividends, plus interest, equals total return.

EXPECTED SOURCE OF HEALTH CARE PAYMENTS: These payer categories are used to indicate the type of entity or organization expected to pay or did pay the greatest share of the patient's bill:

- Medicare—A federally administered third-party reimbursement program authorized by Title XVIII of the Social Security Act. Includes crossovers to secondary payers.
- Medi-Cal—A state administered third-party reimbursement program authorized by Title XIX of the Social Security Act.
- Private Coverage—Payment covered by private, nonprofit, or commercial health plans, whether insurance or other coverage, or organizations. Included are payments by local or organized charities, such as the Cerebral Palsy Foundation, Easter Seals, March of Dimes, and Shriners.
- Workers' Compensation—Payment from workers' compensation insurance, government or privately sponsored.
- County Indigent Programs—Patients covered under Welfare and Institutions Code Section 17000. Includes programs funded in whole or in part by County Medical Services Program (CMSP), California Health Care for Indigent Program (CHIP), and/or Realignment Funds whether or not a bill is rendered.
- Other Government—Any form of payment from American government agencies, whether local, state, federal, or foreign, except those included in the Medicare, Medi-Cal, Workers' Compensation, or County Indigent Programs categories listed above. Includes California Children Services (CCS), the Civilian Health and Medical Program of the Uniformed Services (TRICARE), and the Veterans Administration.
- Other Indigent—Patients receiving care pursuant to Hill-Burton obligations or who meet the standards for charity care pursuant to the hospital's established charity care policy. Includes indigent patients, except those described in the County Indigent Programs above.

- Self-Pay—Payment directly by the patient, personal guarantor, relatives, or friends. The greatest share of a patient's bill is not paid by insurance or health plan.
- Other Payer—Any third-party payment not included in the above categories. Included are cases where no payment will be required by the facility, such as special research or courtesy patients.

EXPECTED UTILITY: The average health care utility from all possible outcomes.

EXPECTED VALUE: A measure of estimated probability distribution return of some health care good or service output.

EXPENDITURE: Monetary disbursement for goods, services, assets, and other economic inputs, usually expected to be used in the short-term. The issuance of checks, disbursement of cash, or electronic transfer of funds made to liquidate an expense regardless of the fiscal year a medical service was provided or the expense was incurred. Medical expenditures refer to funds spent as reported by State Medicaid Programs.

EXPENDITURE CAPITAL: The amount of money paid for a fixed asset.

EXPENSE: The decrease in stockholder or owner's equity from using assets or increasing liabilities in the course of delivering health care goods or services. Funds actually spent or incurred providing goods, rendering medical services, or carrying out other health mission related activities during a period. Expenses are computed using accrual accounting techniques that recognize costs when incurred and revenues when earned and include the effect of accounts receivable and accounts payable on determining annual income. The overhead cost involved in running the health care business, aside from losses of claims.

EXPENSE ALLOWANCE: Compensation or reimbursement in excess of prescribed salary or commissions for overhead, and so forth. It includes money paid by an insurer to an agent or agency head for incurred expenses.

EXPENSE BUDGET: The pro forma budget used to forecast health care operational expenses.

EXPENSE CONSTANT: A flat health insurance charge added in the computation of the premium in which the pure premium is so low that the cost of issuing and servicing the policy cannot be recovered.

EXPENSE COST VARIANCE: The difference between estimated and actual variable expenses.

EXPENSE FACTOR: A load or sales commission.

EXPENSE INCURRED: Expenses paid and expected to be paid.

EXPENSE LIABILITIES: Taxes and expenses incurred due to normal business operating activities.

EXPENSE PAID: Money paid out related to normal operating expenses, but not the cost of health care claims payments. It includes money disbursed by the health insurance company for conducting business other than for the purpose of paying claims.

EXPENSE PER DAY: Total health care expenses of the facility exclusive of ancillary expenses divided by patient days.

EXPENSE PER DISCHARGE (HOSPITAL): Adjusted inpatient expenses divided by discharges (excluding nursery).

EXPENSE PER UNIT OF SERVICE: The average cost to the hospital of providing one unit of service.

EXPENSE RATIO: Percentage of a portfolio or mutual fund efficiency calculated by dividing expenses by net assets. The cost of a mutual fund, variable annuity subaccount, or portfolio to conduct business as a percent of its assets. Expense ratios are calculated or found in prospectuses.

EXPENSE RESERVE: A fund set aside to pay future expenses, for example, a health insurance company is responsible for incurred-but-unpaid expenses.

EXPENSE RISK: The liability of a managed-care or health insurance company for higher costs than charged for in the policy premiums.

EXPENSE VOLUME VARIANCE: The total high or low variance from actual volume compared with budgeted or forecasted volume.

EXPERIENCE GOOD: A good or service for which valuation or worth determination is difficult or even blind, prior to purchase or consumption, such as health care services or medical care.

EXPIRATION: The day of cessation for the life of an option contract.

EXPIRATION DATE: The date which an option contract must be exercised. The date on which an option and the right to exercise it cease to exist.

EXPIRATION MONTH: The month in which an option ceases to exist.

EXPIRY: The day of cessation for a derivative security.

EXPLANATION OF BENEFITS (EOB): A statement of insurance coverage that lists any health services that have been provided as well as the amount billed and payment made by the health plan for those services.

EXPLICIT COST: Money paid to an outside (outsourced) vendor for health care inputs or resources.

EXPOSURE: Extent of assumed risk.

EXPOSURE DRAFT: AICPA, FASB, and GASB document inviting public comment before a final pronouncement is issued.

EXTENDIBLE SECURITY: Debt or bond whose maturity date may extend well into the future.

EXTENSION: An informal method of reorganization where creditors voluntarily postpone payment on past due invoices and obligations. It also includes time granted by a taxing authority, such as the IRS, state, or city, which allows a taxpayer to file tax returns later than the original due date.

EXTENT OF TESTS OF CONTROL: Evidence about whether a company's internal control over financial reporting is operating effectively.

EXTERNAL BENEFIT: Health care services accruing to patients other than actual buyers. *See also* spillover benefit.

EXTERNAL COST: Health care costs not borne by the provider, but by other members of a cohort. *See also* spillover cost.

EXTERNAL DISECONOMICS: Factors outside the control of a health care entity that raises its average total costs, as health care industry output rises over time.

EXTERNAL DISECONOMY: The uncompensated cost from a patient or health care entity resulting from the consumption or output of another patient's or entity's benefits.

EXTERNAL ECONOMICS: Factors outside the control of a health care entity that lowers its average total costs, as health care industry output rises over time.

EXTERNAL ECONOMY: The uncompensated benefit from a patient or health care entity resulting from the consumption or output of another patient's benefits.

EXTERNAL FUNDS: Money brought in from outside a company, usually in the form of debt.

EXTERNAL REPORTING: Reporting to stockholders and the public, as opposed to internal reporting for medical management's decision making.

EXTERNALITIES: Effects of a program that impose costs on persons or groups who are not targets. The cost or benefits of health care market transactions that are not reflected in the prices buyers and sellers use to make their decisions. For example, the existence of spillover externalities may work to make health care entities choose efficient tax rates within the context of infinitely repeated tax competition decisions. Moreover, given the increased potential of capital mobility, local governments are concerned with the spill-in effects of public health goods from surrounding regions, which might entail reducing local incentive to deviate from an efficient external reporting outcome

EXTINGUISHMENT OF DEBT: To pay a liability or bring it to an end.

EXTRA DIVIDEND: A dividend in addition to a regular recurring dividend.

EXTRA ORDINARY ITEM: An irregular, rare, or infrequent revenue or expense occurrence. It is reported separately, less applicable income taxes, in the entity's statement of income or operations.

EXTRANEOUS COSTS: Expenses not related to a specific health care product, department, procedure, intervention, drug, patient, or service and includes step-down, direct, and indirect costs.

EXTRINSIC VALUE: Time-value component of an option premium.

F

F: Commodity futures symbol for a January delivery month.

FACE AMOUNT CERTIFICATE COMPANY (FACC): An investment company that issues a debt instrument obligation itself to pay a stated sum of money (face amount) on a date fixed more than 24 months after issuance, usually in return for deposits made by an investor in periodic installments.

FACE VALUE: The redemption value of a bond or preferred stock and sometimes referred to as par value.

FACILITY CHARGE: Service fee submitted for payment by a health care facility, such as a clinic, hospital, or ambulatory care center.

FACILITY PAYMENT: Service fee received for payment by a health care facility, such as a clinic, hospital, or ambulatory care center.

FACTOR MARKET: A health care exchange in which units of medical service production are purchased and provided.

FACTORING: The sale of medical accounts receivable at a discount.

FACTORS OF PRODUCTION: Economic inputs, such as capital, equipment and facilities, health care labor, nurses and physicians, and so forth.

FAIL: Transaction between two securities brokers or dealers on which delivery does not take place on the settlement date. A transaction in which a dealer has yet to deliver securities is referred to as a "fail to deliver," and a transaction in which a dealer has not yet received securities is referred to as a "fail to receive."

FAIL SAFE: The Medicare Preservation Act of 1995.

FAIL TO DELIVER/RECEIVE: Failure of a sell side broker/dealer to deliver securities, or the failure of a buy side broker/dealer to receive securities.

FAIR CREDIT BILLING LAW: The law that protects the rights of people who receive erroneous bills from creditors.

FAIR CREDIT REPORTING ACT (FCRA): A consumer protection law that regulates the disclosure of consumer credit reports by consumer/credit reporting agencies and establishes procedures for correcting mistakes on one's credit record.

FAIR CREDIT REPORTING LAW: The right to review credit history and have errors corrected.

FAIR DEBT COLLECTION PRACTICE: Protection from unfair or deceptive debt collection practices.

FAIR MARKET VALUE (FMV): A legal term generally meaning the price at which a willing buyer will buy and a willing seller will sell an asset in an open free market with full disclosure. Book value is accounting value.

FAIR RETURN PRICE: The price of a health care product or service that enables its medical producers to receive a normal profit.

FAIR VALUE: Value that is reasonable and consistent with all of the known facts.

FAIRNESS OPINION: Opinion whether the monetary consideration in a health care business transaction is fair from an economic and financial perspective.

FALLACY OF COMPOSITION: Incorrect suggestion that what is good for an individual patient is also good for a population cohort. *See also* utilitarianism.

FALLEN ANGEL: The quality deterioration of a former investment grade security.

FALSE CLAIMS ACT: A Civil War-era law increasingly popular with prosecutors who pursue inappropriate billing mishaps by physicians. This is because, in 1990, the health care industry accounted for about 10% of all false claims penalties recovered by the federal government. By 2000, the health care share was 40%. This Act allows a private citizen, such as a patient, employee, or a competing provider, to bring a health care fraud claim against an organization or an individual, on behalf of and in the name of the United States of America. The "realtor" who initiates the claim is rewarded by sharing in a percentage of the recovery from the health care provider. Essentially, this Act allows informers to receive up to 30% of any judgment recovered against government contractors, including Medicare, Medicaid, Civilian Health and Medical Program of the Uniform Services (CHAMPUS), prison systems, American Indian reservations, or the Veterans' Association (VA) systems. With a low burden of proof, triple damages, and penalties up to $11,000 for each wrongful claims submission, this law is a favorite among prosecutors pursuing health care fraud. All that must be proven is that improper claims were submitted with a reckless disregard of the truth. Intentional fraud is irrelevant to these cases, even if submitted by a third party, such as a billing company. Therefore, it is imperative that the attending physicians understand the concepts of proper documentation and basic billing requirements.

FALSE STATEMENT: Anyone who knowingly and willfully falsifies or conceals a material fact or makes a material false fictitious or fraudulent statement in connection with the delivery of or payment for health care benefits, items, or services may face fines and up to 5 years imprisonment. This pertains to any untruth in health care matters, especially financial.

FAMILY INCOME: The total income earned by a family unit and used for family maintenance, includes income earned by more than one family member, such as when both spouses are employed.

FAMILY OF FUNDS: Groups of mutual funds managed by the same company. Owning a number of funds within the same family often can make it easier to switch money among funds.

FAST MARKET: A rapidly changing and volatile securities market.

FAVORABLE VARIANCE: When health care business revenues or expenses are higher or lower than expected. It is an excess of actual revenue over projected health care revenues or actual medical costs over a projected costing time period.

FEASABILITY STUDY: A report detailing the economic practicality and the need for a proposed capital program. The feasibility study may include estimates of revenues that will be generated and details of the physical, operating, economic, or engineering aspects of the proposed project, as in a proposed hospital economic feasibility study. *See also* Certificate of Need (CON).

FEATHERBEDDING: Payment for health care products or services not rendered.

FEDERAL DEFICIT: Federal government spending in excess of revenues.

FEDERAL DEPOSIT INSURANCE CORPORATION (FDIC): An agency of the U.S. government that insures deposits up to $100,000 in federally and state-chartered banks. The insurance is financed by a fee paid by the insured institutions. The FDIC promotes the safety and soundness of insured depository institutions and the U.S. financial system by identifying, monitoring, and addressing risks to the deposit insurance funds. The FDIC also is the primary federal regulator of about 6,000 state-chartered "nonmember" banks (commercial and savings banks that are not members of the Federal Reserve System).

FEDERAL DEPOSITORY INSURANCE: A program of the FDIC that insures depositors in federally- and state-chartered banks.

FEDERAL FUNDS: Immediately available funds representing non-interest-bearing deposits at Federal Reserve banks. Federal funds are actively traded among commercial bank members of the Federal Reserve System. Federal funds are the primary payment mode for government securities and are often used to pay for new issues of municipal securities and for secondary market transactions in certain types of securities.

FEDERAL FUNDS RATE: The interest rate on federal funds. The rate of interest paid on overnight loans of excess reserves made between commercial banks. Movements of this rate are considered an important indicator of the future direction of interest rates.

FEDERAL HOME LOAN MORTGAGE CORPORATION (FHLMC): A publicly chartered agency that purchases mortgages from federally insured lenders and then repackages and resells them on the open market, such as Freddie Mac.

FEDERAL INSURANCE CONTRIBUTIONS ACT (FICA): The Social Security tax that employers and employees pay, based on the employee's gross salary. The current FICA tax rate is 7.65% each, for employer and employee.

FEDERAL MANAGERS' FINANCIAL INTEGRITY ACT (FMFIA): A program to identify management inefficiencies and areas vulnerable to fraud and abuse and to correct such weaknesses with improved internal controls.

FEDERAL MEDICAID MANAGED CARE WAIVER PROGRAM: The process used by states to receive permission to implement managed care programs for Medicaid or other categorically eligible beneficiaries.

FEDERAL MEDICAL ASSISTANCE PERCENTAGE (FMAP): The portion of the Medicaid program that is paid by the federal government.

FEDERAL NATIONAL MORTGAGE ASSOCIATION (FNMA): A government-sponsored private corporation that purchases mortgages from lenders and resells them to investors, such as Fannie Mae.

FEDERAL OPEN MARKET COMMITTEE (FOMC): Group that sends instructions to the Federal Reserve Bank of New York to sell or buy government securities on the open market.

FEDERAL POVERTY LEVEL (FPL): The amount of income determined by the Federal Department of Health and Human Services to provide a minimum for food, clothing, transportation, shelter, and other necessities.

FEDERAL REGISTER (FR): Governmental publication listing health care changes and mandated standards such as HCPCS (HCFA Common Procedure Coding System) and ICD-9-CMs.

FEDERAL RESERVE: The U.S. central bank.

FEDERALLY QUALIFIED HMO: Health maintenance organization that meets the standards of the Federal Health Maintenance Organization Act (FHMOA).

FEE: A charge or price for professional services, such as medical care.

FEE ALLOWANCE: A fee schedule for medical or health care services rendered.

FEE DISCLOSURE: Physicians discussing or submitting professional charges prior to medical treatment.

FEE FOR SERVICE: (a) Method of reimbursement based on payment for medical services rendered by practitioners. The payment may be by an insurance company, patient, or government program, such as Medicare or Medicaid. (b) Refers to payment in specific amounts for specific services rendered—as opposed to retainer, salary, or other contract arrangements. In relation to the patient, it refers to payment in specific amounts for specific services received, in contrast to the advance payment of an insurance premium or membership fee for coverage, through which the services or payment to the supplier are provided.

FEE SCHEDULE: A listing of accepted fees or established allowances for specified medical procedures. As used in medical care plans, it usually represents the maximum amounts the program will pay for the specified procedures.

FEE SCHEDULE INDEX: Primary care provider fee schedule listing reimbursement, bonus, incentive, penalty, and withhold rate indices for clinically appropriate and economically cost-effective care.

FEE SCHEDULE PAYMENT AREA: A geographic area where payment for a given service, under the Medicare Fee Schedule, does not vary.

FEE SPLITTING: Unethical or illegal "kickback" or return of a portion of fees for a referral or other patient care or intervention.

FELLOW OF THE INSTITUTE OF ACTUARIES (FIA): A designation for an individual who has been examined by and becomes a member of the Institute of Actuaries. It may be health care specific.

FETTER, TREVOR: Chairman and CEO of Broadlane in San Francisco, California.

FEWNESS: A small number of buyers or sellers.

FFS EQUIVALENCY: A benchmark of the difference between traditional commercial fee-for-service physician compensation to an alternative system such as seen with HMOs, MCOs, PPOs, PHOs, discounted FFS, Medicare, Medicaid, CHAMPUS, fixed payments, capitations, and so forth. It is an economic comparison.

FFS INCENTIVES: The incentive to do additional diagnostic tests and procedures or to deliver more than an appropriate amount of care in order to increase medical provider or health care facility compensation, in a traditional commercial fee-for-service payment system.

FFS WITHHOLD: A percentage of salary, bonus plan, or hold-back percentage which may or may not be paid to a medical provider or health care facility for medical care utilization.

FHA PROGRAM: Mortgage insurance from the Federal Housing Administration for principle and interest on a loan.

FIDELITY BOND: A bond that guarantees the faithful performance in life and health insurance matters, among others. Also known as a fiduciary bond.

FIDUCIARY: Relating to, or founded upon, a trust or confidence. A fiduciary relationship exists where an individual or organization has an explicit or implicit obligation to act in behalf of another person or organization's interests in matters that affect the other person or organization. This fiduciary is also obligated to act in the other person's best interest with total disregard for any interests of the fiduciary. Traditionally, it was generally believed that a physician had a fiduciary relationship with patients. This is being questioned in the era of managed care as the public becomes aware of the other influences that are effecting physician decisions. Doctors are provided incentives by managed care companies to provide less care, by pharmaceutical companies to order certain drugs, and by hospitals to refer to their hospitals. With the pervasive monetary incentives influencing doctor decisions, consumer advocates are concerned because the patient no longer has an unencumbered fiduciary. On the other hand, a commissioned stockbroker salesperson or financial advisor does not have such an obligation to clients.

FIDUCIARY BOND: A bond that guarantees the faithful performance in life and health insurance matters. Also known as a fidelity bond.

FIELD WAREHOUSE: Inventory financing method where a "physical warehouse" is located at the health care facility.

50–50 RULE: Adequate clinical quality and fiscal soundness is encouraged when a third-party HMO, MCO, commercial insurance plan, and so forth, does not have more than 50% of its insureds in a combined status. One federal payer patient per commercial patient.

FILING: Registration of securities, as with the State or Securities Exchange Commission.

FILING DATE: Date of new securities registration by an issuing company.

FILING EXTENSION: The additional time period to file an income tax return.

FILING OF RETURNS: Those taxpayers meeting certain statutory requirements must file various returns on prescribed forms and in a timely manner.

FILL: To execute an order on a securities transaction.

FILL OR KILL (FOK) ORDER: A securities order that requires immediate purchase or sale of a specified amount of stock. If the order cannot be filled immediately, it is automatically canceled (killed).

FINAL PRODUCTS: Health care goods or services sold to the end-user patient, and not to be used or resold to others, as in drug samples.

FINAL PROSPECTUS: Legal document that includes material information about a new securities registration, such as price, delivery date, and underwriter's spread.

FINANCE: The study, sources, timing, and channels of private or public funds, and the authority to raise and distribute those funds. The study of economic markets.

FINANCE COMMITTEE: Committee of the board of directors whose duty it is to review financial results, approve budgets, set and approve spending authorities, review the annual audit, and review and approve outside funding sources.

FINANCE DATA: Data regarding the financial status of managed care entities.

FINANCIAL ACCOUNTING: Accounting that focuses on information outside the health care or other entity.

FINANCIAL ACCOUNTING STANDARDS: Official professional standards, FASB which are part of GAAP, in the United States.

FINANCIAL ACCOUNTING STANDARDS BOARD (FASB): The private organization that determines how domestic accounting is practiced. It is an independent, nongovernmental authority for the establishment of accounting principles in the United States.

FINANCIAL ADVISOR: A "consultant" who advises a securities issuer on matters pertinent to the issue, such as structure, timing, marketing, fairness of pricing, terms, and bond ratings. A financial adviser may also be employed to provide advice on subjects unrelated to a new issue of municipal securities, such as advising on cash flow and investment matters. The financial adviser is sometimes referred to as a "fiscal consultant" or "fiscal agent." MSRB Rule G-23 provides that a firm or bank that has acted in a financial advisory capacity with respect to a new issue of municipal securities (pursuant to a written contract) may underwrite the new issue (a) on a negotiated basis after making certain disclosures, obtaining the consent of the issuer and terminating the financial advisory relationship; or, (b) on a competitive basis if the issuer gives written consent before the financial adviser's bid is submitted. A Financial Advisor may also be a stockbroker or commissioned salesperson. Many are not fiduciaries.

FINANCIAL ANALYSIS: The research and study of financial statements.

FINANCIAL ASSETS: Economic asset that is not fixed. Paper claims of a holder.

FINANCIAL BUDGET: Projected cash outflows and inflows, with a period-ending balance sheet and statement of cash flows.

FINANCIAL DATA: Data regarding the financial status of managed care or other entities.

FINANCIAL FORECAST: Estimate of the expected financial position and the results of company operations and cash flows based on expected conditions (see Table 1).

FINANCIAL FUTURES: A contract for the delivery of a financial asset into the future.

FINANCIAL GUARANTY INSURANCE COMPANY (FGIC): A wholly owned subsidiary of FGIC Corporation which offers noncancelable insurance guarantying the full and timely payment of principal and interest due on securities on stated maturity, mandatory sinking fund, and interest payment dates. FGIC writes insurance on (1) new issue tax-exempt securities that may be insured partially or entirely, and (2) unit investment trusts. In the case of unit investment trusts, individual issues may be insured for their entire life or until an issue is sold out of the trust. Bonds insured by FGIC are currently rated AAA by Standard & Poor's and Aaa by Moody's Investors Service, Inc.

FINANCIAL INSTITUTION: Company engaged in any aspects of finance including commercial banks, thrift institutions, investment banks, securities brokers and dealers, credit unions, investment companies, insurance companies, and REITs.

FINANCIAL INTERCHANGE: Provisions of the Railroad Retirement Act (RRA) providing for transfers between the trust funds and the Social Security

Table 1: Hospital Financial Forecast for a Sample Project with Key Ratios

	2007	2008	2009	2010	2011
Admission growth	8.5%	3.6%	3.7%	3.8%	6.0%
Operating margin	10.7%	10.1%	12.2%	4.3%	5.5%
Net margin	12.6%	16.9%	21.3%	10.1%	10.1%
Earnings before interest	11.8%	11.4%	13.3%	12.2%	12.6%
EBID margin	20.1%	19.6%	21.1%	23.4%	22.9%
Debt service coverage	10.7	11.7	14.6	3.4	3.5%
Days of cash on hand	517	567	485	468	491
Debt to total capital	61.7%	58.0%	53.9%	51.3%	48.8%

Equivalent Benefit Account (SSEBA) of the Railroad Retirement program to place each trust fund in the same position as if railroad employment had always been covered under Social Security Insurance (SSI).

FINANCIAL INTERMEDIARY: Person or entity that operates a financial channel between two parties, such as an HMO or health insurance company. A third party that borrows from one group in order to lend to another.

FINANCIAL LEVERAGE: Asset purchase with borrowed funds. Ratio of total debt to assets may be positive or favorable, or negative and unfavorable.

FINANCIAL MARKET: A place of financial, capital, or other asset exchange.

FINANCIAL MIX: The methods in which a health care or other organization provides for its daily working capital and operating needs.

FINANCIAL PLANNER: One who helps devise a financial map with economic goals and objectives in mind.

FINANCIAL POSITION: Balance sheet or related information.

FINANCIAL RATIOS: Financial ratios, with ratio analysis, are the calculation and comparison of mathematic ratios derived from the information in a managed care or other company's financial statements. The level and historical trends of these ratios can be used to make inferences about a hospital or company's financial condition, premiums and payouts, its operations, and its attractiveness as an investment or insurance policy (see Table 2).

Table 2: Sample Median Hospital Financial Ratios Published by Standard & Poor's

	AA	A	BBB	NIG[1]
Net patient revenue	713,572	262,996	102,495	115,620
Maximum debt service coverage	4.1	3.5	2.5	1.5
Operating margin	3.1%	3.5%	1.2%	−1.3%
Profit margin	4.5%	3.2%	1.9%	−0.4%
Days cash on hand	211	159	110	50
Cash to debt	155.9	103.8	71.0	33.4
Debt to total capital	32.8	37.3	44.3	65.3
Days of revenue in accounts receivable	53.8	53.8	55.3	53.5
Capital expenditures to depreciation expense	159.9	147.8	119.6	

[1] Not investment grade, 2004.

FINANCIAL RISK: The degree of uncertainty of future cash flow from a health care business entity due to financial leverage or debt.

FINANCIAL SERVICES MODERNIZATION ACT (GRAMM-LEACH-BLILEY): Act of 1999 that eliminated the distinction between banks, insurance companies, and securities firms. It repealed portions of the Bank Holding Company Act (BHCA) of 1956 and the Glass-Steagall Act (GSA) of 1933.

FINANCIAL STATEMENTS: Business accounting documents that report on monetary amounts from a health care, individual, or other entity. The four formal written accounting records of company status are: (1) Balance Sheet, (2) Income Statement, (3) Cash Flow Statement, and (4) Statement of Changes in Operating Condition.

FINANCIAL STRUCTURE: The right side of a balance sheet indicating the manner in which a health care firm is financed.

FINANCIAL VIABILITY: The survivability of a health care or other business enterprise.

FINANCING ACTIVITIES: Events seen on a Statement of Cash Flows (SCFs), such as borrowing or paying-back loans.

FINANCING MIX: The methods by which a health care organization provides for its daily working-capital and operating needs.

FINKER, STEVEN A., PhD, CPA: Executive Committee member of the International Society for Research in Healthcare Financial Management, Towson, Maryland.

FIRE SALE: The rapid sale of assets or financial positions, without regard to price.

FIREWALL: Financial metaphor for the legal separation between certain economic activities (underwriting versus research and development).

FIRM: A health care or other organization that produces goods or services for sale in an attempt to make a profit. Inputs into outputs.

FIRM COMMITMENT: Financial securities underwriting where the underwriter buys the entire issue from the issuer at an agreed upon price and then proceeds to sell the issue. The issuer has a firm commitment because the entire issue is sold to the underwriter.

FIRM MARKET: In the OTC market, a quotation on a given security rendered by a market maker at which he stands ready and able to trade immediately for 100 shares (a round lot) unless otherwise specified.

FIRM ORDER: A brokerage order confirmed and not subject to cancellation.

FIRM PRICE: A designation that a securities quotation (a bid or an offering price) will not be changed for a specified period of time and will be the price of any transaction executed with the party to whom the quotation is given during that period. The dealer giving a firm quotation also commits itself not to effect a transaction in the securities with any other party during that period. For example, a dealer may give another dealer an offering price on specified securities that is "firm for one hour." If the second dealer wishes to purchase those securities at that price, it would contact the first dealer during that time period and execute the transaction. Firm quotations may sometimes be subject to a "recall," either immediately upon notice or after a specified period.

FIRM QUOTE: Market maker round-lot bid or offer securities price, stated but not identified as a quote.

FIRST DOLLAR COVERAGE: Health insurance plan without a deductible.

FIRST-IN, FIRST-OUT (FIFO): An inventory costing method where the first costs into inventory are the first costs attributed to cost of goods sold. The ending inventory is based on the cost of the most recent purchases. In times of rising prices, a higher total cost inventory is produced with a lower cost of goods sold. This happens because FIFO decreases an expense (cost of goods sold) and increases taxable income. Deflation has the opposite effect. *Note:* Any switch from FIFO to LIFO does not change reality, and although a decrease in reported incomes occurs, it does not increase cash outflows. But, for a taxable health care entity, after tax net cash flow does increase.

FIRST MORTGAGE: A debt or loan that is in first lien position, taking priority over all other liens that are financial encumbrances.

FISCAL: Pertaining to finances.

FISCAL AGENT: Contracted claims agency that processes Medicaid health insurance or other claims.

FISCAL CREDENTIALING: The economic analysis of multiple processes and procedures to gather, allocate, analyze, and interpret meaningful financial information relative to a medical practitioner or venue of economic performance.

FISCAL INTERMEDIARY: The agent (e.g., Blue Cross) that has contracted with medical providers of health service to process claims for reimbursement under health care coverage. In addition to handling financial matters, it may perform other functions such as providing consultative services or serving as a center for communication with providers and making audits of providers' needs.

FISCAL POLICY: Government policy of raising taxes and spending money.

FISCAL SERVICES: The nonrevenue-producing cost centers for those services generally associated with the accounting, credit, collection, and admitting operations of a facility.

FISCAL SOUNDNESS: The required amount of funds that a managed care organization must keep on reserve due to financial risk, as regulated by the Department of Insurance.

FISCAL YEAR: A 12-month period for which an organization plans the use of its funds, such as the federal government's fiscal year (October 1 to September 30). Fiscal years are referred to by the calendar year in which they end. For example, the Federal fiscal year 2007 began October 1, 2006. Hospitals can designate their own fiscal years, and this is reflected in differences in time periods covered by the Medicare Cost Reports. The term is ordinarily used only when the 12-month period is not a regular calendar year.

FISHER, DONALD: President and CEO of the American Medical Group Association in Alexandria, Virginia.

FISHERION CRITERION: Optimal investment by a health care organization or other firm that should be invested in real assets until the marginal internal rate of return equals the appropriately risk-adjusted rate of return on securities.

FITCH INVESTORS SERVICE: An independent service company based in New York City that provides ratings for municipal securities and other financial information to investors.

FIVE HUNDRED DOLLAR RULE: SEC Regulation-T exemption provision for margin account deficiencies of less than $500.

FIXED ANNUITY: Guaranteed insurance investment contract for a given period at a given rate of return.

FIXED ASSET: Nonmovable health care entity assets, such as a gamma knife or MRI.

FIXED ASSET TURNOVER RATIO (FATR): Ratio of dollars generated for each dollar reinvested in a health care or other organization's plant and equipment.

FIXED BUDGET: A financial plan in which specifically allocated amounts do not vary with level of activity or volume. Also known as a static budget.

FIXED CHARGE-COVERAGE RATIO (FCCR): EBIT plus lease payments / interest + lease payments + (debt payments / 1-tax rate).

FIXED COSTS: Health care provider or facility costs that do not change with fluctuations in census, utilization of services, or when a health care or other entity varies its output.

FIXED INCOME SECURITY: A preferred stock or a debt security with a stated percentage or dollar income return.

FIXED INPUT: A health care or other input whose quantity does not change over the short-term.

FIXED INTEREST RATE DEBT: The unchangeable interest rate on the life of a debt based security.

FIXED LABOR BUDGET: A series of income and outflow projections for human labor costs.

FIXED RESOURCE: Any resource quantity that cannot be altered.

FIXED SUPPLIES BUDGET: An expense budget of fixed supply costs that does not vary as a result of the amount of services provided by a health care or other business entity.

FLAT: A transaction involving bonds (most income bonds and all obligations for which interest is not currently being paid) in which accrued interest is not added to the contract price.

FLAT FEE PER CASE: Flat fee paid for a patient's treatment based on diagnosis and/or presenting problem. For this fee the medical provider covers all of the services the patient requires for a specific period of time. Often characterizes "second generation" managed care systems. After an HMO squeezes out costs by discounting fees, this method is often used. If the medical provider is still standing after such a discount blitz, this approach can be good for providers and patients, because it permits much flexibility in meeting patient needs.

FLAT FEE SYSTEM: A single lump sum fee paid for a medical treatment based on diagnosis for a specific period of time.

FLAT MARKET: Stable exchange market malaise characterized by little price movement, low volume, and little activity.

FLAT RATE PRICE: Three types of flat-fixed-rate medical reimbursement models exist: (1) capitation fee, (2) per-diem fee, and (3) per-case fee.

FLEXIBLE BUDGET: An estimate of revenues and expenses over time and a range of health care services.

FLEXIBLE BUDGET VARIANCE: The difference between what a health care entity actually spent at the actual level of output, and what it should have spent to obtain the actual level of output.

FLEXIBLE EXPENSES: Costs and expenditures that can be adjusted, reduced or eliminated.

FLEXIBLE PREMIUM ANNUITY: An annuity that permits additional premium payments into the contract after the original purchase.

FLEXIBLE SPENDING ACCOUNT/HEALTH CARE/DEPENDENT CARE EXPENSES: An employee benefits plan that permits the deferral of pretax earnings, for various purposes, such as un-reimbursed medical expenses.

FLIGHT TO QUALITY: Capital movements to low risk safe-havens in time of economic stress.

FLIP: The purchase of stock shares, especially in an IPO, and immediately selling them for profit.

FLIPPERS: A stock day trader who flips securities.

FLOAT: Time delay in the billing and collecting cycle.

FLOATER: A colloquial term for a security with a floating or variable interest rate.

FLOATING RATE: A variable interest rate on a security that changes at intervals according to an index, formula, or other standard of measurement as stated in the bond contract. One common method is to calculate the interest rate as a percentage of the rate paid on selected issues of Treasury securities on specified dates.

FLOATING RATE NOTES: Bonds with coupons that float and are adjusted periodically. The rate is calculated using an agreed-upon formula in the indenture, generally a spread over Treasury bills. Some floating rate bonds have floors and ceilings, both of which protect the investor's coupon income in a declining rate environment and also limit his or her coupon return when rates increase.

FLOOR: Term that refers to the amount certain deductible expenses must exceed to generate tax savings. For example, medical expenses are deductible, but only to the extent they exceed 7.5% of AGI (floor) do they result in tax savings.

FLOW OF FUNDS: The order and priority of handling, depositing, and disbursing pledged revenues, as set forth in a hospital revenue bond contract. Generally, the revenues are deposited, as received, into a general collection account or revenue fund for disbursement into the other accounts established by the bond contract. Such other accounts generally provide for payment of the costs of debt service, operation and maintenance costs, debt service reserve deposits, redemption, renewal and replacement, and other requirements.

FLOWER BONDS: Older U.S. Bond, accepted at par value at the time of death for estate tax purposes.

FLURRY: Sudden and unexpected increase in securities trading activity.

FOB DESTINATION: Free-on-Board until a travel destination is reached.

FOB SHIPPING: Free-on-Board for destination shipping costs.

FOLEY, MARY: Past president for the American Nurses Association in Washington, D.C.

FOR PROFIT: A health care or other organization where financial profits, if any, can be distributed outside the company.

FORECASTING: Predicting future economic and financial trends based on current data and other estimations. Pro forma estimation.

FORECLOSURE: Seizure of assets and collateral by a creditor when default under a loan or debt agreement occurs.

FOREIGN CORPORATION: Firm not organized under the laws of a territory or state. Taxing of foreign corporations depends on whether the corporation has nexus or effectively connected income in that state.

FOREIGN CURRENCY TRANSLATION: Restating foreign currency in equivalent dollars. Unrealized gains or losses are postponed and carried as Stockholder's Equity until the foreign operation is substantially liquidated.

FOREIGN EXCHANGE MARKET: An overseas market for the purchase or sale of currencies.

FOREIGN TAX CREDIT: U.S. taxpayer that pays or accrues income tax to a foreign country may elect to credit or deduct these taxes in a determinable U.S. dollar amount. This is usually done on an individual tax return with a specific form.

FORFEITURE: The loss of assets or rights due to the failure of contracted terms and conditions.

FORGIONE, DANA A., PhD, CPA, CFE, CME: Director of the School of Accounting, Florida International University and previous coadvisor to the MBA Healthcare Management Program at the Merrick School of Business, University of Baltimore, with a joint appointment at the School of Pharmacy. A consultant to health care organizations who analyzed the financial and operating performance of more than 5,500 hospitals throughout the United States and used twice by the U.S. Congress in national health care policy deliberations, and by the Texas Attorney General in landmark hospital charity care legislation. Founder and director of the International

Society for Research in Healthcare Financial Management, Ltd.; managing editor of *Research in Healthcare Financial Management*; and a columnist for the *Journal of Health Care Finance*. He has conducted professional training programs on Medicare regulation, fraud and abuse regulations, physician self-referral prohibitions, governmental auditing, forensic accounting, electronic data recovery, and related issues to hundreds of accountants, auditors, regulators, fraud examiners, IRS agents, physicians, surgeons, allied health care professionals, and VA inspectors general.

FORGONE BENEFIT: A cost accounting value not achieved because of a different course of action.

FORM 3: SEC required form for all holders of 10% or more of a company stock, and by all directors and officers.

FORM 4: SEC required form for holding changes for all stockholders of 10% or more of a company stock, and by all directors and officers, even if no change has taken place.

FORM 8-K: SEC required form for material financial events of public companies.

FORM 1040: The general tax form used by individual taxpayers.

FORM 1065: The general tax form used by partnerships to report profits and losses.

FORM 1120S: The general tax form used by S Corporations to report profits and losses.

FORM 2106: The general tax form used by individual taxpayers to report miscellaneous itemized deductions (e.g., hospital employee business expenses).

FORM 4562: The general tax form used to report depreciation and to compute and report the Internal Revenue Code Section 179 expense election.

FORM T: National Association of Securities Dealers (NASD) required form for reporting equity transactions executed after normal market hours.

FORM W-2: The year-end summary of wages/salaries and taxes withheld, provided by the employer to the employee for completion of the employee's income tax return for submission to the IRS.

FORM 10-K AND FORM 10-Q: Annual and quarterly reports, respectively, required by the Securities and Exchange Commission (SEC) of every issuer of a registered security, including all companies listed on the exchanges and those with 500 or more shareholders or more than $1 million in gross assets. Audited financial statements for the fiscal year must include revenues, sales, and pretax operating income, a 5-year history of sales by product line, and a sources and uses of funds statement comparative to the prior year. The quarterly report is not required to be as extensive, nor must it be audited, but it should contain a comparison to the same quarter in the prior year. These reports are available to the general public and are required to be filed on a timely basis.

FORM 13-D: SEC required form for noncontrol equity positions acquired in the ordinary course of business.

FORM 13-G: SEC required short form of Schedule D (noncontrol equity positions acquired in the ordinary course of business).

FORM LETTER: National Association of Securities Dealers (NASD) approved letter for securities sales literature.

FORWARD: A financial market similar to futures in terms of deferred deliveries. Notable differences include a lack of contract standardization, central clearinghouse, and potential for substantial counterparty risk. It does allow contractual term customization and deliveries at times, points, and grades other than those listed for futures contracts.

FORWARD CONTRACT: Commitment to sell or buy an asset at a certain price and time in the future.

FORWARD MARKET: An exchange in which a commitment is made at a quantity and price now, and agreed upon for future delivery, such as fixed rate health insurance or commodities exchange.

FORWARD PRICING: A method to determine the purchase or redemption price after receipt of a mutual fund or variable annuity order from a customer. All bid and asked prices are based on the next computed net asset value after receipt of the order.

FOUR HORSEMEN: Original Jackson Hole Wyoming Group of economists and financial developers of the managed care competitive concept in American medicine: Alain C. Enthoven PhD; Clark Havighurst, PhD; Walter McClure, PhD; and Paul M. Ellwood, MD. Also a slang term of endearment.

FOURTH MARKET: Direct institutional securities trading without the use of an intermediary or brokerage firm.

FRACTIONAL SHARE: A portion of a whole share of stock.

FRAGMENTATION: Medical fee unbundling or separation to increase payment.

FRANCHISE: Legal arrangement whereby the owner of a trade name, the franchisor, contracts with a party to use the name on a nonexclusive basis to sell goods or services, the franchisee. Usually the franchise agreement grants strict supervisory powers to the franchisor over the franchisee which, nevertheless, is an independent business, clinic, medical practice, hospital, and so forth.

FRAUD: A deception that could result in one paying for medical services it should not. For example, if a medical provider files a claim for a service (tooth extraction) that wasn't provided. It is willful misrepresentation by one person of a fact inflicting damage on another person.

FRAUD ALERT: Warning from the Office of the Inspector General (OIG) to medical providers that warns of fraud and abuse law violations.

FRAUD AND ABUSE: Federal and state, Medicare and Medicaid, violations of the Internal Revenue Code, Stark I and II laws, or other codes that proscribe patient referrals to entities in which a family member has a financial interest. Abuse is unneeded, harmful, or poor quality health care delivery or services.

FRAUD AND ABUSE LEGISLATION: The original Social Security Act, Congressional legislation of 1977, 1981, 1987, OBRA, Stark I, Stark II and HIPAA, and so forth.

FRAUDULENT HEALTH CARE MODELS: A silent, faux, or "mirror" preferred provider organization (PPO), health maintenance organization (HMO), or other provider model that is not a formalized managed care organization (MCO) at all. Rather, it is an intermediary that attempts to negotiate practitioner fees downward by promising practitioners a higher volume of patients in exchange for the discounted fee structure. The intermediary then resells the packaged contract product to any willing insurance company, HMO, PPO, or other payer and pockets the difference as a nice profit. Sometimes, these virtual organizations are indemnity companies in disguise. Physicians should not fall for this ploy because pricing pressure will be forced even lower in the next round of "real" PPO negotiations! Occasionally, an insurer, financial planner, or accountant (or a bold insurance agent) will enter a market and tell the medical practitioners in that market that it has signed up all the local, or many major, employers. Then, the insurer, financial planner, or accountant goes to the employers and tells them the same story about signing up all the major providers. In fact, neither group signed up, and a Ponzi-like situation is created. Certified Financial Planners©, Certified Medical Planners©, and all ethical financial professionals and health law attorneys should be aware of this deception and protect their clients.

FREE CASH FLOW: Cash flow after health care entity or other business operating expenses. The amount of free cash flow is a good indicator of profit levels.

FREE CASH FLOW PER SHARE: Corporate net income, plus all noncash expenses such as depreciation, less dividends, and capital expenditures, on a per share basis. It is a benchmark of financial flexibility.

FREE LOOK: A letter to potential mutual fund investors or insurance purchasers explaining plan sales charges and fees, allowing them to terminate the plan without cost.

FREE MARKET: The situation that exists when there are no restrictions or limits preventing buyers or sellers from entering or exiting a market. *See also* capitalism.

FREE RIDE: One who consumes public goods or services, such as health care, without contributing to payments or costs.

FREE RIDING & WITHHOLDING: The failure of a broker/dealer to make a bona fide public offer of a hot issue, also called "withholding."

FREE TRADE: The unrestricted or unimpeded process of conducting business or transactions. *See also* capitalism.

FREEDOM OF CHOICE: The decreasing economic ability to seek medical care from a provider or facility of choice. *See also* managed care.

FREEDOM OF ENTERPRISE: The ability to start a legal business and sell products or services in a market of choice.

FREEZE OUT: Minority shareholders pressure to sell securities.

FRICTIONAL UNEMPLOYMENT: Unemployed health care or other workers that are between jobs or in transition.

FRIEDMAN, EMILY, PhD: Independent economist and health policy analyst in Chicago, Illinois.

FRIEDMAN RULE: A cash model monetary system that tends toward deflation so that it is not costly to patients who have money to continue to hold it.

FRINGE BENEFITS: Employment benefits beyond salary, cash, or wages, such as health or life insurance, pension plans, vacation time, and so forth.

FRIST, WILLIAM, MD: U.S. Senator for Tennessee in Washington, D.C. He is a ranking member on the public health subcommittee, and a member of the Health, Education, Labor, and Pensions Committee.

FRONT END LOAD: Funds paid at the outset of the direct participation program that do not contribute materially to the actual investment vehicle. Front-end load typically consists of distributions to general partners, organizational fees, or acquisition fees. See also commission.

FRONT RUNNING: Form of market manipulation where a broker/dealer delays processing of a large customer trade in an underlying security until the firm can execute an options trade in that security in anticipation of the client's trade impact on the underlying security.

FRONTIER ANALYSIS: Mathematical evaluation of a health care firm's efficiency in an attempt to quantify best and worst practices, and augment or improve them.

FRONTIER STUDY: Relationship of real health care outputs and costs, compared to theoretically best practices and outputs.

FROZEN ACCOUNT: Cash account where a customer fails to pay for a purchase within the allowable Regulation-T period and no extension has been obtained. Prior payment is required before any further purchase executions for 90 days thereafter. Margin accounts are never frozen.

FULL CAPACITY SALES (FCS): Actual sales divided by percent of capacity of fixed-asset operations.

FULL CAPITATION: The health plan or primary care case manager is paid for providing services to enrollees through a combination of capitation and fee for service reimbursements.

FULL CHARGE: Fee-for-service medical reimbursement.

FULL COST: Expense that includes all associated costs. See also fully allocated costs.

FULL DISCLOSURE LAWS: State or federal laws that mandate public health care or other companies to disclose financial and other information that may affect the value of their securities.

FULL EMPLOYMENT: The use of all available human resources and labor to produce health care products and services.

FULL INTEREST PAYMENT: Loan or debt payment option that satisfies the minimum amount and all regular monthly interest due.

FULL PERSONAL CAPITATION: Advanced method of fixed rate individual capitation for a primary care physician gate keeper who subcapitates medical specialists. See also contact capitation; global capitation.

FULL PRINCIPAL AND INTEREST PAYMENT: Loan payment option that includes all the interest due and reduces principal.

FULL PRODUCTION: The maximum amount of medical goods and services produced from the employed resources of an economic sector, such as health care.

FULL RISK CAPITATION: The complete acceptance of all fiscal risk by a health care plan, facility, or medical provider for the plan's members, in return for greater compensation. Providers are paid a single per member per month rate to cover all health care (professional, facilities and technical) services for a population of people (patients).

FULL SERVICE BROKER: A licensed stockbroker salesman (registered representative of a brokerage firm) with a research department and other products and services to supply clients with incidental investing advice, but not a fiduciary.

FULL TIME EMPLOYEE (EQUIVALENT) (FTE): Generally, employees of an employer who work for 1,000 or more hours in a 12-month period, as defined for pension plan purposes in the Employees Retirement Income Security Act (ERISA).

FULLY ALLOCATED COSTS: Medical service costs after considering all directed and fair share costs.

FULLY CAPITATED: All-risk, fixed-rate, per patient global capitation reimbursement by contract, including medical, surgical, ancillary, and facility specialists. Providers are paid a single per member per month rate to cover all health care services for a population of patients. Global capitation of all downstream health care provider and facility costs.

FULLY DEPRECIATED: Fixed asset which has lost all depreciation (noncash) expense deductions that the U.S. tax law allows.

FULLY FUNDED PLAN: A health plan under which an insurer or managed care organization bears the financial responsibility of guaranteeing claim payments and paying for all incurred covered benefits and administration costs.

FULLY LOADED: All marketing, sales, and administrative fees of a mutual fund or brokerage account. This includes life insurance, health insurance, or managed care contract, including agent commissions.

FULLY REGISTERED: A security that has been registered as to both principal and interest. Such securities are payable only to the owner, or to order of the owner, whose name is noted on records of the issuer or its agent.

FUNCTIONAL COSTS: Operating costs classified by function or purpose.

FUND: Collection of assets set aside for a defined purpose.

FUND ACCOUNTING: Nonprofit health care or governmental accounting method that views an organization as a collection of funds.

FUND AVAILABILITY: The dollar amount or time period represented by checks that have been deposited but have not cleared.

FUND BALANCE: Excess of assets over liabilities and fund reserves.

FUNDAMENTAL ANALYSIS: Uses a quantitative (using numbers) approach to securities market forecasting based on an analysis of corporate balance sheets and income statements. A corporation's strengths and weaknesses, as shown by arithmetic formulas and other measurements of economic and industry trends, are used to predict future price movements of its stocks and bonds. It is the opposite of Technical Analysis (TA).

FUNDED DEBT: Longer-term debt.

FUNDING: The replacement of short-term debt with long-term securities.

FUNDING LEVEL: Amount of revenue required to finance a medical care or other program.

FUNDING METHOD: System for employers to pay for a health benefit plan. Most common methods are prospective and/or retrospective premium payment, shared risk arrangement, self-funded, or refunding products.

FUNDING VEHICLE: The fully funded account into which the money that an employer and/or employees pay in premiums to an insurer or managed care organization, and is deposited until the money is paid out.

FUNGIBLE: The ability of a security to change, or be substituted or exchanged.

FUTURE COSTS: A decision-making and forward looking directive relevant to an alternate selection expense charge process. There are two types:

- *Avoidable Future Costs:* can be eliminated or saved if the activity in question is saved, eliminated, or discontinued. For example, salary and administration costs might be reduced in a hospital if 40% of the beds were taken out of service.
- *Incremental Future Costs:* are a change from a specific management activity (e.g., starting or expanding a service, closing or opening a department, acquiring new equipment). For example, the incremental costs for signing a capitated managed care contract would generate 100 new patients next year.

FUTURE SUM OF AN ANNUITY: The compound value of the sum of an equal number of periodic payments.

FUTURE VALUE (FV): The amount of money that an invested lump sum or series of payments will be worth, at some point in the future.

FUTURE VALUE ANNUITY: The future worth of an annuity payment stream based on its terms and conditions.

FUTURE VALUE FACTOR (FVF): A multiplier for an invested lump sum of money or payment stream used to estimate its future value.

FUTURES CONTRACT: A contract calling for the delivery of a specific quantity of a physical good or a financial instrument (or the cash value) at some specific date in the future. There are exchange-traded futures contracts with standardized terms, and there are over-the-counter futures contracts with negotiated terms.

FUTURES MARKET: A stock exchange where futures options and contracts are traded.

G

G: Commodity futures symbol for a February delivery month.

G-7: A Group of Seven Nations: Britain, Canada, France, Germany, Italy, Japan, and the United States. These countries represent 66.5% of the world economy and representatives from them meet annually to discuss economic, political, and health care policy issues though numerous subsidiary meetings and/or medical or other policy research collaborative efforts.

G-8 FINANCE MINISTERS: Ministers of Finance for the eight largest industrial countries in the world. G 7–8.

GAIN/LOSS: Difference between the amounts of money received when selling an asset and its book's value, or the difference between sale and purchase price of a security.

GALBRAITH, JOHN KENNETH, PhD (1908–2006): Berkeley-trained economist who was considered a renegade because of his first theory of price control with anti-inflationary health economic implications, and his second theory that argued that success arose not out of "getting the prices right," but rather of "getting the prices wrong" and allowing health care and other industrial concentration to develop. Regarded as successful only when there is a countervailing power against potential abuse in the form of medical unions, supplier and consumer organizations, and government regulations. He also provided early critical economic commentary on competitive markets and marketing.

GALBRAITH, JOHN KENNETH, EFFECT: Marketing and advertising effects of health care products, goods, or medical services. Direct-to-consumer marketing of pharmaceuticals is a modern competitive example.

GAP OPENING: Opening stock price significantly different (higher or lower) than the previous day.

GARNISHMENT: Creditor access to a debtor's wages in order to satisfy a debt or overdue account.

GEARING: A measure of quantity exposure for warrants.

GENERAL ACCOUNT: The account into which premium revenues received by an insurance company are deposited. These funds are usually invested in high quality and safe securities issues. A stockbroker or brokerage firm's customer's margin or credit account.

GENERAL ACCOUNTING OFFICE (GAO): Accounting and auditing office of the U.S. government. An independent agency that reviews federal financial transactions and reports directly to Congress.

GENERAL AND ADMINISTRATIVE EXPENSES: Health care or other entity's operating expenses not found in the supply and labor budgets.

GENERAL FUND: Liabilities and assets of a nonprofit health care organization that are not set aside for a specified purpose.

GENERAL JOURNAL: The journal used to record all transactions that do not fit into a special journal.

GENERAL LEDGER: Ledger of accounts reported in financial statements.

GENERAL OBLIGATION BOND: A bond that is secured by the full faith and credit of an issuer with taxing power. General obligation bonds issued by local units of government are typically secured by a pledge of the issuer's ad-valorem taxing power. General obligation bonds issued by states are generally based upon appropriations made by the state legislature for the purposes specified. Ad-valorem taxes necessary to pay debt service on general obligation bonds are often not subject to the constitutional property tax millage limits. Such bonds constitute debts of the issuer and normally require approval by election prior to issuance. In the event of default, the holders of general obligation bonds have the right to compel a tax levy or legislative appropriation, by mandamus or injunction, in order to satisfy the issuer's obligation on the defaulted bonds.

GENERAL OPERATING EXPENSES: Expenses of an insurance or other company other than commissions and taxes. The administrative costs of running a business.

GENERAL PARTNER: An investor and a partner for the purposes of profits, losses, and the liabilities of the partnership. A general partner materially participates in the day-to-day management of the partnership and is jointly and severally liable for the actions and debts of the partnership.

GENERAL REVENUE: Income to the supplemental medical insurance trust fund from the general fund of the U.S. Treasury. Only a very small percentage of total SMI trust fund income each year is attributable to general revenue.

GENERAL SECURITIES REPRESENTATIVE EXAMINATION: The Series seven (7) securities licensing and sales examination.

GENERALLY ACCEPTED ACCOUNTING PRINCIPLES (GAAP): Accounting guidelines formulated by the Financial Accounting Standards Board (FASB) which govern how accountants measure, process, communicate, and record financial information.

GENERALLY ACCEPTED AUDITING STANDARDS (GAAS): Standards set by the AICPA that concern auditor qualities and judgment in the performance of professional reports.

GEOGRAPHIC ADJUSTMENT FACTOR (GAF): Third-party factor to neutralize geographic financial differences in health care provider costs and resources prices (i.e., Medicare).

GEOMETRIC MEAN: The Nth root of the product of "n" numbers.

GEOMETRIC MEAN LENGTH OF STAY (GMLOS): A mathematical component that determines DRG reimbursement for a hospital length of stay.

GEPHARDT, RICHARD: U.S. representative (D-Mo.) and minority leader.

GERBERDING, JULIE, MD: Director of the U.S. Centers for Disease Control and Prevention in Atlanta, Georgia.

GHOST: One who works with two or more market makers to manipulate stock prices. This is unethical behavior.

GIBRAT'S LAW: Relationship between health care business size and growth which suggests that unit size and growth percentages are statistically independent.

GIFFEN GOOD: Theoretical construct that suggests a health care good or service that experiences increased demand when price rises, and decreased demand when prices fall.

GILT EDGE SECURITY: A well known legacy company with a rock solid history of dividend payments and bond performance. Analogous to a "blue chip" stock in the equities market.

GINI COEFFICIENT: A number between zero and one that is a measure of health care inequality. The concentration of medical providers in a health care market or the industry.

GINNIE MAE PASS-THROUGH CERTIFICATE: Fixed income debt security that represents an undivided portion of a pool of insured mortgages whose principal and interest payments are guaranteed by the Government National Mortgage Association (GNMA).

GINSBURG, PAUL: President of the Center for Studying Health System Change in Washington, D.C.

GLAMOR STOCK: Equities with wide public exposure, owned by institutions, and followed by many stock analysts with high growth rate potential.

GLASS-STEAGALL ACT OF 1933: Federal law that separated commercial banks, investment banks, and insurance companies. It was designed to confront the problem that banks in the Great Depression collapsed because they held vast amounts of common stock.

GLOBAL BUDGETING: Limits placed on categories of health spending. A method of hospital cost containment in which participating hospitals must share a prospectively set budget. Method for allocating funds among hospitals may vary, but the key is that the participating hospitals agree to an aggregate cap on revenues that they will receive each year. Global budgeting may also be mandated under a universal health insurance system.

GLOBAL CAPITATION: Providers are paid a single per member per month rate to cover all health care (professional, facilities, and technical) services for a population of people (patients). The complete acceptance of all fiscal risk by a health care plan, facility, or provider for plan members, in return for greater compensation.

GLOBAL CASE RATES: Providers are paid a lump sum upon referral to cover all health care (professionals, facilities, and technical) services, specific to a defined illness episode.

GLOBAL FEE: A total charge for a specific set of services, such as obstetrical services that encompass prenatal, delivery, and post-natal care. Managed care organizations will often seek contracts with hospitals that contain set global fees for certain sets of services. Outliers and carve-outs will be those services not included in the global negotiated rates.

GLOBAL FUND: A mutual fund (open or closed) whose holdings include outside the United States.

GLOBAL PER DIEM FEE: All prospective medical reimbursement payments for a hospitalized patient, fixed per day.

GLOBAL SURGERY PACKAGE: Code for a normal surgical procedure, including all elements and without complications, submitted and accepted for reimbursement.

GNOME: Maturity length of 15 years for certain government securities.

GNP DEFLATOR: The ratio of real to nominal GNP as an index of average prices used to deflate GNP.

GODFATHER OFFER: Munificent and highly beneficial takeover offer that cannot be refused by management.

GOING AHEAD: Stockbroker trading in front (before) of a customer's orders. This is an unethical practice

GOING CONCERN: A continuous health care or other business enterprise currently in operations. A reasonable assumption that a medical practice, clinic, hospital, or business can remain in operation long enough for all of its current plans to be carried out.

GOING CONCERN VALUE: The value of a continuous health care or other business enterprise entity that is expected to continue into the future, and derived from patients, vendors, and HMO insurance contracts, a trained and assembled workforce, tangible and intangible assets, degrees, certifications, accreditations, licenses, and so forth.

GOING LONG: Purchasing and owning securities outright for potential profit.

GOING PUBLIC: Selling private corporate shares to the public for the first time, usually in the over-the-counter or auction markets.

GOING SHORT: Selling securities otherwise not owned.

GOLDEN HANDCUFFS: A munificent and abundant employment contract that ties an executive to a corporation.

GOLDEN PARACHUTE: Munificent and lavish executive contract with abundant fringe benefits resulting from a job loss.

GOLDSMITH, JEFFREY: President of Health Futures in Charlottesville, Virginia.

GOLLIER, CHRISTIAN, PhD: Professor at the University of Toulouse in Anatole, France and Fédération Française des Sociétés d'Assurances (FFSA) Chair of Insurance at the Industrial Economics Institute. He is a financial expert on life insurance, health risk management, and insurance.

GOOD DELIVERY: Proper securities delivery by a selling firm to the purchaser's office of certificates that are negotiable without additional documentation and that are in units acceptable under the Uniform Practice Code (UPC).

GOOD DELIVERY MUNICIPAL SECURITIES: The presentation by a seller of securities previously sold to a purchaser that are in acceptable form for delivery purposes as defined in MSRB Rules G-12(e) (with respect to interdealer deliveries) and G-15(c) (with respect to deliveries to customers). The delivery standards specified in those rules cover such matters as the criteria for fundability of securities, denominations, the attachment of legal opinions and other required documents, the presentation of interest payment checks in certain circumstances, and other similar matters.

GOOD FAITH DEPOSIT: A sum of money provided to an issuer of a new issue of municipal securities sold at competitive bid by an underwriter or underwriting syndicate as an assurance of performance on its bid. The good faith deposit is usually in an amount from 1% to 5% of the par value of the issue, and generally is provided in the form of a certified or cashier's check. The check is returned to the bidder if its bid is not accepted, but the check of the successful bidder is retained until the issue is delivered. In the event the winning bidder fails to pay for the new issue on the delivery date, the check is usually retained as full or partial liquidated damages.

GOOD FAITH ESTIMATE: A written estimate of financial closing costs which a lender must provide within 3 days of submitting a loan application.

GOOD-TILL-CANCELED ORDER: A limit securities order that remains valid indefinitely, until executed or canceled by the customer.

GOODMAN, ALLEN C., PhD: Health care economist and pioneer of high-deductible health insurance plans from Wayne State University in Detroit, Michigan.

GOODS AND SERVICES: All the valuable products and services that the health care industry produces. Medical care output.

GOODS MARKET: An exchange where health care products and services are purchased and provided.

GOODWILL: (1) The value and economic benefit attributed to the good name in the community, above and beyond the norm for a similar health care entity, void of their brand recognition. (2) The excess fee, price, or cost of a medical service, health care firm, or operating unit over the current fair market value of the net assets of the firm, or unit. (3) The ability of a health care business entity to generate income in excess of a normal rate on assets due to superior doctors, managerial skills, market position, new product technology, and so forth. There are two types of goodwill:

- *Business Goodwill* is the difference between the book value of assets on the health care business's balance sheet and what the business or practice would sell for; or, as the going-concern value that results from an organized assemblage of revenue-producing assets, such as the propensity of patients, doctors, payers, and contractors (and their revenue streams) to return to the business in the future.
- *Personal* or *Doctor Goodwill* results from the charisma, knowledge, skill, and reputation of a specific doctor, owner, or manager, and various doctor-associates. Personal Goodwill is generated by the reputation and personal attributes of the doctors that accrue to that individual shareholder. Because these attributes "go to the grave" with that specific doctor or shareholder, and therefore can't be sold, they have no economic value. Personal doctor goodwill is not transferable. Even with long transition periods of introduction for a new acquiring doctor-owner, the charisma, skills, reputation, and personal attributes of the doctor-seller cannot, by definition, be transferred.

GOTTLIEB, GARY, MD: President of the Brigham and Women's Hospital in Boston, Massachusetts.

GOVERNING DOCUMENTS: Official legal documents that dictate how an entity is operated, including articles of incorporation, bylaws, partnership agreement, trust agreement, or trust indenture. A LLC includes the articles of organization and operating agreement.

GOVERNMENT ACCOUNTING STANDARDS BOARD (GASB): Organization that has the authority to establish standards of financial reporting for all units of state and local government.

GOVERNMENT AGENCY ISSUES: Government agency bonds are used to finance various entities created by the U.S. Congress, such as public hospitals or clinics, and therefore the government has a moral obligation (but is not guaranteed) to pay interest and principal. As noted, while most government agency bonds are composed of pools of mortgages, they also exist for other types of loans. Some common examples are Federal Farm Credit Bank (FFCB), Federal Home Loan Bank (FHLB), Federal National Marketing Association (FNMA),

Student Loan Marketing Association (SLMA), Federal Home Loan Mortgage Corporation (FHLMC), and Refinancing Corporation (REFCORP). The minimum size of these bonds is generally $10,000, and multiples of $5,000 are available. Some lesser-known issues can be in smaller minimum sizes. Four major types fall within the general category of federal agency issues:

- Federal agency discount notes are issued in maturities of less than one year, similar to treasury bills. They trade in increments of $10,000, and because they lack a coupon they are bought and sold on a discount yield basis.
- Fixed-rate debentures pay interest every 6 months and return the principal upon maturity at par.
- Floating-rate notes are issued with varying maturity options and reset features for the coupon.
- Mortgage-backed issues pay monthly principal and interest. Three agencies issue these instruments: Government National Mortgage Association (Ginnie Mae), the Federal National Mortgage Association (Fannie Mae), and the Federal Home Loan Mortgage Corporation (Freddie Mac). Government agencies also issue zero coupon bonds.

GOVERNMENT NATIONAL MORTGAGE ASSOCIATION (GNMA): A government-owned corporation that acquires packages and resells mortgages and mortgage purchase commitments in the form of mortgage-backed securities, such as Ginnie Mae.

GRACE PERIOD: Period of time during which a depositor can withdraw funds from a certificate of deposit without being penalized. It is also the period of time during which a loan payment may be paid after its due date during which no late charge or other penalty is assessed. There is a similar concept in the insurance industry.

GRADE: A quality rating system for debt, equities, or commodities.

GRADUATED SECURITY: Upgraded securities listing (i.e., from the OTC to the NYSE).

GRAHAM (BENJAMIN)-DODD (DAVID) INVESTING: Conservative and fundamental investing methodology based on undervalued assets.

GRAMM-LEACH-BLILEY ACT: The Financial Services Modernization Act of 1999 that eliminated the distinction between banks, insurance companies, and securities firms.

GRANTEE: Person to whom property is transferred.

GRANTOR: The party who initially sells, writes, or grants an option. (1) The person who transfers property. (2) The person who creates a trust.

GRANTOR RETAINED ANNUITY TRUST (GRAT): A trust in which the grantor retains the right to a fixed dollar amount (the annuity) for a fixed term. If the grantor survives until the end of the annuity term, all of the trust principal will pass to others and escape the grantor's estate for death tax purposes.

GRANTOR RETAINED INCOME TRUST (GRIT): A trust in which the grantor retains the right to receive the income. To satisfy all gift and estate tax law requirements, the GRIT must be either a GRAT or a GRUT.

GRANTOR RETAINED UNI-TRUST (GRUT): A GRUT is similar to a GRAT, except that with a GRUT the grantor retains the right to receive a fixed percentage of the value of the trust annually. Thus, the total annual payments will fluctuate in direct proportion to the value of the trust.

GRANTS: The funds given to a health care or other entity for a special project, and usually for a certain time period, along with various other terms and conditions.

GRASSLEY, CHARLES: U.S. Senator (R-Iowa) and ranking member of the Finance Committee.

GRAVEYARD MARKET: Bear (depressed) market with substantial investor loss.

GREENMAIL: Premium price paid to a corporate raider through a proxy contest with shareholders.

GREENSHOE: Underwriting allotment option in excess of the first stipulated share amount. Depending on demand and/or market stabilizing functions, an underwriter can exercise this option for additional shares. Usually, the greenshoe is limited to an additional 15% of new shares.

GRESHAM'S (SIR THOMAS) LAW: Economic theory that suggests bad (worn) money drives good (new) currency out of circulation.

GRIDLOCK: A condition where securities trading activity stops when the spreads between bids and offers widen dramatically and volume diminishes.

GROSS: Business data that is usually financial, and not yet subject to deductions, reductions, discounts, charge-offs, and so forth.

GROSS CHARGES PER 1,000: An indicator calculated by taking the gross health care charges incurred by a specific group for a specific period of time, dividing it by the average number of covered members or lives in that group during the same period, and multiplying the result by 1,000. It is calculated in the aggregate and by modality of treatment, for example, inpatient, residential, partial hospitalization, and outpatient. It is a measure used to evaluate utilization management performance.

GROSS COSTS PER 1,000: An indicator calculated by taking the gross costs incurred for health care services received by a specific group for a specific period of time, dividing it by the average number of covered members or lives in that group during the same period, and multiplying the result by 1,000. This is calculated in the aggregate and by modality of treatment, for example, inpatient, residential, partial hospitalization, and outpatient. It is a measure used to evaluate utilization management performance. This is the key concept for the medical provider. In managed care, this indicator should be below collections per 1,000.

GROSS DOMESTIC PRODUCT (GDP): The total current market value of all goods and services produced domestically during a given period. It differs from the Gross National Product (GNP) by excluding net income that residents earn abroad.

GROSS EARNING: Total earnings, before deduction of taxes and expenses.

GROSS EXPENSE PER DISCHARGE: The average expense incurred by hospitals to provide inpatient care, including room and board, patient care services, and goods sold, from admission to discharge. It is gross inpatient expenses, divided by discharges, and excluding nursery discharges.

GROSS EXPENSE PER VISIT: The average expense incurred by a hospital to provide care for one outpatient visit. It is gross outpatient expenses divided by outpatient visits.

GROSS INCOME: Income, from whatever personal or business source derived, before taxes are deducted.

GROSS INPATIENT EXPENSES: Operating expenses related to providing inpatient services. Excludes nonoperating expenses and income taxes but includes physician professional component expenses. Gross inpatient expenses are determined by allocating total operating expenses using the ratio of gross inpatient revenue to the total gross patient revenue.

GROSS INPATIENT REVENUE: Total inpatient charges at the hospital's full established rates for services rendered and goods sold, including revenue from daily hospital services, inpatient ambulatory services, and inpatient ancillary services. Also includes charges related to hospital-based physician professional services. Other operating revenue and non-operating revenue are excluded.

GROSS INVESTMENT: Money spent on replacing depreciated capital and on net additions to corporate capital stock.

GROSS MARGIN: Excess of sales revenues over cost of health care products, services, or goods sold.

GROSS MARGIN METHOD: An estimation of inventory profit, based on a cost of goods sold model: Beginning inventory, plus net purchases equals cost of DME goods available for sale. Cost of goods available for sale, minus cost of goods sold equals ending inventory.

GROSS NATIONAL PRODUCT (GNP): The total current market value of all goods and services produced domestically during a given period. It differs from the Gross Domestic Product (GDP) by including net income that residents earn abroad.

GROSS OUTPATIENT EXPENSES: Total operating expenses relating to outpatient health care services. Excludes nonoperating expenses and income taxes, but includes physician professional component expenses. Gross outpatient expenses are determined by allocating total operating expenses using the ratio of gross outpatient revenue to total gross revenue.

GROSS OUTPATIENT REVENUE: Total outpatient charges at a hospital or clinic established rates for outpatient ambulatory and outpatient ancillary services rendered and goods sold. Also includes charges related to hospital-based physician professional services. Other operating revenue and nonoperating revenue are excluded.

GROSS PATIENT REVENUE: The total charges at a hospital's or clinic's established rates for the provision of patient care services before deductions from revenue are applied. Includes charges related to hospital-based physician professional services. Other operating revenue and nonoperating revenue are excluded.

- Gross Inpatient Revenue—Gross revenue for daily hospital services and inpatient ancillary services before deductions from revenue are applied.
- Gross Outpatient Revenue—Gross revenue for outpatient ancillary services before deductions from revenue are applied.

GROSS PATIENT SERVICE REVENUE: The total charges at a health care facility's established rates for the provision of patient care before deductions from revenue are applied. It is the total amount of monies a health care organization earns, at full retail price, for its medical services.

GROSS PRIVATE DOMESTIC HEALTH CARE INVESTMENT: Investment purchases and private expenditures of health care firms, the value of related construction, and the change in inventory during the year.

GROSS REVENUE PER DAY: The average amount charged by a hospital for 1 day of inpatient care (gross inpatient revenue divided by patient-census days).

GROSS REVENUE PER DISCHARGE: The average amount charged by a hospital to treat an inpatient from admission to discharge (gross inpatient revenue divided by discharges).

GROSS REVENUE PER VISIT: The average amount charged by a hospital for an outpatient visit (gross outpatient revenue divided by outpatient visits).

GROSS SALES: Sales revenue at total value, without discounts, bad debt, or other adjustments.

GROSS WORKING CAPITAL: Same as current assets (CAs).

GROUP NET ORDER: A securities order submitted to an underwriting syndicate for a new municipal issue that, if allocated, is allocated at the public offering price without deducting the concession or takedown. A group net order benefits all members of the syndicate according to their percentage participation in the account, and consequently is normally accorded the highest priority of all orders received during the order period.

GROUP SALES: Sales of securities by a syndicate manager to institutional purchasers.

GROUPER: Software that assigns DRGs and components for health care reimbursement.

GROWTH FUND: A mutual fund whose primary investment objective is long-term growth of capital. It invests principally in common stocks with growth potential.

GROWTH INCOME FUND: A mutual fund whose aim is to provide for a degree of both income and long-term growth.

GROWTH INVESTING: A style of investing that tries to outperform the market by investing in companies that are experiencing growth patterns in earnings, cash flows, sales, capitalization, and so forth.

GROWTH RATE: The percentage rate at which the economy, securities, or some other benchmark are increasing in value.

GROWTH STOCK: A stock that has a record of relatively fast earnings growth, usually 1 1/2 to 2 times the average for the market as a whole. If the growth is expected to continue, the stock carries a higher price/earnings multiple than the average for the market. See also emerging health care organization (EHO).

GTC: Good Till Canceled, or an open order for securities purchase.

GUARANTEED INVESTMENT CONTRACT (GIC): A debt-based fixed instrument sold to retirement plans in large denominations and amounts.

GUARANTY: Legal arrangement involving a promise by one person to perform the obligations of a second person to a third person, in the event the second person fails to perform.

GUARDIAN: Financial fiduciary or manager of another's assets, on their behalf.

GUIDELINE COMPANIES: Companies that have investment characteristics comparable to those of the company being valued, as in the health care sector. Ideal guideline companies are in the same industry as the company being valued, however, if there is insufficient transaction evidence available in the same industry, it may be necessary to select companies with other similarities such as companies serving the same markets, having similar products, growth, and cyclical variability.

GUIDELINE PUBLIC COMPANY METHOD: A valuation method for public health care or other companies based on the comparable values for business of same or similar enterprise.

GUIDING FUNCTION OF PRICE: The ability of health care price changes to bring about quantity changes in inputs and outputs demanded and supplied.

GUN JUMPING: Securities trading on nonpublicly disclosed information; unethical.

GUNSLINGER: An aggressive portfolio manager prone to risk taking in order to achieve higher investment returns.

GUSTAFSON, RICHARD: Senior partner of Heidrick & Struggles in Chicago, Illinois.

GUTS: Purchase or the sale of two in-the-money options. A long-guts position consists of the purchase of a low strike call and the purchase of a high strike put. A short-guts position consists of the sale of the high strike put and the sale of the low strike call.

H

H: Commodity futures symbol for a March delivery month.

HAIRCUT: Slang term for a very steep broker commission or securities transaction cost.

HALAMKA, JOHN: Chief Information Officer of CareGroup in Boston, Massachusetts.

HAMMERING THE MARKET: An intense stock market sell-off period.

HANDS OFF: An investor willing to take a passive role in the investment process, or one who delegates roles.

HANDS ON: An investor unwilling to take a passive role in the investment process, or one who does not delegate roles and may be controlling.

HARRIS, BARRY C., PhD: Principal and Board Chairman of Economist, Incorporated in Washington, D.C. He earned his PhD from the University of Pennsylvania.

HARROD NEUTRAL: Synonym for a health care production function in which human capital and labor (doctors and nurses) is a more effective variable than capital.

HART-SCOTT-RODINO ACT: Mandates premerger FTC and DOJ notification if an acquiring health care entity has net annual sales of a proscribed amount, or if the acquired health care entity has net assets of less than proscribed amounts, or vice versa. 15-USC., 18a; Section 7A of the Clayton Act.

HAVIGHURST, CLARK: Attorney and health care economist and one of the original Four Horsemen of managed medical care from the Jackson Hole Group. He is now the William Neal Reynolds Professor of Law at Duke University in Durham, North Carolina.

HCFA: Health Care Financing Administration (older term; it is now Centers for Medicare and Medicaid Services).

HCFA-1450: HCFA's (older term, now CMS) name for the institutional uniform claim form, or UB-92.

HCFA 1500: HCFA's (older term, now CMS) standard form for submitting physician service claims to third-party (insurance) companies.

HEAD AND SHOULDERS: A technical theory founded on the belief that a market trend may be predicted by plotting price fluctuations of securities on graph paper. A "top" indicates a bearish future as prices have topped, while a "bottom" is bullish as the market has bottomed.

HEAD OF HOUSEHOLD: One entitled to special tax rates that fall midway between single rates and married filing joint rates, if they fit qualifying profiles.

HEALTH CARE: Medical products, goods, and services used as economic inputs to produce certain health care outputs.

HEALTH CARE CLEARINGHOUSE: A public or private entity that does the following, including but not limited to, billing services, repricing companies, community health management information systems or community health information systems, and "value-added" networks and switches are health care clearinghouses if they perform these functions: (1) Processes or facilitates the processing of information received from another entity in a nonstandard format or containing nonstandard data content into standard data elements or a standard transaction; (2) Receives a standard transaction from another entity and processes or facilitates the processing of information into nonstandard format or nonstandard data content for a receiving entity.

HEALTH CARE COMMON PROCEDURAL CODING SYSTEM (HCPCS): Medicare and other payer codes to describe medical procedures and supplies for payment:

- Level I CPT: Payment for a wide spectrum of medical services and procedures.
- Level II CPT: Alphanumeric and initiated by a single letter with four numbers.
- Level III CPT: Local and regional codes phased out in 2003.
- CDT: *Current Dental Terminology* codes.

HEALTH CARE COMMON PROCEDUREAL CODING SYSTEM MODIFIERS: Codes that identify and/or augment circumstances that change HCPCS supply or medical service descriptions, for payment.

HEALTH CARE ECONOMICS: The study of medical services scarcity, and its financing, accounting, production, value, distribution, cost, and consumption.

HEALTH CARE FINANCING ADMINISTRATION (HCFA): The former agency within the Department of Health and Human Services that administered federal health financing and related regulatory programs, principally the Medicare, Medicaid, and Peer Review Organization. The newer agency is called the Centers for Medicare and Medicaid Services (CMS).

HEALTH CARE FRAUD AND ABUSE CONTROL PROGRAM (HFACP): A joint project between the OIG and the Department of Justice (DOJ). The primary functions are to coordinate federal, state, and local enforcement in controlling health care fraud, to conduct investigations relating to delivery and payment of health care services, and to oversee Medicare and Medicaid exclusions, civil money penalties, and the antikickback law. The program is also designed to provide opinions, alerts, and a means for reporting and disclosing final adverse actions against health care providers. HIPAA established the Health Care Fraud and Abuse Control Account within the Medicare Part A Trust Fund and funds DOJ and HHS activities for operation of CMS (HCFAC). In addition to federal appropriations, the program receives a portion of funds collected from health care fraud and abuse penalties and fines. HIPAA also authorizes funds from general revenues for the FBI to combat health care fraud and abuse.

HEALTH CARE FRAUD AND ABUSE DATA COLLECTION PROGRAM: The Health Care Integrity and Protection Data Bank (HIPDB) was created to coordinate information with the National Practitioner Data Bank (NPDB). Currently, health plans, health maintenance organizations, and federal and state agencies are required to report final adverse actions taken against health care providers on a monthly basis. This database operates under the auspices of the Department of Health and Human Services, the Health Resources and Services Administration, and the Bureau of Health Professions. The Secretary of HHS is responsible for operating this data bank in the same fashion as the NPDB. There are five types of final adverse actions against a health care provider, supplier, or practitioner that are reported into this data bank:

- civil judgments in federal/state court related to the delivery of a health care item or service;
- federal or state criminal convictions related to the delivery of a health care item or service;
- actions by federal or state agencies responsible for licensing and certification;
- exclusions from participation in a federal or state health care program; and
- any other adjudicated actions or decisions that the secretary of HHS establishes by regulations.

These actions must be reported, regardless of whether the subject of the report is appealing the action. Federal and state agencies, hospitals, and health plans are permitted to query the HIPDB. This will also lead to increased activities by other Federal agencies, including the Internal Revenue Service and the Federal Trade Commission, which can lead to civil and criminal penalties.

HEALTH CARE PREPAYMENT PLAN (HCPP): (1) Plans that receive payment for their reasonable costs of providing Medicare Part B services to Medicare enrollees. (2) A health plan with a Medicare cost contract to provide only Medicare Part B benefits. Some administrative requirements for these plans are less stringent than those of risk contracts or other cost contracts.

HEALTH CARE SECTOR COSTS: Payments and revenue received by physicians and health care entities that represent the cost of business for the government, insurance industry, or paying sector. Generally, the paying sector includes hospital inpatients and outpatients, medical providers, skilled nursing facilities, and home health care agencies, all of which are annually indexed for inflation.

HEALTH CARE SYSTEMS INTERNATIONAL PAYMENT TOPOLOGY: Refers to a broad system of international macroeconomic health care benefits and financial payment methodologies among developed countries:

- *Mixed systems:* Hybrid of traditional sickness insurance and national health coverage: Iceland, Ireland, Japan, Australia, Switzerland, and the United States.
- *National health services:* State provided funding: Italy, Greece, Denmark, New Zealand, Turkey, Portugal, and the United Kingdom.
- *National health insurance:* Country provided health insurance system: Finland, Canada, Spain, Norway, and Sweden.
- *Traditional sickness insurance:* State subsidy of the private insurance industry: Belgium, France, Austria, Luxembourg, the Netherlands, and Germany.

HEALTH MAINTENANCE ORGANIZATION (HMO): A legal corporation that offers health insurance and medical care. HMOs typically offer a range of health care services at a fixed price (see capitation). Types of HMOs:

- Staff Model—Organization owns its clinics and employs its doctors.
- Group Model—Contract with medical groups for services.
- IPA Model—Contract with an IPA that contracts individual physicians.
- Direct Contract Model—Contracts directly with individual physicians.
- Mixed Model—Members get options ranging from staff to IPA models.

HEALTH PLAN FLEXIBLE SPENDING ACCOUNT (HPFSA): A fund to which employees contribute pretax money to pay for health insurance premiums and/or un-reimbursed medical costs. Exclusions exist on a use-it-or-lose-it basis.

HEALTH SAVINGS ACCOUNT (HSA): Tax-free accounts that are paired with a variety of high-deductible health insurance plans (traditional, managed care, HMO, PPO, etc.) that empower employees and patients to have greater control over their health care and treatment decisions. Started in 2004, HSAs have been approved as part of the Medicare Act of 2003 and may augment or replace MSAs by political or competitive fiat. HSAs are very similar to MSAs, but they are less restrictive. HSAs are open to all employers, while MSAs are only available to the self-employed or businesses with 50 or fewer employees. In addition, the deductibles for HSAs are lower than the deductibles for MSAs. For HSAs, a high-deductible plan is one in which the deductible is about $1,050 for individuals and $2,100 for a family. The maximum contribution for an HSA is the full amount of the deductible rather than the percentages allowed by MSAs. The maximum savings portion for a family in 2006 was $5,450, with an individual contribution up to $2,700, both indexed for inflation. Catch-up provisions are available for those older than 55 years. Assuming all conditions established by the IRS are met, contributions to the HSA are tax deductible (as an adjustment that will reduce gross income on page one of Form 1040). Limitations for eligible individuals with family coverage include a maximum monthly contribution of 1/12 of the lesser of the annual deductible of the high-deductible plan. The maximum monthly contribution for eligible individuals with self-only coverage is 1/12 of the lesser of the annual deductible of the high-deductible plan. Contributions for a year may be made until the tax return due date (without extensions). Distributions from the account used to pay qualified medical expenses are not taxable, but other distributions are taxable and subject to a 10% penalty tax. The activity of an HSA is reported by a trustee. Contributions to the plan are reported on IRS Forms 5498-SA, and distributions from the plan are reported on IRS Form 1099-SA. HSAs are administered by actuarial firms and insurance companies. Amounts in HSAs not distributed by the end of the year may be rolled over into the next year.

HEAVY MARKET: A falling market due to a large supply of offers to sell, rather than to buy, the relevant securities.

HEDGE: A security that has offsetting qualities or the attempt to "hedge" against inflation by the purchase of securities whose values should respond to inflationary developments. Securities having these qualities are "inflation hedges." Purchase of a call option may be used as a hedge on a short sale.

HEDGE FUND: A mutual fund or investment company that, as a regular policy, "hedges" its market commitments. It does this by holding securities it believes are likely to increase in value and at the same time is "short" other securities it believes are likely to decrease in value. The sole objective is capital appreciation. This type of fund is highly aggressive.

HEDGE FUND TYPES: Reflect different investment styles, product lines, and geographic regions, such as:

- Bond Arbitrage
- Convertible Securities

- Currencies and Major Foreign Markets
- Emerging Markets
- Equities
- Macro or Mixed Products and Strategies
- Mortgage Backed Securities
- Stocks and Bonds

HEDGING: Offsetting investment risk by using a security that is expected to move in the opposite direction. Options and short selling are commonly used to hedge stock positions.

HEDGING PARADOX: Favorable basis movements that do not guarantee a favorable global result for a hedge. It occurs when the basis behavior is unfavorable yet the hedge is still beneficial.

HEIR: One who inherits a portion, or all of an estate, by being named in a will or a direct line of the decedent.

HELPPIE, RICHARD D.: Former Chief Executive Officer, financier, economist and Founder of the Superior Consultant Company, Inc (SUPC-NASD). He is currently a health care financial futurist and was former Managing Director of Affiliated Computer Services, Inc. (NYSE:ACS), a premier provider of diversified business process and information technology outsourcing solutions to commercial and government health care clients worldwide.

HERFINDAHL-HIRSCHMAN INDEX (HHI): A measure of industry competitiveness. It is the sum of the squared market share of individual health care companies.

HERZLINGER, REGINA E., PhD: A Manhattan Institute Center for Medical Progress Senior Fellow who writes on health care economics issues. She is a Nancy R. McPherson Professor of Business Administration Chair and the first woman to be tenured and chaired at Harvard Business School. She is widely recognized for innovative research and early predictions of the demise of managed care, and coined the terms "consumer-driven health care" and "health-care-focused factories" in the belief that a managed care economic backlash is giving control back to physicians, patients, and medical providers.

HETEROSKEDASTICITY/HETEROSCEDASTICITY: Condition where residual variance is not constant; as in cross-sectional analyses. It also occurs in various consumer, income, risk, and size of firm studies.

HICKS-KALDOR CRITERION: A cost-benefit analysis economic support model for public projects, such as hospitals. It is positive when total gains from the project exceed total losses.

HIDDEN LOAD: A stockbroker's sales commission not immediately visible (transparent) to an investor; such as with municipal hospital revenue bonds; a built-in commission charge.

HIERARCHY: The order or rank of codes, for medical reimbursement.

HIGH: The most value a security achieved in a given period.

HIGH FLYER: Speculative and high priced security that has recently jumped in price.

HIGH YIELD BONDS: Bonds issued by U.S. corporations that carry less than investment-grade ratings, which are referred to as junk bonds. For purposes of high-yield bonds, below investment grade means Ba or lower by Moody's and BB or lower by Standard & Poor's. The market for high-yield bonds is large. A high-yield security compensates the bondholder for the added risk by offering a higher coupon than could be obtained from investment-grade corporate bonds. Several types of bonds fall within the high-yield sector, including zero coupons, split coupon, increasing rate, floating rate, pay-in-kind, first mortgage, and equipment trust certificates. These are structured just like other bonds bearing the same name. The only difference is the investment quality of the corporation issuing the debt. Because of the higher coupon, there is a potential for higher total returns to the bondholder. Because of their inherent risk, these bonds are an alternative for more aggressive fixed-income investors. They may also be attractive to equity investors who are willing to assume the risk of the lower investment quality. Such investors recognize that as the underlying credit quality of the issuer improves, the value of its bonds should increase as well.

HIGH YIELD SECURITY: Noninvestment grade debt security that is offering a high rate of return due to its grave risk. These are often referred to as junk bonds.

HIGHLY CONFIDENT LETTER: Investment banking letter of intimidation suggesting certainty in the ability to arrange financing (junk bond debt) for a securities deal (usually a hostile takeover) or leveraged buy-out (LBO).

HILL, EDWARD, MD: Past President of the American Medical Association in Chicago, Illinois.

HILL BURTON ACT: 1946 Federal legislation that provides subsidies of indigent and charity medical care, especially in rural areas and related and hospital projects.

HIPAA (HEALTH INSURANCE PORTABILITY AND ACCOUNTABILITY ACT OF 1996): Also known as the Kennedy-Kassebaum Act, HIPAA is federal legislation that mandates the electronic (1) connectivity, (2) transmission, (3) storage/retrieval, and (4) confidentiality of all health care information. The shift to Electronic Data Interchange (EDI) has been planned by the federal government and the Health Care Financing Administration for more than a decade. Its goal is to reduce the 17% administrative cost of health care through the standardization of electronic transactions into a single format, replacing the 400-plus disparate platforms currently used. Implementation of the EDI was scheduled for 2006. For purposes of HIPAA, the definition of a covered entity includes three classes:

- Individual health care providers, pharmacies, hospitals, skilled nursing facilities (SNFs), and home health care agencies.
- Medicare, Medicaid, insurance companies, HMOs, MCOs, and other health plans.
- Health care vendors, clearinghouses, billing firms, internet service providers (ISPs), Web servers and hosting companies, as well as computer software and hardware companies and other third-party vendors facilitating EDI.

Although nonpunitive in nature, civil penalties may be as high as $100 per violation, with a cap of $25,000 per year. Criminal penalties include fines of up to $250,000 and/or imprisonment for up to 10 years.

HIPPA COSTS: Expenses and charges required of covered entities (CEs) to implement, comply and maintain the regulations of HIPAA privacy and transmission rules, as described below:

- Privacy Official Costs: Requires a designated privacy official responsible for the development and implementation of privacy policies and procedures. The cost of this function is the personnel-hours to train and develop detailed policies and procedures, as well as the oversight management between departments, evaluating procedures and assuring compliance. Depending on the size of the hospital, clinic, medical office, or covered entity, and the diversity of activities involving privacy issues, staff involved with privacy related issues need to devote significant economic resources to ensure compliance with this effort.
- Internal Complaints Costs: Requires each covered entity, clinic, or hospital to have an internal process to allow an individual to file a complaint concerning the covered entity's compliance with its privacy policies and procedures. This requires CEs to designate a contact person who is responsible for receiving and documenting the complaint as well as the disposition.
- Disclosure Tracking and History Costs: Requires CEs and providers to be able to produce a record of all disclosures of protected health information, except for such items as treatment, payment, health care operations, or disclosures to individuals. This requires a note in the electronic or manual record of when, to whom, and what information was disclosed, as well as the purpose of the disclosure. It was estimated that 15% of all

patient records would have annual disclosures and that most hospitals already track patient disclosures. However, it required many hospitals and CEs to update their software systems to assure full compliance.

- De-identification of Certain Information Costs: Requires CEs to assess what information is needed to be de-identified, such as information related to driver's license numbers, specific age, and research data. This requires hospitals to review and modify existing agreements and/or reprogram automated systems to remove key information that needs to be excluded.

- Policy and Procedures Development Costs: Requires CEs to develop policies and procedures to establish and maintain compliance with the regulation, such as copying medical records or amending records. Depending on the number of existing policies and procedures previously written and the size of the organization (i.e., multihospital systems or university settings), fees are paid to outside consultants to assist in developing tailored or customized policies and procedures for internal operations may be considerable.

- Training Costs: Requires each CE to develop training programs for its staff based on the size of the facility, number of staff, types of operations, worker turnover, and in general the experience of the work force.

- Notice Costs: Requires hospitals and CEs to provide a notice at each admission, regardless of how many visits an individual had to the hospital in a given year. The initial cost is training the staff and the ongoing cost related to printing the notices.

- Consent Costs: Requires all hospitals and CEs to obtain an individual's consent for use or disclosure of protected health information for treatment, payment, or health care operations. Because most hospitals and CEs have already been obtaining consents from patients therefore, the only additional cost is in changing document language to conform to the rules.

- Business Associates Costs: Requires all CEs to obtain a written contract or arrangement that documents satisfactory assurance that business associates will appropriately safeguard protected health information in order to disclose it to a business associate, based on such an arrangement. An example of a business associate would be a hospital contract with a billing firm. Depending on the size of the hospital or CE, more extensive relationships and agreements might be affected.

- Inspection and Copying Costs: A significant cost to all hospitals and CEs as the degree of inspection and copying of medical records is not expected to change in the future. Most states have given patients rights (in varying degrees) to access medical information. The primary cost to the CEs is to develop the procedures identifying what information

is accessible and who has the right to request that information and the affiliated copying costs.
- Law Enforcement and Judicial and Administrative Proceedings Costs: Allows disclosure of protected health information without patient authorization under four circumstances: (1) Legal process or required by law; (2) To locate or identify a suspect, fugitive, material witness, or missing person; (3) Conditions related to a victim of crime; and (4) Protected health information that may be related to a crime committed on its premises.

HIRSCH, GIGI, MD: Former psychiatrist, emergency room physician, internist, health care economist and Harvard Medical School faculty member who founded MD IntelliNet, LLC (MDI), a provider of exclusive access to carefully selected service partners with special expertise and commitment to the unique economic career challenges of physicians.

HISTORIC COST: FASB rule requiring financial statements to list assets at original or acquisition cost; original cost of an asset to an entity.

HISTORIC VOLATILITY: A statistical measurement of securities price variability over some defined time frame such as 10, 20 30, 50, 60, 75, or 90 days.

HIT: Slang term for an impending significant business development with a major negative impact on the current market value of related securities.

HOGAN, JOHN: President and CEO of GE Medical Systems in Waukesha, Wisconsin.

HO-LEE OPTION MODEL: Arbitrage Free Model (AFM) that uses an estimated spot curve to evaluate embedded options in credit or fixed income securities.

HOLD: An opinion to neither buy nor sell a particular security.

HOLDBACK: An amount, usually a set fee or percentage of billed medical service charges, kept by the preferred provider organization or third-party administrator to cover losses.

HOLDER: The (long) owner of a security.

HOLDER OF RECORD: Securities owner listed in the issuing company's corporate records.

HOLDING COMPANY: A corporation designed to hold the stock of other companies.

HOLDING PERIOD: The length of time an asset or investment is held by its owner.

HOLDING PERIOD RETURN: Total investment return for a specific time period, divided by investment cost.

HOLDING STREET NAME: A securities account, held by a broker-dealer (nominal owner), on behalf of the owner customer (beneficial owner).

HOLE: Medicare Part D (2006) basic plan that requires patients pay all medications costs from $2,251–$5,100 resulting in a "hole" or coverage gap. After medication costs exceed $5,100, patients pay about 5% of the remainder (indexed annually); slang term.

HOLMER, ALAN: President and CEO of Pharmaceutical Research and Manufacturers of America in Washington, D.C.

HOME EQUITY LINE OF CREDIT: A line of credit allowing borrowed funds at the time and in the amount of choice up to a maximum credit limit qualified. Repayment is secured by the home or business equity. Simple interest (interest-only payments on the outstanding balance) is usually tax-deductible. Often used for improvements, major purchases or expenses, and debt consolidation.

HOME EQUITY LOAN: Fixed or adjustable rate loan obtained for a variety of purposes, secured by home equity. Interest paid is usually tax-deductible. It is often used for home improvement or freeing-up of equity for investment in other real estate or investments. Recommended by many to replace or substitute for consumer loans whose interest is not tax-deductible, such as auto or boat loans, credit card debt, medical debt, and education.

HOME RUN: Slang term for a short-term but very large investment gain.

HOMOSKEDASTICITY: Condition where residual variance is constant.

HORIZONTAL ANALYSIS: The percentage change of a line item financial statement value for a given time period.

HORIZONTAL MERGER: Occurs when competing health care sellers in the same market combine to form a single large business enterprise.

HORIZONTAL SPREAD: Differential composed of two puts or two calls on the same underlying instrument. It is horizontal because both options have the same strike or exercise price but two different expiration dates. Generally, the trade is placed with the nearby option sold and the deferred option purchased, as an attempt to capitalize on the acceleration in time value decay for the nearby relative to the deferred contract month.

HOSPITAL AUDIT COMPANIES: Retrospective medical audit providers that typically achieve a 15–20% savings of billed health care claims.

HOSPITAL-BASED PHYSICIAN: The term *hospitalist* for a hospital-based physician was coined in 1996 by Dr. Robert M. Wachter of the University of California at San Francisco. It denotes a specialist in inpatient medicine. Inpatient care in this country used to be provided to hospitalized patients by their primary care or admitting physician. Although this model has the advantage of continuity, and perhaps personalization, it often suffered because of the physician's limited knowledge base and unfamiliarity with the available internal and external resources of the hospital. Furthermore, the limited time the physician spent with individual patients prevented the physician from becoming the quality leader in this setting. These shortcomings have led hundreds of hospitals around the country to turn to hospitalists as dedicated inpatient specialists. At the center of a hospitalist-based medical group is the concept of low cost and comprehensive, broad-based care in the hospital, hospice, or extended care setting. The benefits of a well-designed hospitalist program far outweigh the patient inefficiencies that such a program entails. The National Association of Inpatient Physicians (NAIP) estimates that there are approximately 3,000 hospitalists in the United States. It is estimated that the number could increase tenfold in a couple of years if the hospitalist program were fully adopted.

HOSPITAL CAPITATION: Prospective and fixed payment system for hospitals and inpatient facilities, on a per member basis, for a given number of patients and by contract.

HOSPITAL DAY: A term to describe any 24 hour period commencing at 12:00 A.M., or 12:00 P.M., whichever is used by a hospital to determine a hospital day, during which a patient receives hospital services at the hospital.

HOSPITAL DAYS (PER 1,000): A measurement of the number of days of hospital care HMO members use in a year. It is calculated as follows: Total number of days spent in a hospital by members divided by total members. This information is available through Department of Health and Human Services (DHHS), Office of Health Maintenance Organizations (OHMO), and a variety of other sources.

HOSPITAL DRG RISK POOL: Hospital standardized risk pool with various other arrangements based on diagnostic-related group schedules and with bonus distributions for cost savings.

HOSPITAL EXPENSE INSURANCE: Basic medical expense insurance that provides benefits subject to a specified daily maximum for hospital room and board charges, plus lab, ambulance, and operating room costs. Also referred to as hospitalization insurance or basic hospital insurance.

HOSPITAL INCREMENTAL COST OF CARE: The expenses above fixed costs that need to be financially recovered by a facility, in relation to actual services rendered and supplies used as patients are treated. *See also* hospital DRG risk pool.

HOSPITAL INCOME INSURANCE: A form of insurance that provides a stated weekly or monthly payment while the insured is hospitalized, regardless of expenses incurred and regardless of whether or not other insurance is in force. The insured can use the weekly or monthly benefit as he chooses, for hospital or other expenses.

HOSPITAL INFLATION INDEX: Nominal hospital expenditures per inpatient divided by real hospital expenditures per patient.

HOSPITAL RISK POOL: Any monetary set-aside to provide bonuses or economic incentives from hospital or health facility care savings. *See also* hospital variable cost-risk pool.

HOSPITAL SUBCAPITATION: A secondary and subordinate prospective fixed payment method used by hospitals, for a contracted package of inpatient services, usually paid monthly as a global responsibility of the primary care medical provider and with bonus incentives for cost efficient care. It is an alternate system to per diem hospital payments.

HOSPITAL VARIABLE COST-RISK POOL: Financial risk-sharing arrangement between medical groups and hospitals with an economic incentive for reducing utilization and cost efficient care; usually fixed-costs are covered and followed by variable-cost coverage in contracted agreements with break-even analysis, budget pro forma projections, actuarial variance estimations, and so forth.

HOSTILE: The unsolicited bid by an acquiring company. It may be either accepted or rejected by the target company.

HOSTILE TAKEOVER: Corporate shareholder transfer (takeover) against the wishes of management and directors, and usually financed by debt, such as junk bonds (low investment grade debt), and as in a leveraged buy-out (LBO) situation.

HOT ISSUE: A security that is expected to trade in the aftermarket at a premium over the public offering price.

HOT STOCK: Stolen illegal stock "ownership."

HR 10 PLAN: A Keogh plan.

HUMAN CAPITAL INVESTMENT: Any action taken to improve the production efficiency of human labor; doctors and nurses, and so forth.

HUMAN HEALTH CARE CAPITAL: The skills, conscientious industry, and qualifications of cognitive workers such as doctors, nurses, and medical technicians.

HUMAN RESOURCE COST: Typical labor charges or expenses as indicated below:

- Idle Time Labor Costs: represents the cost of an office employee (direct office labor) who is unable to perform his or her assignments due to power failures, slack time, and the like.
- Overtime Premium Costs: the overtime premium paid to all health care office workers (direct and indirect labor) is considered part of the general office overhead.
- Fringe Benefit Costs: are typically made up of employment-related costs paid by the office. These costs may be handled in two different ways: as indirect labor added to general overhead costs or as fringe benefits added to direct labor costs.

HUMPED: A yield curve that exhibits a "bump-rise" in its middle and would have a concave appearance.

HUNG UP: A large drop in securities prices to below their purchase value with the potential for real loss.

HUNKER DOWN: Slang term for the attempt to sell a large number of securities, or large block position, by a stockbroker (work hard to make a sale).

HUNTER, DAVID: CEO of Hunter Group in St. Petersburg, Florida.

HURDLE RATE: The cost of capital or interest rate.

HYBRID: A security with mixed debt-equity characteristics, such as a convertible bond with a coupon that pays interest and behaves like a credit instrument, even as it has a conversion feature that gives it equity characteristics.

HYBRID COST: Expenses with both fixed and variable components. *See also* mixed cost.

HYBRID PENSION PLAN: A pension plan that has features of both a defined contribution plan and a defined benefit plan:

- Money purchase plan: A plan in which an employer agrees to contribute a specified amount to the plan on behalf of each employee. The amount available at any time is determined by the contributions and how well the investments perform.
- Target benefit plan: A plan in which an employer agrees to contribute a specified amount to the plan. This plan features a formula that sets up a target benefit for each employee. The target benefit plan is meant to be similar to a defined benefit plan, but without the actual guarantee of the final benefit. The final benefit ultimately is determined by how well the investments perform.

HYBRID PER DIEM: Health care reimbursement arrangement system that combines multiple service lines such as surgery, obstetrics, emergency room, radiology, pathology and GI, and so forth, and averages their payments together into an estimated blended rate, per day, for general pricing purposes.

HYBRIDIZATION: The creation of a new financial instrument that has two or more credit, equity, currency, or commodity characteristics.

HYPERBOLIC DISCOUNTING: Accounting model for the differences in patient preferences over health care consumption now, versus consumption in the future.

HYPERINFLATION: A very high rate of inflation sustained for at least a single year.

HYPOTHECATION AGREEMENT: A document giving a stockbroker the right to pledge securities to a bank in order to provide funds for lending (margin-credit) capacity.

HYSTERESIS, PHYSICIAN LABOR: A hypothesized property of physician unemployment rates that suggest there is a ratcheting effect, so a short-term rise in medical unemployment rates tends to linger.

I

I-BONDS: Inflation indexed (variable interest rate) U.S. savings bonds. They are purchased for face value but accumulate interest calculated monthly and compounded semiannually for 30 years. Series I-bonds are issued only in registered form and are not transferable. The bonds may be either in book-entry or definitive form.

IBNR CALCULATION METHODS: The three IRS accepted methods for estimating IBNRs are:

- Actuarial Data Analysis: IBNRs are calculated with demographic data, insurance reports, statistical and risk dampening stochastic probabilities, utilization data, and past payment claims data to estimate IBNRs. This costly method is most appropriate for newer organizations without a significant claims history.
- Historic Cost Analysis: This method of estimation is most appropriate for established organizations, and is based on the actual number of past claims on a per/member, per/month basis.
- Open Referral Analysis: This method estimates the cost of all open referral authorizations on file (in and out of network). Essentially, it assumes a traditional open referral accounting structure in a restricted gatekeeper controlled environment. Then, the average cost per medical service segment is estimated and multiplied against the average cost per segment. In this manner, cost estimates are matched with medical service segments over time, and IBNR claims are mitigated.

IDENTIFIABLE PROBLEM: Inability to distinguish between two economic relationships with similar variables (i.e., health care supply and demand).

IGNAGNI, KAREN: President and CEO of the American Association of Health Plans in Washington, D.C.

ILLEGAL DIVIDEND: Corporate stock dividend declared in violation of state law or its charter.

ILLIQUID: A dearth of cash flow to meet current obligations and/or maturing debt.

***i*MBA INDEX©:** Ratio of health care service costs paid by consumers (coinsurance) compared to amounts paid by health insurance and managed care plans. It is the average aggregate affordability ratio currently undergoing economic compression (see Figure 2).

IMMEDIATE ANNUITY: An insurance contract that begins payouts to the owner (annuitant) immediately.

IMMEDIATE OR CANCEL (IOC) ORDER: A purchase order for securities that requires immediate execution at a specified price of all or part of a specified

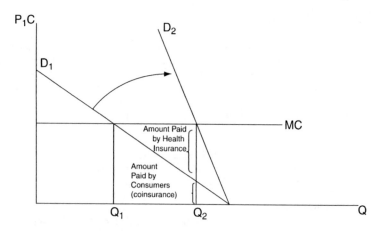

Figure 2: Health Care Services.

amount of stock, with the unexecuted portion required to be canceled by the broker.

IMMEDIATE WRITE-OFF: Fixed asset cost recognition in the period acquired.

IMMELT, JEFFERY: Chairman and CEO of General Electric Co., in Fairfield, Connecticut. He is the former president and CEO of GE Medical Systems in Waukesha, Wisconsin.

IMPAIRED CAPITAL: Situation when health or other insurance company liabilities and claims consume a company's surplus and the capital is impaired. Suspension of the right to do business ultimately follows.

IMPAIRED CREDIT: A reduction in the credit rating of a health care or other organization that increases the cost of capital.

IMPERFECT COMPETITION: Occurs when more than one seller competes for sales with other sellers of competitive health care products or services, each of whom has some price control.

IMPLICIT COST: The cost of nonpurchased inputs, imputed at cash value.

IMPLICIT OPTION: An embedded option.

IMPLICIT RENT: Money that a health care firm pays itself for the use of its durable inputs.

IMPLIED PRICE: Securities price computed by a model that considers a comparable benchmark, volatility, and spread adjustment and is used in the absence of a current market price.

IMPLIED REPO RATE: Reposition repurchase rate influenced by the cost of funds, tax rates, deductibility of carry-charges, yields, the time to expiration and organizational constraints. It indicates the implied rate of return for specified repurchase investments.

IMPLIED VOLATILITY: Current volatility required to generate an option premium given a known market price, an interest rate, an expiration date, and a strike price.

IMPOUND ACCOUNT: An escrow account.

IMPREST SYSTEM: Method to maintain a constant balance petty cash account.

IMPROPER ACCUMULATION: The retained earnings of a health care or other entity done to help stockholders avoid personal income taxation.

IMPUTED COST: Opportunity cost that does not require an actual expenditure of cash.

IMPUTED INTEREST: Rate or amount of interest considered to have been paid, although not actually paid.

IMPUTED VALUE: Logical or common sense value that is not recorded or determined mathematically.

INACTIVE ACCOUNT: Any account that has not had any transactions for an extended period of time.

INCENTIVE: Economic and financial motivators to health care entities and medical providers to deliver cost-effective and appropriate care.

INCENTIVE FEE: Additional commission to sell an inferior financial product or security.

INCENTIVE STOCK OPTION: A hospital or other employee benefit plan that allows certain employees the right to purchase employer securities at a favorable price once they have increased in value subsequent to the date the options were granted. Exercising options under an ISO does not result in current income tax consequences to the employee.

INCENTIVE STRUCTURE: Arrangements to induce the health care labor force into certain actions.

INCOME: Money derived from a health care business entity, before taxation.

INCOME ADJUSTMENT BONDS: Long-term debt obligations offered in which the interest will be paid by the corporation only when, as, and if earned.

INCOME APPROACH: Valuation method that converts future estimated financial and economic benefits into a current, single present-value amount.

INCOME BENEFICIARY: One who receives the income generated by a trust fund's principal.

INCOME BOND: A debt that pays interest only if earned.

INCOME EARNING ABILITY: The ability of an individual to earn an income or wage. The three major threats to income earning ability are death, disability, and old age, all of which may be protected against by life and health insurance.

INCOME EFFECT: The change in consumption of health care products or services, *only* as a result of variation in the purchasing power of money funds induced by a price change. Also referred to as a health care substitution effect.

INCOME ELASTICITY: Synonymous with health care consumption, income elasticity = (I / C) * (dC / dI), where I = patient income and C = patient consumption (see Table 3).

INCOME ELASTICITY OF DEMAND: A patient-consumer or purchase-sensitivity measurement that is compared to each 1% change in income.

INCOME FROM INVESTMENTS: Unrestricted income, gains, and dividends from sales of investments.

INCOME FROM OPERATIONS: Accounting difference between revenues and expenses, or the net sales of a health care or other entity.

INCOME FUND: An investment company (mutual fund) that stresses higher than average current income distributions.

INCOME, GROSS: Before-tax earnings.

INCOME IN RESPECT OF DECEDENT: Amounts due and payable to a decedent at his or her death because of some right to income. [IRC §691(c)(2)]

INCOME INVESTMENT COMPANY: An income-producing mutual fund (investment) company.

INCOME LOSS FROM HEALTH CARE OPERATIONS: Gross patient service revenue plus other operating revenues, minus deductions from revenue and total health care expenses.

INCOME STATEMENT: One of four major types of financial statements used by businesses. It is primarily a flow report that lists a company's income or revenues and its expenses for a certain period of time in order to summarize a company's financial operations.

INCOME STOCK: Stock purchased for its income and dividend producing ability rather than its growth potential.

Table 3: Income Elasticity of Selected Health Services

Services	Income Elasticity
All health care expenditures	.25–1.2
Hospital services	.02–.04
Dental services	.61–3.20
Physician services	.01–.85
Nursing home	.60–.90

Compiled Source: Foland, Goodman & Stano. (2001). *The economics of health and health care.* New York: Prentice-Hall.

INCOME TAX: A local, state, or federal surcharge imposed on personal or corporate income.

INCOME TAX BASIS: (1) A concept to determine the proper amount of gain to report when an asset is sold. It is generally the cost paid for an asset plus the amounts paid to improve the asset less deductions taken against the asset, such as depreciation. (2) Consistent accounting that uses income tax accounting rules while GAAP does not.

INCORPORATION: State charter that allows a health care organization or other business and its owners to operate as a company.

INCREASE IN DEMAND: Augmentation of the quantity demanded of a health care good or service at every price level.

INCREASE IN SUPPLY: Augmentation of the quantity supplied of a health care good or service at every price level.

INCREASING COST INDUSTRY: A space where the price of at least some inputs increases as a direct result of the expansion of the industry, such as health care, due to aging demographics.

INCREASING MARGINAL RETURNS: Marginal product or service of the last health care worker hired, which exceeds the marginal product or health care service of the second last worker hired.

INCREASING RATE BOND: Debt whose coupon interest rate rises over time.

INCREASING RETURN: Increase in the marginal product of a health care or other resource input as additional units are used.

INCREASING RETURNS TO SCALE: The percentage increase in a health care firm's output, when it exceeds a percentage increase in its inputs. *See also* economies of scale.

INCREMENTAL ANALYSIS: Business decision-making tool that focuses on adoptable altered items.

INCREMENTAL CASH FLOW: The marginal cash flow differences between projects.

INCREMENTAL COST: Incurred cost if an additional activity is undertaken.

INCREMENTAL COST OF CAPITAL: The average cost of supplemental capital raised in a given year.

INCURRED: The exact date and time when medical services are rendered to a patient.

INCURRED BUT NOT REPORTED (IBNR): Refers to health care claims that reflect services already delivered, but, not yet reimbursed, reported, or captured as a liability by the insurance company. These are bills "in the pipeline" and a crucial concept for proactive (prospective) medical providers who explore arrangements that put them in the role of adjudicating claims and operating in a subcapitated payment system. Failure to account for these potential claims may lead to bad financial decisions because of liability underestimation. Good health administrative operations have fairly sophisticated mathematical models to estimate this amount at any given time.

INCURRED CLAIM: A situation where insurance premium payment may be demanded under the provisions of the policy, or all claims with dates of service within a specified period.

INCURRED CLAIMS COST: For an IBNR initiative, if the net present value of an IBNR claim is greater than zero, the claims initiative will make money. If it is less than zero, it will not. NPV calculation for IBNR claim costs inputs include:

- Investment costs: money expended for the IBNR initiative at the beginning.
- IBNR claims costs: potential revenues accrued as a result of the initiative over a period. This can be one time or recurring revenue.
- Accrual costs: built as a result of the initiative over a period. This can be one time or a recurring item.
- Discount rate cost: the actuary, accountant, or finance department reduction rate.
- Time period costs: the time interval to compute the NPV of IBNR claims.

INCURRED CLAIMS LOSS RATIO: Incurred claims divided by premiums. Medical expenses not yet paid by a managed care or health insurance company. It is a type of medical loss ratio.

INCURRED CLAIMS NPV: The cumulative differential between the potential IBNR revenue and cost streams discounted at the discounted rate minus the investment:

$$NPV = \Sigma \, ((R_t - C_t) / (1 + r)^t) - I$$
$$t = 1$$

Given: where t represents time, n represents the number of time periods, R is revenue impacts, C is cost impacts, r is the discount rate, and I is the IBNR Investment.

INCURRED EXPENSES: Health care service or other expenses paid or to be paid.

INCURRED LOSS: Managed care or health insurance losses occurring within a fixed period, whether or not adjusted and paid during the same period. Obtained by adding to losses paid during a given year those losses still outstanding at the end-of-the-year, less losses outstanding at the beginning of the year.

INCURRED LOSS RATIO: The ratio, fraction, or percentage of losses incurred, relative to premiums earned. Relationship of incurred losses to health insurance premiums, experienced by the insuring entity.

INDEFEASABLE TITLE: Ownership that can not be declared void.

INDEMNIFY: To financially compensate for loss or damages. To make economically whole again.

INDEMNITY: Latin term for unhurt *(indemnis)*. Indemnity health insurance renders a patient economically unhurt by a random accident or illness.

INDEMNITY PLAN: Traditional fee-for-service health insurance.

INDENTURE: A written agreement between issuer and creditors by which the terms of a debt issue are set forth, such as rate of interest, means of payment, maturity date, terms of prior payment of principal, collateral, priorities of claims, trustee, and so forth.

INDEPENDENT GOODS: Health care or other products or services that have no relationship between price and demand.

INDEPENDENT STANDARDS BOARD (ISB): A private standard-setting body governing the independence of auditors from their public company clients.

INDEPENDENT VARIABLE: Data point that induces a change in some other dependent point.

INDEX: A statistical measure of change in the health care or general economy. In the case of financial markets it is essentially an imaginary portfolio of securities representing a particular market or a portion of it. Each index has its own calculation methodology and is usually expressed in terms of a change from a base value. It is also a percentage upon which future interest rates for adjustable rate debts are based. Common indexes include the major bank Prime rate, the CMT (Constant Maturity Treasury, usually a 1-year term), COFI (Cost of Funds for the Eleventh District financial institutions), and the MTA or average rate of a 1 year Government Treasury Security.

INDEX FUND: The duplication of specific securities indices by a mutual fund. Index funds are designed to take advantage of the average long-term growth of the market segment tracked by the index rather than attempting to beat the market. The cost of managing an index fund is usually less than managing other types of funds that require more frequent trading. Popular indices are: S&P 500, S&P 100, EAFE, targeted average maturity dates, and various bond indices such as the Lehman Aggregate Bond Index.

INDEX MULTIPLIER: The amount specified in the option contract by which the in-the-money difference of the option is multiplied to arrive at the cash settlement upon exercise.

INDEX OPTION: An option whose underlying entity is an index. Generally index options are cash-settled.

INDEXING: Tying health care economics or financial amounts to some benchmark, such as the Consumer Price Index, Consumer Medical Price Index, or Producer Price Index.

INDICATED YIELD: Dividend or interest rate as a percentage of the current market price of a security.

INDICATION OF INTEREST (IOI): An expression of consideration by an underwriter's customers for investment in a new security expected to be offered soon, generated from the dissemination of a *Red Herring* prospectus. It is not a binding commitment on the customer or the underwriter.

INDIFFERENCE CURVE: An illustration of various health care markets, or other baskets of goods or services, that provides patients-consumers with similar utility.

INDIGENT: The state of having sparse or no income, savings, or assets to meet health care payment needs. *See also* insolvency.

INDIRECT BUSINESS TAX: Surcharges, such as general or excise taxes, imposed indirectly on a health care business entity rather than on its products, goods, and services.

INDIRECT COST: Health care cost not traced to specific patient or medical service. It is the opposite of a direct cost.

INDIRECT LABOR: Human cost difficult to trace to specific products or health care services.

INDIRECT MATERIAL: Material costs difficult to trace to a specific finished product, good, or service.

INDIRECT METHOD: Operating activities format for the Statement of Cash flows that commence with net income and demonstrate the reconciliation from net income to operating cash flows.

INDIVIDUAL HEALTH CARE DEMAND: The demand curve or demand schedule of a single patient.

INDIVIDUAL INCENTIVE: Bonus or additional payments to medical providers and facilities for providing cost efficient care. It may also be applied as patient incentives for a healthy lifestyle (regular exercise, no smoking, no drug use, body weight limits, etc.) in the form of insurance premium fee reductions.

INDIVIDUAL RATIONAL ALLOCATION: A health care economic allocation is personal if no patient is worse off in that allocation scheme than with his own endowment fund.

INDIVIDUAL RETIREMENT ACCOUNT (IRA): An arrangement that permits individuals to receive income tax deductions for limited amounts that are set aside for retirement savings (indexed):

- *Regular Deductible/Nondeductible IRA:* Are either deductible or nondeductible for individual income tax purposes. Earnings are tax deferred, meaning that taxes on earnings are paid at the time of withdrawal. An IRA that is not a Roth IRA or a SIMPLE IRA. Individual taxpayers are allowed to contribute 100% of compensation (self-employment income for sole doctors, proprietors, and partners) up to a specified maximum dollar amount to a traditional IRA. Contributions to a traditional IRA may be tax-deductible depending on income, tax-filing status, and coverage by an employer-sponsored retirement plan ($4,000 limit in 2006, with $5,000 over 50 catch-up provisions; indexed annually).

- *Roth IRA:* Amounts of contributions to Roth IRAs are nondeductible. Earnings on Roth IRAs are never taxable ($4,000 limit in 2006, with 5,000 over 50 catch-up provisions; indexed annually).
- *Educational IRA:* Are nondeductible, however, earnings are not taxable if withdrawn to pay qualified educational expenses. Anyone may contribute up to $500 per year to an Educational IRA for a child under age 18, provided the total contribution does not exceed $500 per year. The account must be designated as an Educational IRA from its inception. The annual contribution limit for a Coverdell Education Savings Account (ESA) is $2,000. The Modified Adjusted Gross Income qualification limits for the ESA phase out between $95,000 and $110,000 for individuals and between $190,000 and $220,000 for married couples filing jointly. Under the regulations enacted in 2002, a child may contribute to his/her own ESA, even if he/she does not have earned income.
- *Conduit IRA:* A rollover IRA consisting only of a single qualified plan that may be rolled into another qualified pension plan.
- *Inherited IRA:* An IRA of a deceased person.
- *Rollover IRA:* An IRA consisting of a qualified plan(s) that has been "rolled over" into it.
- *SIMPLE IRA:* $10,000 contribution limit for 2006, with $2,500 over 50 catch-up provisions. It is indexed annually, and an employee may elect to have up to 100% annual compensation deferred into the account. An employer must match contributions dollar-for-dollar, up to 3% of compensation. A separate Simple IRA is also available to a spouse or family member if they have received at least $5,000 in compensation during any 2 years proceeding the current calendar year and are reasonably expected to earn at least $5,000 during the current calendar year.
- *SEP IRA:* For self-employed doctors, medical professionals, or other individuals. Indexed annually, a SEP IRA owner may contribute up to 25% of compensation, as much as $42,000 for 2005 ($44,000 for 2006). However, the maximum compensation upon which SEP contributions can be based is $210,000 ($220,000 for 2006). The term "compensation" for self-employed physicians, medical professionals, and individuals refers to earned income. A spouse and children may participate in the plan and open their own SEP IRAs as long as they are employees of the company.

- *Spousal IRA:* Allows a married person to make a self-directed IRA contribution for his/her spouse. A couple can contribute up to 100% of combined earned income or $8,000 whichever is less, for tax year 2006 (plus an extra $500 per person under the "catch-up" provision, if both individuals are age 50+, bringing the total to $9,000). Children can also have an IRA account if they have income.

INDIVIDUAL SPECIALIST CAPITATION: Fixed payments to medical specialists that are often economically problematic due to geographic undesirability, economies of scale, availability, flexibility, and contract size.

INDUCED CONSUMPTION: Annual health care purchases that respond to a change in disposable income, currently as seen with lifestyle drug use.

INDUSTRIAL DEVELOPMENT BOND: In general, securities issued by a state, a local government, or development agency to finance the construction or purchase of industrial, commercial, or manufacturing facilities to be purchased by or leased to a private user. IDBs are backed by the credit of the private user and generally are not considered liabilities of the governmental issuer (although in some jurisdictions they may also be backed by an issuer with taxing power). Hospitals usually float revenue bonds.

INEFFICIENT MARKETS: Securities or commodities that do not reflect the risk-return relationship, allowing for profit or loss.

INEFFICIENT PORTFOLIO: A securities portfolio that does not maximize the risk-return relationship.

INELASTIC: Economic concept of the inability to quickly adjust supply or demand despite changes in market conditions.

INELASTIC DEMAND: Occurs when the price elasticity of demand for health care or other services is equal to, or greater than zero but less than one (1).

INELASTIC SUPPLY: Occurs when the price elasticity of supply for health care or other services is equal to, or greater than zero but less than one (1).

INFERIOR GOOD: A health care product or service whose demand decreases when income increases.

INFLATION: A persistent upward movement in the general price level of health care or other goods and services, which results in a decline in the purchasing power of money.

INFLATION FACTOR: A premium load to provide for future increases in medical costs and loss payments resulting from inflation. A loading to provide for future increases resulting from inflation in medical costs and loss payments.

INFLATION RISK: The uncertainty over the future value (FV) of money or an investment asset. Lost purchasing power risk.

INHERITANCE: Property acquired through laws of descent and distribution from a person who dies without leaving a will. The value of property inherited is excluded from a taxpayer's gross income, but if the property inherited produces income it is included in gross income. A taxpayer's basis in inherited property is the fair market value at the time of death.

INHERITANCE TAX: A tax on property received from someone who has died. An inheritance tax is owed by the recipient, as a legal matter, but is usually paid by the estate. Most states levy inheritance taxes.

INITIAL COVERAGE: The first company following and reporting of a particular security by a financial analyst(s).

INITIAL MARGIN: Amount of funds and/or securities required to establish a position.

INITIAL PUBLIC OFFERING (IPO): A corporation's first offering of stock to the public, "going public."

INJUNCTION: A legal prohibition against certain actions.

INNOVATION: The first commercial applicability of a health care or other product, invention, test, new technology, and so forth.

INPUTS: The land, instruments, vehicles, labor, cognitive resources, and so forth, that are used and combined to produce health care goods, products, or services.

INQUIRY: Procedure of seeking information, both financial and nonfinancial, of knowledgeable persons throughout the company. It is used in an audit and often is complementary to performing other procedures. This procedure may range from formal written inquiries to informal oral inquiries.

INSIDE INFORMATION: Slang term referring to privileged information concerning a health care or other corporation.

INSIDE MARKET: The inside market is normally the highest bid and the lowest asked prices and is displayed on Level One (I) of NASDAQ.

INSIDER: Technically, an officer or director of a company or anyone owning 10% of a company's stock. The broader definition includes anyone with nonpublic information about a company. It is a slang term.

INSIDER TRADING: The act, in violation of SEC Rule 10b-5 and the Insiders Trading Act of 1988, of purchasing or selling securities (or derivative instruments based on those securities) based on information known to the party purchasing or selling the securities in his capacity as an insider (i.e., as an employee of the issuer of the securities) or as a result of information illicitly provided to him by an insider. Extensive case law exists concerning the varieties of acts that may be considered to be insider trading or the circumstances in which a person may be considered to be an insider or to be trading illegally on the basis of inside information.

INSOLVENCY: A legal determination occurring when a managed care plan no longer has the financial reserves or other arrangements to meet its contractual obligations to patients and subcontractors.

INSOLVENCY CLAUSE: A reinsurance clause that holds the reinsurer liable for its share of loss assumed under the treaty, even though the primary insurer is insolvent.

INSOLVENCY CONDITION: Mutual agreement between contracted parties such as HMOs and PPOs, to terminate health care, medical insurance payments, treatment facility care, and so forth, on the date of corporate inability to pay liabilities as a going-concern-entity. It is the coordination or transfer of health care agreement duties in order to maintain quality patient care at a time of fiscal inability.

INSOLVENT: Refers to a situation in which an entity's liabilities exceed the fair market value of its assets and/or that condition where the entity is not able to pay debts or service debt when due or on a timely basis.

INSTALLMENT: Partial or incomplete payment.

INSTALLMENT BASIS: Purchase or sale paid for fractionally over time.

INSTALLMENT DEBT: A debt or loan that is repaid in successive payments over a period of time.

INSTALLMENT METHOD: Accounting method of reporting gains on the sale of assets exchanged for a receivable. The gain is reported as a note is paid.

***INSTITUTE* OF MEDICAL BUSINESS ADVISORS©, INC. (*i*MBA):** The *Institute* of Medical Business Advisors, Inc., (www.MedicalBusinessAdvisors. com) is a leader in promoting and integrating personal financial planning and medical practice management principles through its online CERTI-FIED MEDICAL PLANNER© professional designation program (www. CertifiedMedicalPlanner.com). The CMP© marks provide a symbol of excellence for financial service professionals to validate their economic commitment and financial advisory expertise to medical providers and the health care industrial complex. *i*MBA, Inc., also offers a wide range of books, white papers, CD-ROMs, thought leadership essays, lectures, and adult learning opportunities and referral services that keep pace with rapid changes in the domestic health care administration space. Through its broad-based virtual structure and competitive research and development projects, *i*MBA, Inc., ensures that all stakeholders are represented in establishing an informed, ethical and meaningful voice with fiduciary accountability for the health industry

INSTITUTIONAL BROKER: Stockbroker who purchases and sells securities for institutions rather than individual investors.

INSTITUTIONAL INVESTORS: Banks, insurance companies, pensions, and mutual funds that buy and sell securities and other investments in large volumes.

INSTITUTIONAL SALES: Sales of securities to hospitals, banks, financial institutions, mutual funds, insurance companies, or other business organizations (institutional investors) that possess or control considerable assets for large scale investing.

INSTRUMENT: Contractual financial legal document with attached terms and conditions usually purchased as an investment for profit vehicle.

INSUBSTANTIAL RIGHTS: Right to use donated property that is retained by a donor when the retained rights do not interfere with the donee-charity's unrestricted use or full ownership of the donated property. [George v. U.S. 11/30/61, DC-MI]

INSURANCE RESERVES: The present value of future claims, minus the present value of future premiums. Reserves are balance sheet accounts set up to reflect actual and potential liabilities under outstanding insurance contracts. There are two main types of insurance reserves: premium reserves and loss (or claim) reserves.

INSURED BONDS: Bonds that are insured privately and guarantee the prompt payment of principal and interest. Generally, insured bonds have an AAA rating by Moody's.

INSURED MUNICIPAL BONDS: Municipal bonds that are insured against default to guarantee the prompt payment of principal and interest, which is usually tax exempt.

INTANGIBLE ASSET: A nonphysical business asset that grants certain rights and privileges (copyright, trade names, services marks, brand names, etc.) that have business enterprise economic value for owners. It is an asset without physical form, such as a patent, trademark, physician goodwill, or copyright. *See also* intellectual property.

INTELLECTUAL PROPERTY: Nonphysical assets such as copyrights, trademarks, and patents. Logos or special colors may also be intellectual properties for health care or other entities. *See also* intangible asset.

INTENSITY: A measure of health care or other resource used by an organization for operations.

INTENSIVE MARGIN: The degree to which a health care resource is utilized or applied to medical care, such as the work effort put in by a doctor or the number of hours a nurse might work.

INTEREST: The rent paid for borrowed money or received for loaned money. Ownership in property or business, and so forth. Standard computations are:

- Interest Compounded Annually: Amount = $(1 + \text{interest rate})*t$; where i is the interest rate and t is expressed decimally (0.05 for 5%). Also, t is the time and 0.5 refers to 1/2 of a year, 2 equals 2 years, and 7.75 equals 7 3/4 years.
- Interest Compounded Continuously: Amount = eit; where e is equal to 2.7183, i is the interest rate and t is expressed decimally (0.05 for 5%). Also, t is the time and 0.5 refers to 1/2 of a year, 2 equals 2 years, and 7.75 equals 7 3/4 years.
- Interest Discounted Annually (Present Value of Reversion): Amount = $(1 + \text{interest rate}) - t$ or, Amount = $1 / (1 + i) t$; where i is the interest rate and t is expressed decimally (0.05 for 5%). Also, t is the time and 0.5 refers to 1/2 of a year, 2 equals 2 years, and 7.75 equals 7 3/4 years.

- Interest Discounted Continuously: Amount = e-it; where e is equal to 2.7183, i is the interest rate and t is expressed decimally (0.05 for 5%). Also, t is the time and 0.5 refers to 1/2 of a year, 2 equals 2 years, and 7.75 equals 7 3/4 years.
- Interest Impact on Accumulation of 1 Per Period: Amount = [(1 + i) t − 1]/I; where i is the interest rate and t is expressed decimally (0.05 for 5%). Also, t is the time and 0.5 refers to 1/2 of a year, 2 equals 2 years, and 7.75 equals 7 3/4 years.
- Interest Impact on Installment to Amortize or Amortization: Amount = i / [1 − (1 / 1 + i) t]; where i is the interest rate and t is expressed decimally (0.05 for 5%). Also, t is the time and 0.5 refers to 1/2 of a year, 2 equals 2 years, and 7.75 equals 7 3/4 years.
- Interest Impact on Present Value of Ordinary Annuity of 1 Per Period: Amount = 1 − [1 / (1 + i) t] / i: where i is the interest rate and t is expressed decimally (0.05 for 5%). Also, t is the time and 0.5 refers to 1/2 of a year, 2 equals 2 years, and 7.75 equals 7 3/4 years.
- Interest Impact on Sinking Fund Factor: Amount = i / z (1 + i) t − 1; where i is the interest rate and t is expressed decimally (0.05 for 5%). Also, t is the time and 0.5 refers to 1/2 of a year, 2 equals 2 years, and 7.75 equals 7 3/4 years.

Such formulae are based on calculating values basis 1 unit of currency (U.S. Dollar [USD]). To adjust for other amounts such as $1,000, multiply the resulting factor by 1,000.

INTEREST ACCRUED: Interest earned but not yet payable.

INTEREST ADJUSTED COST METHOD: An insurance method of comparing the costs of similar policies by using an index that takes into account the time value of money due at different times through interest adjustments to the annual premiums, dividends, and cash value increases at an assumed interest rate.

INTEREST EXACT: The interest that is computed on the basis of 365 days of the year.

INTEREST FACTOR: One of three factors taken into consideration by an insurance company when calculating premium rates. This is an estimate of the overall average interest that will be earned by the insurer on invested premium payments.

INTEREST RATE: That percentage of a principal sum earned from investment or charged upon a loan.

INTEREST RATE RISK: Interest rate risk is the most important risk presented by bonds and long-term debt. As interest rates rise, the price of debt and bonds typically fall. As a result, the market value of a bond may be higher or lower at any point in time. However, an investor does not realize any gain or loss on a bond unless it is sold before maturity.

INTERFUND BORROWING: The borrowing of assets by a trust fund (OASI, DI, HI, or SMI) from another of the trust funds when one of the funds is in danger of exhaustion.

INTERMEDIARY: A third-party empowered to make financial, investment, business, managerial, economic, personal, or similar decisions for others.

INTERMEDIATE PRODUCTS: Health care goods and/or DME for resale by another company.

INTERMEDIATION: Place of money or assets with a third party.

INTERNAL AUDIT: A check of managerial financial control processes. It is performed within an entity by its staff rather than an independent certified public accountant.

INTERNAL CONTROL (IC): Process designed to provide reasonable assurance regarding achievement of various management objectives, such as the reliability of financial reports. It is a system which safeguards assets and accurate and reliable accounting records.

INTERNAL CONTROL OVER FINANCIAL REPORTING: A process designed to provide reasonable assurance regarding the reliability of financial reporting and the preparation of financial statements for external purposes in accordance with GAAP.

INTERNAL ECONOMICS OF HEALTH CARE: The reduction in the marketing and cost of a health care product or service that results from the increased output of the company.

INTERNAL RATE OF RETURN (IRR): Rate at which the net present value of an investment is zero. A percentage return on investment.

INTERNAL REVENUE CODE (IRC): The legislation that defines tax deductions and liabilities for tax payers in the United States. It is a collection of tax rules of the federal government, and Title 26 of the United States Code.

INTERNAL REVENUE SERVICE (IRS): Federal agency that administers the IRC. It is part of the U.S. Treasury Department.

INTERNALIZATION OF EXTERNALITIES: Occurs when the marginal cost or benefit of a health care or other product or service is adjusted so that market sales results in efficient output.

INTERNATIONAL ACCOUNTING STANDARDS COMMITTEE (IASC): Independent private sector formed in 1973, with the objective of harmonizing the accounting principles used in medical organizations and other businesses for financial reporting around the world.

INTERNATIONAL CLASSIFICATION OF DISEASES, NINTH EDITION: Numeric (usually) codes used for statistical and payment reporting in the United States.

INTERNATIONAL CLASSIFICATION OF DISEASES, TENTH EDITION: Alphanumeric codes used for statistical reporting by the World Health Organization (WHO), but not the United States.

INTERNATIONAL CLASSIFICATION OF DISEASES, TENTH EDITION-CLINICAL MODIFICATION: Clinical modifications of ICD-10 codes developed for the United States.

INTERNATIONAL FUND: A portfolio that buys securities of companies headquartered outside of the U.S. These are global funds that invest in securities of both the United States and foreign countries.

INTERNATIONAL HEALTH ECONOMICS ASSOCIATION (iHEA): Global society formed to increase communication among health economists, foster a higher standard of debate in the application of economics to health and health care systems, and assist young researchers at the start of their careers; in Philadelphia, Pennsylvania.

INTERPOSITIONING: An unethical and unfair practice by a broker/dealer of needlessly employing a third party between the customer and the best available market so that the customer pays more on a purchase or receives less on a sale than he should.

INTERSTATE OFFERING: Securities Exchange Commission registered securities offered by states to residents outside of the issuing state.

INTER-VIVOS TRUST: A trust created while the grantor (settlor or creator) is alive. It may be either revocable or irrevocable. *Inter-vivos* is a Latin phrase meaning "living."

IN-THE-MONEY: An option is said to be in-the-money when it has intrinsic value. A *call option* is in-the-money if the underlying security's price is greater than the option's exercise price. A *put option* is in-the-money if the underlying security's price is lower than the option's exercise price.

IN-THE TANK: Slang term for a fast dropping financial market.

INTRA DAY: Within the financial market's trading day.

INTRA STATE EXEMPTION: An exemption under the 1933 Act from SEC registration for offerings whose issuer, offers, and purchasers are in one state and meet certain other requirements.

INTRINSIC VALUE: A *call option* is said to have intrinsic value when the market price of the underlying health care security is greater than the exercise price. A *put option* is said to have intrinsic value when the market price of the underlying health care security falls below the exercise price, OR, the value of a health care business enterprise that an investor considers real and will become apparent to others reaching the same conclusion.

INVENTORY: The quantity or balance in a physical asset account, such as Durable Medical Equipment (DME).

INVENTORY CONVERSION PERIOD (ICP): Inventory / Sales / 360 days.

INVENTORY FINANCING: Loan and debt based financing backed by the value of inventory, goods-in-progress, DME, and so forth.

INVENTORY PRODUCT COSTS: All GAAP product costs regarded as an asset for external finance reporting purposes.

INVENTORY PROFIT: Gross margin difference determined between Last in, First out (LIFO) and First in, First out (FIFO) basis.

INVENTORY TURNOVER: The speed at which DME or other inventory is sold or dispensed.

INVERSE FLOATER: A financial instrument where the required interest payment, or coupon, will change inversely to rates prevailing at the time of the reset.

INVERTED YIELD CURVE: Graphical and real market condition where short-term interest rates are higher than longer-term rates, that is, the 1-year rate is greater than the 5-year rate, or the spot (overnight) rate is higher than the 30-year long-bond rate. It may be a recession indicator.

INVESTED CAPITAL: The amount of equity and debt invested in a health care business entity.

INVESTING ACTIVITIES: The actions that decrease or increase long term assets available to a health care organization.

INVESTMENT: The process of adding to, or replenishing capital stock. The purchase of an asset in anticipation of its rise in value.

INVESTMENT ADVISOR: A person in the business of rendering advice or analysis regarding securities for compensation. Persons meeting this definition must register as advisers with the SEC under the Investment Adviser's Act of 1940. The term does NOT include attorneys and accountants giving advice as an incidental part of their professional practice. The person is not necessarily a fiduciary.

INVESTMENT BANK: A broker/dealer organization that provides a service to industry through counseling and underwriting of securities.

INVESTMENT BANKER: One from a broker/dealer organization that provides a service to industry through counseling and underwriting of securities.

INVESTMENT CLIMATE: Financial and investing conditions currently in place, that is, the economic milieu.

INVESTMENT COMPANY: An institution engaged primarily in the business of investing and trading in securities for others including face amount certificate companies, unit trust companies, and management companies, both open-end and closed-end.

INVESTMENT COMPANY ACT OF 1940: Federal statute enacted for the registration and regulation of investment companies. It requires that companies that invest in securities and interstate commerce be registered with the SEC.

INVESTMENT COMPANY ACT OF 1970: Amendment to the ICA of 1940 requiring a registered investment company that issues contractual plans to offer all purchasers withdrawal rights, and purchasers of front end loaded plans surrender rights.

INVESTMENT CONTRACT: A court-defined concept where funds are pooled in the expectation of making profits from the efforts of a third party or promoter.

An investor in such an offering has bought a security, as regulated by the SEC and the states.

INVESTMENT CURVE: Graphical relationship between money funds and economic investments at different levels.

INVESTMENT DEMAND CURVE: Graphical relationship between interest rates and economic investments at different levels.

INVESTMENT DEMAND SCHEDULE: Timeline relationship between interest rates and economic investments at different levels.

INVESTMENT GRADE: The broad credit designation given bonds that have a high probability of being paid and minor, if any, speculative features. Bonds rated BBB or higher by Standard & Poor's Corporation or Baa or higher by Moody's Investors Service, Inc., are deemed by those agencies to be "investment grade."

INVESTMENT GRADE BOND: A bond with one of the top four credit ratings (AAA, AA, A, BBB) of independent bond-rating agencies, such as Moody's or Standard & Poor's (see Table 4).

INVESTMENT INCOME: Gross or total amount of dividends, interest, and so forth received from an investment company's investments before deduction of any expenses. It is the net balance of gross income after payment of operating expenses, including management fees, legal and accounting costs, and so forth. If at least 98% is distributed to shareholders, tax is only paid on the undistributed income.

INVESTMENT INTEREST: Payment for the use of funds used to acquire assets that produce investment income.

INVESTMENT LETTER: A written agreement between a securities seller and buyer, in a private placement of securities, stating that the buyer's intentions

Table 4: Bond Rating Service Company Comparisons

	Standard & Poor's	Moody's	Fitch's
Investment Grade	AAA	Aaa	AAA
	AA	Aa	AA
	A	A	A
	BBB	Baa	BBB
Speculative Grade	BB	Ba	BB
	B	B	B
	CCC	Caa	CCC
	CC	Ca	CC
	C	C	C

are for investment only and that he does not intend to re-offer the securities publicly.

INVESTMENT MANAGER: The person or organization that is responsible for the management of an investment company under contract. Its services usually include general administrative activities and advice and recommendations as to the purchase, holding, or sale of portfolio securities.

INVESTMENT POLICY STATEMENT (IPS): A document drafted between a financial advisor and client that outlines general rules for the advisor. It provides the general goals and objectives and describes the strategies that the advisor should employ to meet them. Specific information on matters such as asset allocation, benchmarks, risk tolerance, reporting, and liquidity requirements would be included in an IPS.

INVESTMENT TAX CREDIT: A direct tax reduction for plant or equipment investments.

INVESTMENT VALUE AS DEBT: Convertible security valuable appraised as if it were nonconvertible debt.

INVESTOR: One who gives financial capital to another with the expectation of financial return.

INVESTOR OWNED: An ownership group that includes health facilities that are partnerships, sole proprietorships, and corporations, or divisions of corporations that issue stock.

INVISIBLE HAND: Tendency for patients, people, and health care or other entities to seek self-interest gratifying activities in competitive markets to further the interest of society or other groups, as a whole. Adam Smith philosophy.

INVOICE: A bill or seller's (health care provider or entity) request for payment from a purchaser (patient or insurer).

INVOLUNTARY CONVERSIONS: Property that is in whole or part destroyed, stolen, seized, requisitioned, or condemned (or where there is a threat or imminence of requisition or condemnation).

IRREGULAR DIVIDENDS: Nonperiodic dividend payments in time and/or amount.

IRREVOCABLE TRUST: A trust that cannot be changed or canceled by its grantor (settlor or creator).

ISOQUANT: All the input and other factors producing a constant level of health care output.

ISSUE: Any of a company's class of securities, or the act of distributing them.

ISSUED AND OUTSTANDING STOCK: That portion of authorized stock distributed among investors by a corporation.

ISSUER: A health care or other corporation, municipality, state, trust, or association engaged in the distribution of its securities and registered under Section 12 of the Securities Exchange Act of 1934. An issuer is required to file reports under Section 15(d) of that Act. Or an issuer must have filed a registration statement with the SEC that has not yet become effective under the Securities Act of 1933 and that it has not withdrawn.

ITEMIZED BILL: A bill or invoice for medical or other goods and services rendered and the charges for each item.

ITEMIZED DEDUCTIONS: Certain personal expenses such as medical expenses. These include various state, local, and foreign taxes, home mortgage interest, investment interest, charitable contributions, and miscellaneous expenses.

J

J: Commodity futures symbol for an April delivery month.

JAMES, BRENT, MD: Executive Director of the Institute for Health Care Delivery Research at Intermountain Health Care in Salt Lake City, Utah.

JANUARY EFFECT: The historic tendency of smaller stocks to rise in early January each year.

JEFFORDS, JAMES: U.S. Senator (I-Vt.) and member of the Health, Education, Labor, and Pensions Committee.

JEL CLASSIFICATION CODES: A system for books and journals relevant to health care economics research and nomenclature. Three levels of precision exist: categories A–Z, subcategories A0–A2 (classify books), and subsubcategories such as A10–A14 (classify journal articles).

JENSEN INDEX (JI): Performance measurement comparing absolute realized investment returns with risk adjusted returns.

JENSEN, MICHAEL, MEASURE: Takes advantage of the CAPM equation to identify a statistically significant excess return or alpha on a portfolio basket of securities. In an efficient market, the CAPM equation is as follows:

$$E(R_j) = R_f + |E(R_m) - R_f| \beta_j$$

However, if a portfolio has been able to consistently add value above the excess return expected as a result of its beta, then the alpha (α_p) of the equation below should be positive and (hopefully) statistically significant. Thus, the alpha term from a regression of the portfolio's returns versus the market portfolio (i.e., typically the S&P 500 in practice) is a measure of risk-adjusted performance.

$$R_j - R_f = \alpha_j + |R_m - R_f| \beta; + \varepsilon_j$$

JEOPARDY: The financial danger of an account being uncollected.

JESSE, WILLIAM: President and CEO of the Medical Group Management Association in Englewood, Colorado.

JOHNSON, NANCY: U.S. Representative (R-Conn.) and chairwoman for the House Ways and Means health subcommittee.

JOINT ACCOUNT (JA): An account in which two or more individuals possess control and may transact business.

JOINT COST (JC): Common health care or other costs.

JOINT MANAGER: Any member of a management group, although the term is often used to refer to a member other than the lead manager.

JOINT RETURN: A return filed by married taxpayers or surviving spouses.

JOINT TENANTS IN COMMON (JTC): Form of joint account or asset ownership where a deceased tenant's fractional account ownership share is retained by his or her estate.

JOINT TENANTS BY ENTIRETY (JTE): Joint ownership method allowed for married couples only. It may offer some protection for the innocent spouse against creditor claims.

JOINT TENANTS WITH RIGHT OF SURVIVORSHIP: Form of joint account ownership where a deceased tenant's fractional account ownership share reverts to the surviving tenant.

JOINT VENTURE (JV): Economic risk sharing arrangement between one or more other health care entities, for profit.

JOURNAL: The chronological accounting record of an organization's transactions. It consists of the original entries of daily financial transactions.

JOURNAL ENTRY: Documentation of the chronological accounting record of an organization's transactions.

JOURNALIZING: The process of documenting the chronological accounting record of an organization's transactions.

JUICE: Slang term for power, as in electrical, economic, financial, political, social, and so forth.

JUMP: Slang term for a market that experiences a significant departure from a price level, whether higher or lower.

JUMP BONDS: Slang term for debt issues that are conditioned, triggering a predetermined movement to another payment arrangement.

JUNIOR SECURITIES: Common stocks and other issues whose claims to assets and earnings are contingent upon the satisfaction of the claims of prior obligations.

JUNK BOND: A speculative security with a rating of BB or lower. It is a "high-yield" security.

JUST IN TIME: Scheduling or production system based on scheduling needs.

JUST IN TIME COSTING: System that starts with completed output and then assigns manufacturing or others costs to units or services-sold, and to inventory.

JUST IN TIME INVENTORY (JITI): Inventory acquisition systems with the following characteristics:

- Fewer inventory accounts or accounts payable
- Reduction or elimination of work-in-progress or handling activities
- Overhead and direct labor costs are not traced

JITI medical systems need a dependable working relationship with suppliers and the precise calculation of inventory needs, especially for:

- Sterile surgical packs
- GI and GU instrumentation
- Orthopedic and OB-GYN inventory
- Invasive heart and lung equipment
- Radio isotopes and trace radiographic materials
- Almost all prescheduled medical interventions and procedures

JUST IN TIME METHOD (JITM): Inventory costing method which means DME is delivered as soon as needed by the health care organization, its prescribing doctor, or patient. In the JITM, inventory is "pulled" through the flow process. This is contrasted to the "push" approach used by traditional operations. In the push system, DME is on-site, with little regard to when it is actually needed. In the JITM pull system, the overriding concern is to keep a minimum cost inventory. The key elements of the JITM consist of six parts:

- A few dependable vendors/suppliers willing to ship with little advanced notice
- Total sharing of demand information throughout the supply chain
- More frequent orders
- Smaller size of individual orders
- Improved physical plant (hospital/clinic) layout to reduce travel flow distance
- Use of a total quality control system to reduce flawed medical products

In other words, inventory is delivered when needed, rather than in advance, saving handling and storage costs. The health care entity never needs to stockpile inventory, and cash flow is enhanced.

JUSTIFIED PRICE: The informed and fair market value of securities.

K

K: Commodity futures symbol for a May delivery month.

K PERCENT RULE: A monetary policy for keeping the growth of money at some fixed rate level, per year.

KAHN, CHARLES "CHIP": President of the Federation of American Hospitals in Washington, D.C.

KAHNEMAN, DANIEL, PhD: Psychologist from University of California at Berkeley and Eugene Higgins Professor of Psychology and Professor of Public Affairs in the Woodrow Wilson School of Public and International Affairs at Princeton University. He shared the 2002 Nobel Prize in Economics (formally known as the Bank of Sweden Prize in Economic Sciences in Memory of Alfred Nobel) with Vernon L. Smith (George Mason University, Fairfax, Virginia). His main findings concerned decision making under uncertainty, where human decisions may systematically depart from those predicted by standard economic theory.

KAPLAN, GARY, MD: Chairman and CEO of the Virginia Mason Medical Center in Seattle, Washington.

KAPPA: Volatility measurement and pricing model for financial derivatives. Synonymous with lambda, sigma, or vega. It is a letter in the Greek alphabet.

KEIRETSU SYSTEM: Maintaining long-term economic and business relationships with medical partners, facilities, vendors, and patients. A disadvantage of this system is slow reaction times, because all are partially protected from external market competition. It is a Japanese concept.

KENNEDY, EDWARD: U.S. Senator (D-Mass.) and chairman on the Health, Education, Labor, and Pensions Committee.

KENNEDY-KASEBAUM HEALTH COVERAGE BILL: Also known as the Health Insurance Portability and Accountability Act of 1996. It includes legislature that allowed portable and high-deductible health insurance plans with low premium payments combined with a savings plan, such as HSAs and MSAs.

KEOGH (HR-10) PLAN: An arrangement that permits self-employed individuals and partners of partnerships to receive income tax deductions for amounts they set aside for savings. It is a tax-deferred trust savings account that allows self-employed individuals or those who own their own incorporated businesses to save for their retirement. Savers place a portion of their income each year in their Keogh account until they reach at least age 59 1/2. Federal income tax on the deposited funds and the interest they earn is deferred until withdrawals are begun, presumably when the saver has retired, and is, therefore, in a lower tax bracket. Employers who establish a Keogh plan for themselves must also make the benefit available to qualified employees.

KEY COMPONENT: One of three components (history, physical examination, and medical decision making) used to select the correct level of evaluation-and-management coding for reimbursement purposes.

KEY EMPLOYEE: A key employee (including former or deceased employees) is one who at any time during the prior pension plan year was:

- an officer whose annual compensation from the employer exceeds $130,000; or

- an employee owning more than 5% of the business; or
- an employee owning more than 1% of the business, and whose compensation exceeds $150,000 for the plan year.

KEY PERSON DISCOUNT: Reduction in business enterprise ownership value from the actual or real loss of an owner or key person.

KEYNESIAN ECONOMICS: Macroeconomic principles that suggest that a capitalistic society does not always utilize its assets efficiency and that fiscal and monetary policy can be used to promote fuller employment levels.

KIBBE, DAVID, MD: Director of the Center for Health Information Technology at the American Academy of Family Physicians in Washington, D.C.

KICKBACK: The federal antikickback statute makes it a crime to knowingly and willfully offer, pay, solicit, or receive any remuneration to induce a person to: (a) refer an individual to a person for the furnishing of any item or service covered under a federal health care program; or (b) to purchase, lease, order, arrange for, or recommend any good, facility, service, or item covered under a federal health care program. The term *any remuneration* encompasses any bribe, or rebate; direct or indirect; overt or covert; cash or in kind; and any ownership interest or compensation interest.

KICKER: Slang term for a debt offering with the added bonus of equity participation under the given terms and conditions of the loan.

KILLER BEES: Slang term for financial and other advisors who assist in preventing a corporate takeover event.

KING, GRAHAM: President of Information Solutions at McKesson Corp., in San Francisco, California.

KINKED DEMAND CURVE: Graphical representations demonstrating that market competitors may follow a price decrease but not a price increase.

KITING: Unethical act of driving securities prices higher through financial market manipulations or taking advantage of check cashing float time.

KIZER, KENNETH, MD: President and CEO of the National Quality Forum in Washington, D.C.

KLOSS, LINDA: Executive Vice President and CEO of the American Health Information Management Association in Chicago, Illinois.

KNOCK'IN: Slang term for an option feature that triggers the activation of an option contract. Down-and-In and Up-and-In option feature.

KNOCKOUT: Slang term for an option feature that triggers the cessation of an option contract. Down-and-Out and Up-and-Out option feature.

KNOCKOUT OPTION: Slang term for the derivative option right, but not the obligation, to, but the underlying position at a given price.

KOLB, MARVIN, MD: President of the American College of Physician Executives in Tampa, Florida.

KOLODNER, ROBERT, MD: Chief Health Informatics Officer of the Veterans Health Administration in Irving, Texas.

KONDRATIEF (NIKOLAI) WAVE: Russian economist who suggested that financial market cycles can be very long, up to 50 years in length.

KONGSTVEDT, PETER R., MD: A partner in the Health & Life Sciences Division of Accenture Corporation. He is a futurist who helped health care organizations assess and implement HIPAA rules and regulations. He is also a medical pay-for-performance and managed care expert.

KURTOSIS: Statistic that describes the degree of peak or flatness of a probability distribution curve relative to its benchmark normal distribution. Leptokurtic (Leptokurtosis) and Platykurtic (Platykurtosis).

L

LABOR: The physical and cognitive efforts of human beings to produce health care products, goods, services or other outputs, as in doctors, nurses, and ancillary workers.

LABOR BUDGET: An expense projection of a health care entity's fixed, variable, and other costs of its labor pool.

LABOR FORCE: Those medical workers employed and unemployed in the health care space.

LABOR LEISURE TRADEOFF: The ratio or combination of health care labor time versus free time of medical workers.

LABOR PRODUCTIVITY (HEALTH CARE): Total health care industrial complex output divided by total health care human labor force. It is the average health care output unit, per worker, per hour.

LABOR VALUE: Suggestion that only health care laborers can produce something of value in the medical and health care marketplace.

LACY, CLIFTON, MD: President and CEO of the Robert Wood Johnson University Hospital in New Brunswick, New Jersey.

LADDER: A series of increasingly longer and revolving debt issues to accommodate interest rate risks and changes regardless of economic cycle.

LADY MACBETH STRATEGY: Slang term for a faux white knight in a hostile corporate takeover attempt who joins or becomes the unfriendly bidder or takeover artist.

LAFFER (ARTHUR) CURVE: Visual suggestion that domestic economic output grows with decreased marginal income tax rates.

LAG FACTOR: Accounting concept related to health care IBNRs claims for services incurred but not processed for payment following the end of a specific time or accounting period. It is the float time.

LAG STUDY: Time determination for the aging of medical claims along with monthly payouts. It is similar to an aging schedule for accounts receivable.

LAGGING ECONOMIC INDICATOR: An economic benchmark such as the unemployment rate, which changes after the economy has started to follow a particular trend.

LAISSEZ-FAIRE: French term suggesting that governmental economic intervention in business and finance is kept to a minimum. It is a form of capitalism.

LAMBDA: Option term that may be used as a synonym for vega, kappa, or sigma.

LAPSE: To expire or lose certain rights and privileges.

LARGE CAP STOCK: Companies with a large market capitalization rate (share number outstanding times share price), usually in excess of $5 billion.

LASPEYRES INDEX: A medical price index calculated from a set ("basket") of fixed medical quantities and units of a finite list of health care goods and services.

LAST-IN, FIRST-OUT (LIFO): An inventory costing method where the last costs into inventory are the first costs attributed to cost of goods sold. The ending inventory is based on the cost of the most recent purchases. Older DME and other costs are left in ending inventory. In times of rising prices, a lower total cost inventory is produced with a higher cost of goods sold. The last items purchased are the most expensive and used first for the calculation. This happens because LIFO increases an expense (cost of goods sold) and decreases taxable income. Given the same revenue, higher expenses mean less profit. Deflation has the opposite effect.

LAST TRADING DAY: The final day for settlement of futures contracts.

LAUNDER: Slang term meaning to make illicitly acquired cash appear legitimate.

LAVIZZO-MOUREY, RISA, MD: President and CEO of the Robert Wood Johnson Foundation in Princeton, New Jersey.

LAW OF DEMAND: Principle that the lower the price of a health care good or service, the greater the quantity patient-consumers are able to purchase over time.

LAW OF DIMINISHING MARGINAL RATE OF SUBSTITUTION: Principle suggesting that the marginal rate of substitution of capital for health care labor falls as the amount of capital and the amount of labor increases.

LAW OF DIMINISHING MARGINAL RETURNS: Principle suggesting that the extra production obtained from increases in variable health care inputs will eventually decline as more variable inputs are used with fixed inputs.

LAW OF DIMINISHING MARGINAL UTILITY: Principle suggesting that the marginal utility of any health care item or service tends to decline as more is consumed over a given period.

LAW OF DIMINISHING RETURNS: The diminished marginal health care product or output of a variable health care input.

LAW OF INCREASING COSTS: Principle suggesting that the opportunity cost of each additional unit of health care output increases over time as more of that good or service is produced.

LAW OF LARGE NUMBERS: Statistical concept where a greater number of units equates to less significance per unit (Poisson's Law). It is the theory of probability that is the basis of insurance and economic risk management, that is, the larger the number of risks or exposures, the more closely will the actual results obtained approach the probable results expected from an infinite number of exposures.

LAW OF SUPPLY: Principle suggesting that the higher the price of a health care good or service, the greater the quantity that sellers are willing and able to make over time.

LAWRENCE, DAVID, MD: Former CEO of Kaiser Permanente in Oakland, California.

LEAD MANAGER: One who generally handles senior negotiations in a negotiated underwriting of a new issue of municipal securities or directs the processes by which a bid is determined for a competitive underwriting. The lead manager also is charged with allocating securities among the members of the syndicate according to the terms of the syndicate agreement and the orders received.

LEADING ECONOMIC INDICATOR: An economic benchmark, such as new housing starts, that changes before the economy has started to follow a particular trend.

LEAKAGE: Diminution of spending or lending potential. Funds lost as commissions or transactions costs.

LEAPE, LUCIAN, MD: Adjunct professor of health policy at the Harvard School of Public Health in Cambridge, Massachusetts.

LEASE: The payment of a specific amount of money, over time, for the use of an asset.

LEDGER: A book of accounts.

LEG: A sustained trend in the financial markets.

LEGAL CAPITAL: Owner or stockholder equity not used for dividends.

LEGAL INVESTMENT: The ability of a particular security to meet the specifications of various states' laws restricting the investment practices of institutions (particularly savings banks) located in the state. This matter is typically addressed in a "legal investment survey" conducted on behalf of the syndicate underwriting the security.

LEGAL LIST: Securities deemed acceptable as holdings for mutual savings banks.

LEGAL OPINION: The written conclusions of bond counsel that the issuance of municipal securities and the proceedings taken in connection therewith comply with applicable laws, and that interest on the securities will be exempt from federal income taxation and, where applicable, from state and local taxation. The legal opinion is generally printed on the securities.

LEGAL RESERVE: Minimum amount of money a health care claim-paying entity must maintain in order to meet future medical insurance claims, debts, liabilities, and obligations, as determined under the various state code guidelines.

LEGISLATIVE RISK: Chance that changes in law might affect the price of certain securities. It can be positive or negative.

LEMON: Slang term for a poor investment.

LENDER: A bank, mortgage company, or mortgage broker offering a loan. Temporarily granting asset use to another in return for interest.

LEPTOKURTIC (LEPTOKURTOSIS): Mathematical description of a peaked condition for a relative distribution statistical curve. It is evaluated against the normal distribution and its attendant bell-shaped curve.

LERNER INDEX: A measure of the health care profitability for a business entity (practice, clinic, or hospital) that provides medical goods, products, and services: (price minus marginal cost) divided by price.

LESSEE: The tenant in a lease or rental agreement.

LESSOR: Property owner in a lease or rental agreement.

LETTER OF CREDIT (LC): Document from a financial institution that guarantees client drafts up to a certain limit amount. It is a conditional bank commitment issued on behalf of a customer to pay a third party in accordance with certain terms and conditions.

LETTER OF INTENT (LI): A pledge to purchase a sufficient amount of open-end investment company shares within a limited period (usually 13 months) to qualify for the reduced selling charge that would apply to a comparable lump sum purchase.

LETTER SECURITY: An unregistered security offered privately in which the purchaser is obliged to sign an investment letter to complete the transaction and to forestall disciplinary action against the seller under the Securities Act of 1933.

LEVEL; 1, 2, or 3: Levels of service for NASDAQ trading firms:

- Level 1—A single average price quote for those not trading OTC.
- Level 2—Level 1 plus trade reports, executions, negotiations, networks, clearing, and bid-ask price quotes for all firms and customers.
- Level 3—Level 1 and 2, plus the ability to enter quotes, execute orders, and send information, for and by market makers.

LEVEL DEBT SERVICE: A maturity schedule in which the combined annual amount of principal and interest payments remains relatively constant over the life of the securities issue.

LEVEL LOAD: A sales commission or charge that remains steady over time.

LEVERAGE: A financial condition brought about by the assumption of a high percentage of debt in relation to the equity in a health care corporation's capital structure. Leverage is the use of borrowed money, or lever. For example:

- For derivative products, little or no margin is required for placing positions.
- For a $100,000 bond bought for cash, a one point in price move would make or lose $1,000. But, for futures, an investor could acquire market performance of the same bond for an initial deposit of only $2,500 and a one point price swing would translate into $1,000, plus or minus.

LEVERAGE FACTOR: Ratio of debt to total assets.

LEVERAGED BUYOUT (LBO): The usually hostile takeover of a company with borrowed funds, such as junk bonds. Assets are then usually stripped to pay the debt.

LEVERAGED LEASE: Transaction where a lessor borrows funds to acquire property which is leased to a third party. Property and lease rentals serve as security for indebtedness.

LEVERAGED STOCK; SECURITIES: Stock or other securities purchased on loan, with debt, or on margin.

LEVERED BETA: The beta reflected in a company whose capital structure includes debt financing.

LEWIN, JACK, MD: CEO and Executive Vice President of the California Medical Association in Sacramento, California.

LIABILITIES: A health care organization's legal obligations to pay creditors. All the outstanding claims for money against a health care corporation: accounts payable, wages and salaries, dividends declared or payable, accrued taxes, fixed- or long-term liabilities such as mortgage bonds, debentures, and bank loans.

LIABILITY: An unclaimed insurance obligation.

LIABILITY DETERMINATION: Determination based on §1879 or §1870 or §1842(L) of the Social Security Act (SSA) of whether the beneficiary and the provider did not and could not have been reasonably expected to know that payment would not be made for services.

LIABILITY PROTECTION: CMS requirement for HMOs that protects a member from financial responsibility of the entity, as well as for liabilities such as physician or hospital fees. Financial reserves are held against possible insolvency.

LIBOR: London Interbank Offered Rate is the rate international banks charge each other and varies throughout each business day reflecting global economic conditions. Standard.

LIBOR INDEX RATES: London Interbank Offered Rate averages that are fixed at a specific time each day and published for various maturity terms.

LICENSE: Federal or state charter granting its holder the right to practice a profession, such as medicine, podiatry, dentistry, law, and so forth.

LIEN: Security interest in an asset of a secured loan. It is a claim against an asset.

LIFE CYCLE BUDGET: The estimated projection of a product's cost and revenues over its useful life.

LIFETIME MAXIMUM: Maximum dollar amount paid toward a medical insurance claim.

LIFT: An increase in securities prices, a sector, or the financial markets.

LIGHTEN UP: Slang term meaning to sell securities for diversification, profit-taking, or other purposes.

LIKE-KIND-EXCHANGE: The swap of two similar assets.

LIMIT ORDER: A securities order in which a customer sets a maximum price as a buyer, and a minimum price to accept as a seller.

LIMITED ACCESS TO BOOKS AND RECORDS: A shareholder's right to inspect financial information made public in accordance with federal, state, exchange, and National Association of Securities Dealers (NASD) regulations.

LIMITED APPRAISAL: The appraisal of a health care or other business entity with restrictions in the analysis, or the scope of project.

LIMITED CHARGE: A Medicare fee limit amount for non-Medicare participating medical providers. Non-PAR reimbursement payment ceiling.

LIMITED CHARGE POLICY: A 1993 Medicare fee limit schedule amount for non-Medicare participating medical providers that disallows charges more than 115% of Medicare Allowable Charges (MAC). Non-PAR reimbursement payment ceiling.

LIMITED LIABILITY COMPANY (LLC): A relatively new form of business entity authorized in more than half of the states. It has certain attributes of both a regular corporation and a partnership. Most notably, its members, and there must be at least two, can operate the business like a general partnership while retaining the limited personal liability that is most often associated with the corporate form.

LIMITED LIABILITY PARTNERSHIP: Association of two or more persons, including one or more general partners (each of whom has unlimited liability), and one or more limited partners (whose individual liability is limited).

LIMITED PARTNERSHIP: Arrangement in which one or more individuals, but not all, have limited liability to creditors of the firm.

LIMITED TAX BOND: A general obligation bond secured by the pledge of a specified tax (usually the property tax) or category of taxes that are limited as to rate or amount.

LIMITING CHARGE: The maximum amount that a nonparticipating physician is permitted to charge a Medicare beneficiary for a service. In effect, it is a limit on balance billing. Starting in 1993 the limiting charge has been set at 115% of the Medicare-allowed charge.

LIMITS: Medical benefits payment ceiling.

LINE ITEM BUDGET: Format that lists expenses and revenues by category, and may be also known as a program or performance budget.

LINE OF CREDIT: A pre-authorized contract between a potential borrower and lender under certain terms and conditions of the contract.

LINEAR HEALTH CARE ECONOMETRIC MODEL: An econometric medical business model expressed in an equation for which the parameters enter serially, whether or not the data require nonlinear transformations to arrive at that financial equation.

LIQUID ASSET: Asset easily and quickly converted to cash without price loss.

LIQUIDATING DIVIDEND: Return of capital to medical suppliers and vendors in the dissolution of a health care or other organization.

LIQUIDATING VALUE: Rock-bottom asset prices for companies or health care entities going out of business.

LIQUIDATION: Refers to the sequence of payouts when health care corporations go bankrupt. The order is as follows:

1. Internal Revenue Service,
2. Secured creditors, including senior bondholders,
3. Unsecured creditors including junior bonds (debentures),
4. Preferred stockholders, and
5. Common stockholders.

LIQUIDATION VALUE: The net amount possibly realized when the assets of a health care or other business enterprise are sold individually, in an orderly but forced fashion. It is the fire sale asset value.

LIQUIDITY: The speed at which an asset can be converted to cash. (1) The ability of the market in a particular security to absorb a reasonable amount of trading at reasonable price changes. Liquidity is one of the most important characteristics of a good market. (2) The easy ability of investors to convert their securities holdings into cash and vice versa.

LIQUIDITY RATIOS: Relationships of short-term obligation payment abilities (i.e., quick ratio, current ratio, etc.).

LISTED FIRM: A company whose stock trades on one of the financial exchanges.

LISTED OPTION: A put or call traded on a national option exchange with standardized terms. In contrast, over-the-counter options usually have nonstandard or negotiated terms.

LISTED PROPERTY: Depreciation limits on certain listed property:

- passenger cars, and other property used as transportation;
- property used for purposes of entertainment, recreation, or amusement;
- computers and peripheral equipment, and cellular telephones.

LISTED SECURITY: An organized exchange traded security.

LISTED STOCK: Stock that trades on one of the registered securities exchanges. "Listed" usually implies listing on the two major exchanges: the New York Stock Exchange (NYSE) and the American Stock Exchange (AMEX, ASE). "Unlisted" companies trade over-the-counter, usually through the National Association of Securities Dealers Automated Quotation System (NASDAQ). Listed stock symbols are three letters; unlisted symbols are four or more letters.

LISTING REQUIREMENTS: The accounting rules and financial regulations required before company stock can be listed on a financial exchange.

LITIGATION SUPPORT: A service that physicians and medical professionals, or financial service professionals such as CMPs©, CFPs©, CFAs©, CPAs, and so forth, provide to attorneys, such as with medical chart review, expert witness testimony about the value of a business or other asset, forensic accounting, health care economics, malpractice, and so forth.

LIVING TRUST: A trust established by a living person who controls the assets contributed to the trust. Such trusts have traditionally been used to avoid probate, but can also provide a vehicle for financial management in the event the creator is incapacitated.

LIVING WILL: A document specifying the kind and extent of medical care a person desires in the event he or she is incapacitated.

LOAD: The amount added to net premiums (risk factor minus interest factor) to cover a company's operating expenses and contingencies. The loading includes the cost of securing new business, collecting premiums, and general management expenses. Precisely, it is the excess of the gross health insurance premiums over net premiums, or a sales commission.

LOAD CHARGE: The additional charge for overhead costs added to health insurance or other net premiums.

LOAD FUND: A mutual fund that charges a sales commission or load.

LOAN AGREEMENT: A legal contract between a debtor and creditor that spells out the terms and conditions of a loan (i.e., indenture).

LOAN AMORTIZATION: To pay back or extinguish a loan, bond, or debt, often presented with a schedule for amortization.

LOAN TERMS: The conditions that specify how a loan will be repaid and a borrower's obligations until the loan is repaid. Some common loan terms include interest rate, fees charged, and the length of the loan.

LOAN TO VALUE RATIO (LTVR): The ratio determined by dividing the balance of a loan by the appraised value of its collateralized asset. For instance, if the balance on a loan is $79,000 and the appraised value of its backed assets is $100,000, the LTV is 79%.

LOAN VALUE: The maximum permissible credit extended on securities in a margin account, presently 50% of the current market value of eligible stock in the account.

LOANED FLAT: A loan without interest rate charges.

LOCK UP PERIOD: Slang term for a 6-month agreement period where insiders do not sell shares following an Initial Public Offering (IPO).

LOCKED MARKET: A very competitive financial market with similar bid and ask prices, and thus low spreads and sales commissions.

LOFTON, KEVIN: Executive Vice President and COO of Catholic Health Initiatives in Denver, Colorado.

LONG: An owned asset or purchased security position. It may also be a party who is bullish on the market.

- Long Coupon: The initial coupon for a municipal security that reflects more than 6 months of accrued interest. The time of accrual is measured from the start of the Dated Date and continues until the end of the initial accrual period, compared to a Short Coupon.

LONG BOND: Government bonds with a maturity time frame greater than 10 years. They are usually 30-year U.S. Treasuries, which suspended issuance in 2001 but were reinstituted on February 9, 2006.

LONG HEDGE: An open futures contract equivalent position. The hedger is long futures against a short actual position.

LONG INDUSTRIALS: Investment grade U.S. corporate bonds with maturities that exceed 10 years.

LONG OPTION: An option that has been purchased.

LONG POSITION: A term used to describe either an open position that is expected to benefit from a rise in the price of the underlying stock (such as long call, short put, or long stock), or an open position resulting from an opening purchase transaction such as long call, long put, or long stock. Securities bought or owned outright.

LONG RUN: An adequate time period for health care producers to vary all inputs required to produce outputs.

LONG RUN AGGREGATE SUPPLY CURVE: Timeline that allows health care or other input prices to be responsive to changes in price level.

LONG RUN AVERAGE COST: Lowest average obtainable output cost when health care inputs can be carried.

LONG RUN COMPETITIVE EQUILIBRIUM: Health care or other industry condition where there is no tendency to enter, leave, expand, or contract the scale of operations.

LONG RUN COST: Minimum expenditure producing any given health care output when all health care inputs are variable.

LONG RUN DEMAND: Price point at which variable quantities of health care products or services are required in for long-term.

LONG RUN SUPPLY: Price point at which variable quantities of health care products or services are available in for long-term.

LONG TERM: An accounting time period of more than 1 year.

LONG TERM ASSET: Any assets other than a current asset. Usually longer than 1 year.

LONG TERM CARE HOSPITAL: This type of entity provides assistance and patient care for the activities of daily living (ADLs), including reminders and standby help for those with physical, mental, or emotional problems. This includes physical disability or other medical problems for 3 months or more (90 days). The criteria of five ADLs may also be used to determine the need for help with the following: meal preparation, shopping, light housework, money management, and telephoning. Other important considerations include taking medications, doing laundry, and getting around outside.

LONG TERM DEBT: Debt for more than a year's term.

LONG TERM EQUITY ANTICIPATION SECURITIES (LEAPS): Options strategy that can extend up to 3 years. It may be either a put or a call typically available for trading in July, with an average 2.5-year lifespan.

LONG TERM INVESTMENTS: Noncurrent assets not used for daily business operations, but for capital appreciation and dividends for more than a year.

LONG TERM LIABILITY: Any liability other than a current liability, and usually longer than 1 year.

LONG TERM REALIZED CAPITAL GAINS: Amount by which the net proceeds from the sale of a security that is held for more than 12 months exceeds its cost of acquisition.

LONG TERM REALIZED CAPITAL LOSSES: Amount by which the acquisition cost of a security that is held for more than 12 months exceeds the net proceeds from its sale.

LONG TERM SOLVENCY: The ability to generate enough cash to pay long term debts as they become due or mature.

LONG THE BASIS: An open cash or spot market position, where the hedger would be long the cash market and short the futures or forward market.

LONGITUDINAL DATA: Financial, economic, business, accounting, or other information for multiple periods.

LOOPHOLE: Circumvention of the spirit, but not letter of the law. Technicality.

LORD, JONATHAN, MD: Senior Vice President and Chief Innovative Officer of Humana in Louisville, Kentucky.

LORENZ CURVE: Visual graph of income enjoyed by each percentage of households, ranked according to income.

LOSS: Excess of business expenses over revenues. Eligible health care expenses that are actually incurred during a contract year and then paid during the 3-month period immediately thereafter.

LOSS PAYABLE: A policy provision that provides for payment of a loss by the health insurance company to someone other than the insured.

LOSS RATIO: The percentage of health or other insurance losses in relation to premiums.

LOSS RESERVE: Estimated liability for unpaid health or other insurance claims or losses that have occurred as of any given valuation date. Usually includes losses incurred but not reported, losses due but not yet paid, and amounts not yet due.

LOT: One contract or unit in the commodities market. It is a singular tangible asset.

LOW: Lowest, or the most minimal value a security holds during a specific time period.

LOW LOAD: A small sales commission on a financial product.

LOW VOLUME DRG: A diagnostic related group with less than five patients per hospital base-year.

LOWER OF COST OR MARKET (LCM) METHOD: Financial statement report of assets at whichever cost is lower: historic cost, or market value.

LOYAL HOSPITAL CONTRACT: Fiscal HMO, MSO, or PHO contracting and negotiations joint-venture legal strategy to maintain economic unity between hospitals and medical providers that forces that payer to accept the facility or not be part of the contract.

LOYAL PROVIDER (PHYSICIAN) CONTRACT: Fiscal contracting and negotiations joint-venture legal strategy to maintain economic unity between hospitals, associated facilities, and medical providers so as to not be separated into smaller units with less bargaining or binding power. It is an "all or nothing" reimbursement contract. It is the reverse of a loyal hospital contract.

LUMP SUM DISTRIBUTION: The withdrawal of an individual's entire balance from an employer-sponsored retirement plan or a Keogh plan. Lump-sum distributions may be eligible for special income tax treatment.

LUXURY GOOD: A health care product or medical service that more affluent patients tend to purchase. It has an income elasticity greater than one.

M

M: (1) Commodity futures symbol for a June delivery month. (2) A designation indicating that a number is to be read in thousands. For example, a transaction for "350M hospital bonds" would involve securities having a par value of $350,000. Numbers in millions are often indicated by the designation "MM."

MAC: Maximum allowable costs (charges) for Medicare.

MAC LIST: Maximum allowable cost or charge schedule for Medicare, usually for generic drugs.

MACAULAY DURATION: Present value of all cash flows from a fixed bond, both principal and interest, weighted by time. It is a measurement of duration expressed in years which is generally less than the stated maturity except for zero coupon bonds. It was established by Frederick Macaulay (1938), whose duration equation is used by portfolio managers as an immunization strategy, and generally demonstrates that:

- The duration of a zero coupon bond is equal to its time to maturity.
- The duration of a coupon bearing bond is less than its time to maturity.
- For bonds with the same coupon rate/yield, a longer maturity has greater duration.
- For bonds with the same yield/maturity, a lower coupon rate has greater duration.

MACROECONOMICS: Economic sector that deals with household, business sector, industry, and major governmental aggregates as a whole.

MACROECONOMIC EQUILIBRIUM: Point where the aggregate quantity demanded for health care products or services equals the aggregate quantity supplied.

MACROHEDGE: Enterprise-wide portfolio risk management offset aimed at the net risk of the aggregated position. Generally, these hedges are more efficient than microhedges for complex portfolios.

MACROHEDGE FUNDS: An alternative investment or hedge fund that is benchmark or index oriented. These funds tend to be industry specific or top-down in approach rather than company specific or bottom-up, and use degrees of leverage to outperform the market indices.

MAIL FLOAT: Time lag between health care payer invoicing and ultimate receipt of payment for medical service rendered.

MAINTENANCE CALL: Demand on a margin account to deposit cash or securities to cover account minimums required by regulatory agencies and the brokerage firm. Because minimums are based on the current value of the securities, maintenance calls can occur as a result of movements in the market price of securities. *See also* margin call.

MAINTENANCE MARGIN: The minimal amount of money in a margin account that triggers a margin call for more funds.

MAINTENANCE REQUIREMENT: Level of margin necessary to support open securities positions given adverse price movements. If the maintenance level is violated, a *variation call* is issued, which would be equal to the amount to restore an account to the initial margin level.

MAJORITY CONTROL: Premium for a health care business entity that exists when provided by a major or majority position of management.

MAJORITY INTEREST: Ownership interest in a health care or other business interest that exceeds 50%.

MAKE MARKETS: To maintain firm offer and bid prices in a given public security by being ready to sell or buy round lots.

MALLON, THOMAS: President of Regent Surgical Health in Weshchester, Illinois. He is a buyer, developer, and manager of surgery centers and surgical hospitals around the country, with expertise in turnaround health care economic situations.

MALMQUIST INDEX: Productivity comparison between an economy industry sector such as health care, or between business X and Y. Named for S. Malmquist, PhD, 1953.

MALONEY ACT: Amendment of the SEC Act of 1934 that provided for Self Regulatory Agencies in the OTC market.

MALPRACTICE EXPENSE: Incurred cost of medical malpractice or liability insurance. It is a specific RVS component.

MANAGED ACCOUNT: A discretionary securities brokerage account managed by a third party on behalf of a client.

MANAGED CARE: Any method of medical care delivery designed to reduce health care costs and improve clinical outcomes, as provided by health maintenance organizations, managed care organizations, and managed health care plans.

MANAGED COMPETITION: *Jackson Hole Group* concept of universal health care with fixed employer contributions for an insurance plan of choice, designed to reduce medical over-utilization, which is transferable and without community ratings.

MANAGED FEE-FOR-SERVICE: The cost of covered services paid by a health insurer after medical care has been rendered. Various managed care tools such as precertification, second surgical opinion, and utilization review.

MANAGED INDEMNITY PLAN: An insurance plan that combines the features of an indemnity plan with cost containment mechanisms; HMO and/or MCO.

MANAGEMENT ACCOUNTING: Non-FASB accounting techniques that focus on information for internal health care business decision makers. *See also* managerial accounting.

MANAGEMENT BUYIN: Large stock purchases by an outside investor to retain existing management.

MANAGEMENT BUYOUT: Large stock purchases by corporate management to take a company private.

MANAGEMENT COMPANY: An investment company that conducts its business in a manner other than as a face amount certificate company or unit investment company.

MANAGEMENT DISCUSSION AND ANALYSIS (MDA): SEC requirement in financial business reporting for an explanation by management of significant changes in operations, assets, and liabilities.

MANAGEMENT EXCEPTION: Focuses on managerial differences between real and budgeted amounts.

MANAGEMENT FEE: Amount paid to a securities portfolio investment manager for its services in the supervision of the investment company's affairs. This fee is set as a percent of the company's net assets. It usually is between .5% and 1% of average annual net assets.

MANAGEMENT REPORT: An annual report of the effectiveness of a company's internal control over financial reporting in addition to its audited financial statements as of the end of the most recent fiscal year.

MANAGER: The member (or members) of a securities underwriting syndicate charged with primary responsibility for conducting the affairs of the syndicate. The manager generally takes the largest underwriting commitment. Also, an organization that serves an open-end investment company as an investment adviser, meaning the entity that manages the securities portfolio.

MANAGERIAL ACCOUNTING: Accounting branch that focuses on information for internal health care business decision makers. It is non-FASB and non-GAAP.

MANAGERIAL ECONOMICS: Non-FASB, non-GAAP, accounting and related allocation resource information for related goods, services, and durable medical equipment. Health care business decision-making information.

MANAGERIAL FINANCE: Health care fiscal and related information used to enhance corporate resource decision making.

MANDATORY REDEMPTION ACCOUNT: A separate account in a sinking fund into which the issuer makes periodic deposits of monies to be used to purchase bonds in the open market or to pay the costs of calling bonds in accordance with the mandatory redemption schedule in the bond contract. It is a bond amortization fund.

MANIPULATION: The creation of false investment activity or investor interest by the frequent buying and selling of a security.

MARGIN: The amount of equity required in an account carried on credit, presently 50% of total cost for eligible stock under Federal Reserve regulations, which is corporate revenues less expenses. The percentage index amount to determine the interest rate for a variable loan, at each adjustment period. For example, if the index is at 5.0, and the margin is 1.5, the interest rate is 6.5%. It is the excess of selling price over unit costs.

MARGIN ACCOUNT: Brokerage account established to extend credit. An account in which a customer uses credit from a broker/dealer to make purchases beyond the actual cash deposited in the account. The extension of credit by broker/dealers is regulated by the Federal Reserve Board under Regulation T as called for in the 1934 Securities Act.

MARGIN CALL (MAINTENANCE MARGIN CALL): A demand to deposit money or securities with a broker/dealer when a purchase is made or when equity in a margin account declines below a minimum standard set by an exchange, the NASD, or the firm.

MARGIN REQUIREMENT: The minimum amount that must be put up in cash to buy securities and established by the Federal Reserve.

MARGIN OF SAFETY: The excess of expected medical sales or health care service revenues over break-even amounts.

MARGIN SECURITY: Any stock, right, or warrant traded on one of the registered stock exchanges in the United States, an OTC stock specifically declared eligible for credit by the Federal Reserve Board, or a debt security traded on one of the registered stock exchanges that either is convertible into margin stock or carries a right or warrant to subscribe to a margin stock. Regulation T of the Federal Reserve Board.

MARGINAL: A one unit, or incremental increase or decrease. Metered.

MARGINAL BENEFIT: The economic dollar value placed on another unit of a health care product or service.

MARGINAL BENEFIT WORK: The extra income received from additional work including nonfinancial satisfaction from health care employment.

MARGINAL COST: The additional cost incurred by increasing the scale of a health care or other program (usually differs from average cost by one unit).

MARGINAL COST LABOR: The amount of total health care human resources labor costs that increase when a health care organization employs one additional unit of labor.

MARGINAL COST PRICE RULE: Suggestion that sets health care product and service price equal to marginal costs.

MARGINAL EFFICIENCY OF CAPITAL: A list of the internal rate of return on invested capital.

MARGINAL EXTERNAL BENEFIT: The additional economic benefit derived from an externality.

MARGINAL EXTERNAL COST: The additional cost involved using one additional unit of health care input.

MARGINAL INPUT COST: The additional cost incurred by using one additional health care or other input unit.

MARGINAL PRIVATE COST: The marginal cost directly incurred by the provider of a health care service or product vendor.

MARGINAL PRODUCT: The increase in total health care product resulting from a one unit increase in a variable health care input.

MARGINAL PRODUCT LABOR: The additional health care output resulting from the addition of an extra input of health care or medical labor.

MARGINAL PROFIT: The change in profit from selling an additional unit of health care product or service. Also, the different between marginal revenue and marginal cost.

MARGINAL PROPENSITY TO CONSUME HEALTH CARE: The percentage of disposable dollars allocated to consume health care services or other purchases.

MARGINAL PROPENSITY TO SAVE HEALTH CARE: The percentage of disposable dollars allocated to save rather than spend on health care related products, goods, DME, and/or services. Insurance HSAs and MSAs.

MARGINAL RATE SUBSTITUTION: The quantity of health care products or services that one would give up for another, if similar.

MARGINAL RATE TECHNICAL SUBSTITUTION: One factor of health care production or output one would give up for another factor, while maintaining the same level of production or output.

MARGINAL RATE OF TRANSFORMATION: A slope of a health care production possibilities curve, and the rate of societal substitution of one health care good for another.

MARGINAL RESPENDING: The additional purchase of health care products or services that results from each extra dollar of income.

MARGINAL REVENUE: The additional revenue obtained by selling an additional unit of product or service.

MARGINAL REVENUE PRODUCT: The change in total revenue obtained by using one additional unit of factor.

MARGINAL TAX RATE: Tax rate paid on the last additional dollar of income.

MARGINAL UTILITY: The additional satisfaction received by consuming an additional health care service or production unit.

MARGINAL UTILITY PER DOLLAR: The marginal health care utility (satisfaction) obtained from the last medical product or service unit consumed, divided by its price.

MARK DOWN: The remuneration received by a dealer or dealer bank selling securities as principal on behalf of a client or a dealer third party. The remuneration consists of the differential between the price of the sale to the third party and the (lower) price paid to the customer by the dealer.

MARK TO MARKET: Occurs when a broker/dealer demands more cash in a down market to maintain minimum requirements. The written notice for such demand is a mark-to-the-market.

MARKUP: The fee charged by a broker/dealer when a security is bought from a market maker and sold to a customer at a higher price. The markup is included in the sale price and is not itemized separately in the confirmation except on a simultaneous (risk less) transaction. Markup is the ratio of medical care price to marginal cost.

MARKUP/MARKDOWN POLICY: An NASD guideline that basically states a markup, markdown, or commission must be fair and reasonable, taking into consideration all relevant factors.

MARKET: An organized public arrangement where buyers and sellers meet to transact business. It is a product or service exchange.

MARKET 2 MARKET: Valuation process that provides an indication of reasonable prices for positions on a daily basis or some other proscribed time frame.

MARKET ACTIVITY: The supplying of health care labor through an exchange or marketplace.

MARKET APPROACH: A comparable value market approach method to appraising a health care firm or business entity based on similar or comparable values of entities in the same or similar health care space.

MARKET BASKET: A varied combination of health care products, goods, and services.

MARKET BASKET INDEX: An index of the annual change in the prices of goods and services providers used to produce health or other goods and services. There are separate market baskets for prospective payment systems (PPSs) hospital operating inputs and capital inputs, and Skilled Nursing Facilities, home health agencies, and renal dialysis facility operating and capital inputs.

MARKET BREAK: A sudden drop in the stock market.

MARKET CAPITALIZATION: The current stock price of a company multiplied by the number of common shares, outstanding. The higher the market capitalization is relative to book value, the more highly the investment community values the company's future.

MARKET CAPITALIZATION OF INVESTED CAPITAL: Market value of equity, plus the market value of the levered debt portion of invested capital.

MARKET CLEARING PRICE: A price at securities or related market equilibrium. Balanced prices.

MARKET CONSTRAINTS: The conditions in which health care firms can sell products and service outputs and purchase inputs.

MARKET DEMAND: The relationship of total health care product or service quantity demand with its price.

MARKET DEMAND CURVE: A curve that is downward sloping to the right showing the relationship between a health care product's price and the quantity demanded of those services.

MARKET DEMAND CURVE FOR LABOR: A curve showing the relationship between the price of health care labor and total amount of labor demanded for those services.

MARKET DEMAND FOR INPUT: The sum of quantity demanded by all health care entities and other employees using that input at any given price level.

MARKET ECONOMY: The coordination of individual health care choices in an exchange between medical service providers and patients.

MARKET EQUILIBRIUM: An economic condition of balanced demand and supply in health care, financial, business, or other markets.

MARKET FAILURE: Inability of the pricing system to allocate health care resources efficiently among buyers and sellers of products or services.

MARKET JITTERS: Uneasy feeling in the financial markets that might induce panic buying or selling.

MARKET MAKER: A NASD broker/dealer ready to provide continuing bids and offers for a given security in the secondary market. An exchange member on the trading floor who buys and sells for his own account and who is responsible for making bids and offers and maintaining a fair and orderly market.

MARKET MULTIPLE: The market value of a health care firm's invested capital or equity divided by a given benchmark measure, such as number of patients, economic benefits, and so forth.

MARKET ON CLOSE (MOC): The purchase or sale of securities as close to the final market bell (day closing) as possible.

MARKET ON OPENING (MOO): An order to buy or sell securities on the opening of a market. Typically, there is a brief period at the commencement of the day's trading which is defined as the opening. This period varies from market-to-market and exchange-to-exchange.

MARKET ORDER: A securities buy order executed immediately at the best available price. A trading instruction from an investor to a broker to immediately buy or sell a security at the best available price.

MARKET PERFORMANCE: A benchmark measure of financial markets, or securities performance.

MARKET PRICE OF RISK: A synonym for the Sharpe Ratio. *See* Sharpe, William, PhD, Ratio.

MARKET RATE: Competitive rate of return.

MARKET RATE INTEREST: The current fair value trade rate for the same or similar securities.

MARKET RISK: The tendency of a securities price to change with the overall marketplace, or systemic risk.

MARKET SHARE: The percentage of health care or other industry sales of a particular health care product, good, service, or company.

MARKET STRUCTURE: The type and number of competing firms in an industry sector, such as the health care industrial complex.

MARKET SUPPLY CURVE: A curve that is downward sloping to the right showing the relationship between a health care product's price and the quantity supplied.

MARKET SUPPLY CURVE; FOR LABOR: A curve showing the relationship between the price of health care labor and the total amount of labor supplied in the market.

MARKET SUPPLY OF INPUT: Ratio between price and quantity and quantity supplied of a health care input.

MARKET SWEEP: Institutional sales offer, after a public tender offer, in order to enhance company control.

MARKET TIMING: Buy and sell strategy based on general outlook, such as economic factors or interest rates, or on technical analysis. It involves trying to predict the gains and declines of the market and then buying at market lows and selling at market highs.

MARKET TONE: Emotional atmosphere of financial markets.

MARKET VALUE (MV): The price of medical or health care services bought or sold on the open market, with transparency, free flow of information, and no coercion.

MARKETABILITY: The ease or difficulty with which securities can be sold in the market. An issue's marketability depends upon many factors, including its interest rate, security provisions, maturity, and credit quality, plus (in the case of the sale of a new issue) the size of the issue, the timing of its issuance, and the volume of comparable issues being sold.

MARKETABILITY DISCOUNT: The dollar amount or percentage that is deducted from an equity interest to reflect a lack of marketability.

MARKETABLE: Easily sold liquid assets.

MARKETABLE SECURITIES: Investments and financial products easily sold and very liquid, such as short term claims that can be sold or bought in the capital markets (T-bills, CDs, short term paper loans), and stocks and other negotiable instruments that can be easily bought and sold on either listed exchanges or over-the-counter markets.

MARKETING: Moving medical goods, products, and services from the producers (doctors, hospitals, clinics, DME, drugs, etc.) to the consumers (patients, Medicare/Medicaid, HMOs, insurance companies, etc.).

MARRIED PUT STRATEGY: The simultaneous purchase of stock and the corresponding number of put options. This is a limited-risk strategy during the life of puts because the stock can be sold at the strike price of the puts.

MARRIED TAXPAYERS: Persons who file a joint tax return combining income and expenses. Individuals will be considered married if:

- They are living as husband and wife;
- They are recognized living together as a common law marriage; or
- They are legally married but separated and living apart, but not legally divorced.

Marriage is determined as of the last day of the tax year.

MARSHALLIAN DEMAND FUNCTION: Denotes $x(p,m)$ as the amount of a health care factor of production that is demanded by a medical care producer given that it costs p per unit and the budget limit that can be spent on all factors is m.

MARTIN ACT: SEC Act of 1934 and 1935 used to combat financial fraud. It grants document subpoena power to the New York Attorney General, to keep an investigation secret or public, to choose between filing civil or criminal charges, and to abrogate the right to counsel or against self-incrimination. In combination, the Act's powers exceed those given regulators in any other state.

MASTER BUDGET: Budgeting financial statements, supporting schedules, and information for an entire health care business enterprise.

MATCHED BOOK: The equalization of borrowing costs and interest rate costs.

MATCHED FUNDING: Asset and liability management technique that offsets fund sources to fund uses.

MATCHED-LOST PROCESS: A "flip of a coin" statistical probability.

MATCHING PRINCIPLE: A fundamental concept of basic accounting that suggests that in a given accounting period, one should try to match revenues with expenses.

MATCHING PRINCIPLE CONVENTION: The identification of expenses incurred during a reporting period in order to measure and match them against revenues in the same period.

MATCHING PRINCIPLE FINANCE: The economic suggestion that short-term financial needs should be addressed and satisfied with short-term resources and products, and long-term needs with long-term resources and financial products.

MATERIAL ITEM: Topic of financial significance in a health care or other business entity that must be noted in financial statements according to GAAP.

MATERIAL WEAKNESS: A significant deficiency or combination of significant deficiencies that results in more than a remote likelihood that a material misstatement of an annual report or interim financial statements will not be prevented or detected.

MATERIALITY: Magnitude of an omission or misstatements of accounting information that, in the light of surrounding circumstances, makes it probable that the judgment of a reasonable person relying on the information would change or be influenced.

MATERIALITY CONCEPT: Suggestion that proper accounting is performed only for items and transactions that are significant to business financial statements.

MATERIALS BALANCE: Place where input supply equals its demand for an intermediate health care product or service.

MATURITY: The date on which a loan, bond, or debenture comes due. Both the principal and any accrued interest due must be paid.

MAVES, MICHAEL, MD: CEO of the American Medical Association in Chicago, Illinois.

MAXIMUM ALLOWABLE CHARGE (MAC): The amount set by an insurance company as the highest amount that can be charged for a particular medical product or service. It is the limit on billed or invoiced charges for Medicare patients by nonparticipating providers.

MAXIMUM ALLOWABLE COST (MAC) LIST: A list of prescriptions where the reimbursement will be based on the cost of the generic product.

MAXIMUM CLAIM LIABILITY: The highest amount of insurance claims for which a group is held liable.

MAXIMUM OUT OF POCKET COST: A predetermined limited amount of money an individual must pay out of pocket, before an insurance company or self-insured employer will pay 100% for an individual's health care expenses.

MAY DAY DECISION: The expiration date of fixed brokerage commission in the United States (May 1, 1975).

MCCLELLAN, MARK, MD: Health care economist and administrator of CMS in Baltimore, Maryland.

MCCLURE, WALTER, PhD: Nationally known health care economist and one of the original Four Horsemen of managed medical care from the Jackson Hole Group, in Wyoming. He is a former President of the Center for Health Policy Studies.

MCGUINNESS, THOMAS P., CPA, CVA, CMP©: Medical practice valuation expert and past president of the National CPA Health Advisory Association (NCPAHAA), in Houston, Texas.

MCGUIRE, WILLIAM: Chairman and CEO of the United Health Care Group in Minnetonka, Minnesota.

MCKENNA, MARK: President of Novation in Irving, Texas.

MEAN (ARITHMETIC): The measure of central location commonly called the average. It is calculated by adding together all the individual values and dividing by the number of values in the group. The simple unweighted mean of four observations, 8, 12, 10, and 14, is 11. This statistic is computed by $(8 + 12 + 10 + 14 = 44)$ 44 divided by 4.

MEAN (GEOMETRIC): The mean or average of a set of data measured on a logarithmic scale. The geometric mean of these four arithmetic mean observations, $8 + 12 + 10 + 14$, is 10.77. It is computed by multiplying each observed value and then deriving the nth root of that number. The geometric mean can only be equal to or less than the comparable arithmetic mean.

MEAN RATE OF RETURN: The return that is between two extreme returns.

MEAN REVERSION: Postulate that short-term rates, appreciation, or volatilities will move toward longer term averages.

MEAN VARIANCE FRAMEWORK: The graphic visual relationship between standard deviation (risk) and the expected return on an investment (rate of return) (see Figure 3).

MEANEY, BRIDGET: Editor of *COR Health Care Market Strategist* in Santa Barbara, California.

MEANS TEST: Income standards above or below certain accepted values. Medicare affluence benchmark.

MECKLENBURG, GARY: President and CEO of Northwestern Memorial Health Care in Chicago, Illinois.

MEDIAN: The measure of central location that divides a set of data into two equal parts.

MEDICAID: A Title 19 Federal program that is managed and partially funded by individual states to provide medical benefits to certain low-income people. Each individual state, under broad federal guidelines, determines what

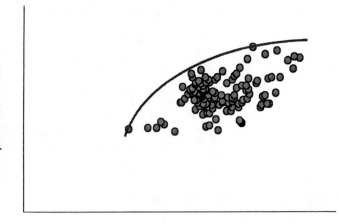

Figure 3: Mean-Variance Framework.

benefits are covered, who is eligible, and how much providers will be paid. Historically, all states but Arizona have Medicaid programs.

- MEDICAID 1115 WAIVER: state administration exemption to speed claims processing.
- MEDICAID 1915(b) WAIVER: alternate local, regional, or state managed care model.

MEDICAL COST RATIO (MCR): Compares the cost of providing a service to the amount paid for the service.

MEDICAL ECONOMIC VALUE ADDED© (MEVA©): Concept that combines finance and accounting income to determine medical practice, clinic, hospital, or other health care business-enterprise entity operations value as an ongoing concern. It is also referred to as economic medical value added.

MEDICAL SAVINGS ACCOUNT (MSA): A health insurance option consisting of a high-deductible insurance policy and a tax-advantaged savings account. Patients pay individually for health care up to the annual deductible by withdrawing from a savings account or paying out of pocket. The policy pays for most covered services once the high deductible is met. Employees can make tax-free contributions but instead of withdrawing the funds at retirement, they are used to pay for certain types of medical care with cheaper pretax dollars. Money accumulates inside the MSA for later use when medical expenses are higher, or saved for retirement. MSAs that are exempt from federal income taxes were part of a demonstration project that began in 1997 and was scheduled to end in 2000, until Congress renewed it through 2011. A number of states also permit employers to establish state tax-exempt MSAs.

MEDICAL SAVINGS ACCOUNT MODEL (MSA-MODEL): A self-employed patient who purchases a high-deductible major medical plan (catastrophic health plan). In 2004, the deductible was set at a minimum of $1,750–2,750 for individual coverage and $3,350–5,050 for family coverage. The family deductible limit was $5,250 in 2005 and $5,450 in 2006 indexed periodically for inflation. Individual owners may make tax-free contributions, but total annual contributions are limited to 65% of the deductible for individuals and 75% of the deductible for families. In addition to the high-deductible health policy, employees may open up a MSA savings/investment account. Contributions are deductible from adjusted gross income, and contributions made by an employer are excluded from income unless part of a cafeteria plan. Contributions may be made for a tax year at any time until the due date of the return for that year. Employer contributions must be reported on the employee's W-2. Earnings of the fund are not included in taxable income for the current year. Funds may be withdrawn from the MSA-models, tax-free, to pay for minor medical expenses. If funds are withdrawn for nonmedical purposes, a 15% penalty is assessed and the funds are taxed as ordinary income. At age 65, the

MSA may be used for any purpose, and pay only the tax on withdrawn funds. *See also* health savings account (HSA); medical savings account (MSA),

MEDICAL SPENDING ACCOUNT: A type of flexible medical savings account, such as a MSA, FSA, and HSA. You must use it or lose it.

MEDICARE: A nationwide, federal health insurance program for those aged 65 and older. It also covers certain people under 65 who are disabled or have chronic kidney disease. Medicare Part A is the hospital insurance program. Part B covers physicians' services. It was created by the 1965 Title 18 amendment to the Social Security Act:

- MEDICARE PART A: Medicare compulsory hospital compensation program, financed through payroll taxes shared by employers and employees alike. Most folks do not pay a premium because they or a spouse have 40 or more quarters of Medicare-covered employment. It is provided free to anyone who qualifies for Medicare benefits but the deductible that pays for inpatient hospital, skilled nursing facility, and some home health care, was $912 in 2005. The Part A deductible is the beneficiary's only cost for up to 60 days of Medicare-covered inpatient hospital care. However, for extended Medicare-covered hospital stays, beneficiaries paid an additional $228 per day for days 61–90 in 2005, and $456 per day for hospital stays beyond the 90th day in a benefit period. For beneficiaries in skilled nursing facilities, the daily coinsurance for days 21–100 was $114 in 2005. However, seniors and certain persons under age 65 with disabilities who have fewer than 30 quarters of coverage may obtain Part A coverage by paying a monthly premium set according to a formula in the Medicare statute at $343 for 2004. In addition, seniors with 30–39 quarters of coverage, and certain disabled persons with 30 or more quarters of coverage, are entitled to pay a reduced premium of $189. All indexed annually (see www.hhs.gov/news/).

  - Coinsurance

    - $228.00 a day for the 61st–90th day each benefit period.
    - $456.00 a day for the 91st–150th day for each lifetime reserve day (total of 60 lifetime reserve days—nonrenewable).

  - *Skilled Nursing Facility Coinsurance:* Up to $114 a day for days 21–100 in each benefit period (indexed annually).

- MEDICARE PART B: Medicare physician compensation program. This is supplementary medical insurance and covers most of what isn't covered by Part A and is paid for by the insured individual via an enrollment program. For 2005 the monthly premium was $78.20, and the coverage also involved a $110 annual deductible and a 20% per service coinsurance (indexed annually).

- MEDICARE PART C: Medicare managed care compensation program, known as *Medicare + Choice* and initiated in 1997. If a beneficiary chooses Part C, it takes the place of Parts A and B. Part C is basically a Medicare HMO plan. In 2000–2004 many carriers ceased offering this type of coverage, and those individuals who had elected to go with a Medicare HMO had to backtrack and re-enroll in the original Medicare fee-for-service program (Parts A and B). This may again change beyond 2005 as traditional Medicare premiums continue to increase. Another name for this program is Medicare Advantage.
- MEDICARE PART D: Medicare Prescription Drug Benefits program which began on January 1, 2006. Most seniors are eligible to participate and most drugs are covered. Economics benefits, premiums, and deductibles will vary and will be indexed annually:

  - *Premium:* Part D premium is $35 per month ($420 annually). This premium is in addition to the Part B premium (automatically deducted from Social Security checks each month, for most patients).
  - *Annual Deductible:* Patients pay the first $250 of prescription drug expenses.
  - *Coinsurance:* Medicare pays 75% of costs between $250 and $2,250. Patients pay the other 25% out of pocket, or a maximum of $500 for coinsurance.
  - *Coverage Gap.* After total prescription drugs expenses reach $2,250, Medicare pays nothing until the patient has spent a total of $3,600 out of pocket (hole). The $3,600 includes the $250 deductible and $500 coinsurance maximum.
  - *Catastrophic Protection:* After spending $3,600, Medicare covers 95% of prescription drug expenses for the remainder of the year.
  - *Low-Income Assistance:* Patients eligible for both Medicare and Medicaid pay no premium, no deductible, and have no gap in coverage. They pay a $1 co-payment per prescription for generic drugs, and a $3 co-payment per prescription for brand name drugs.

MEDICARE APPROVED AMOUNT (MAA): The Medicare payment amount for a covered service that may be less than the actual amount charged.

MEDICARE COST CONTRACT (MCC): A contract between Medicare and a health plan under which the plan is paid on the basis of reasonable costs to provide some or all of Medicare-covered services for enrollees.

MEDICARE COST REPORT (MCR): An annual report required of all institutions participating in the Medicare program. The MCR records each institution's total costs and charges associated with providing services to all patients, the portion of those costs and charges allocated to Medicare patients, and the Medicare payments received.

MEDICARE ECONOMIC INDEX (MEI): An index that tracks changes over time in physician practice costs. From 1975 through the present, increases in prevailing charge screens are limited to increases in the MEI.

MEDICARE FEE SCHEDULE: A list of the costs and payments to medical providers regardless of location or specialty, based on RBRVS. A national total RVU (physician labor, practice expenses, and malpractice liability insurance cost) is assigned for each procedure (HCPCS Level 1 [CPT], Level 2 codes) by a physician (see Table 5).

Table 5: Medicare Costs for Covered Services

Part A: Covered services	What patients pay	Part B: Covered services	What patients pay
Hospital stays: Semiprivate room, meals, general nursing and other hospital services and supplies.	$840 for hospital stay of 1–60 days. $210 per day for days 61–90. $420 per day for days 91–150. All costs beyond 150 days.	**Medical expenses:** Doctors' services, inpatient and outpatient medical and surgical services, supplies, speech, occupational and physical therapy and related medical equipment.	$100 deductible per year. 20% of approved amount after the deductible, except in outpatient setting. 50% for most outpatient mental health. 20% for all ocupational therapy services.
Skilled nursing facility care: Semiprivate room, meals, skilled nursing services and supplies.	$0 for first 20 days. Up to $105 a day for days 21–100. All costs beyond 100th day in benefit period.	**Clinical laboratory services**	$0

(Continued)

Table 5: Continued

Part A: Covered services	What patients pay	Part B: Covered services	What patients pay
Home health care: Intermittent skilled nursing care, physical therapy, speech language pathology services, home health aide services, medical equipment (such as wheelchairs and hospital beds) and supplies and other services.	$0 for home health care services. 20% of approved amount for medical equipment.	**Home health care:** (If you don't have Part A.) Intermittent skilled care, home health aide services and supplies.	$0 for services. 20% of approved medical equipment costs.
Hospice care: Pain and symptom relief and support services. Home care is provided.	Limited costs for outpatient drugs and inpatient respite care.	**Outpatient hospital services:** Services for diagnosis and treatment of illness or injury.	No less than 20% of Medicare payment amount (after deductible).
Blood: From a hospital or skilled nursing facility during a stay.	For first three pints.	**Blood:** As outpatient or as part of Part B covered service.	First three pints plus 20% of approved amount for additional pints (after deductible).

Source: Medicare

MEDICARE INTEGRITY PROGRAM: Allows HHS to contract with nongovernmental organizations, known as Medicare Program Safeguard Contractors, to carry out fraud and abuse detection, cost report audits, utilization review, provider payment determinations, and provider education, and create a list of durable medical equipment subject to prior authorization for reimbursement. Under this program, the Center for Medicare and Medicaid Services (CMS) is required to implement regulations.

MEDICARE MEDICAL SAVINGS ACCOUNT (MMSA): Medicare health insurance with a high deductible, along with a savings account to pay health care expenses and medical bills.

MEDICARE REBATE: Tax-free Medicare deposit option into a modified medical savings account that excludes high-deductible MSAs and high-deductible HSAs.

MEDICARE SECONDARY PAYER: Medicare as a secondary payer when other insurance is available to those over age 65 or with end stage renal disease (ESRD).

MEDICARE SUPPLEMENT: Private insurance that pays health care costs not covered by Medicare.

MEDICARE TRUST FUND: Pay-as-you-go Medicare Part A fund artifice from payroll tax contributions, as hospital costs outpace revenue and contributions.

MEDICHOICE: Medicare+Choice. A Medicare HMO plan.

MEDIGAP: Medicare payment omission and coverage lapses filled by private insurance policies designed to supplement Medicare coverage, called Medigap policies. There are 10 standard Medigap policies designated by the letters A through J. Medigap policies (including Medicare SELECT) can only be sold in 10 standardized plans (see Table 6). The basic benefits included in all plans are:

- *Inpatient Hospital Care:* Covers the Part A coinsurance and the cost of 365 extra days of hospital lifetime care after coverage ends.
- *Medical Costs:* Covers the Part B coinsurance (generally 20% of the Medicare-approved payment amount).
- *Blood:* Covers the first three pints of blood each year.

MELT DOWN: A sharp decline or collapse in financial values. It tends to be used for broader indicators such as market indices or asset classes such as health care REITs or ETFs.

MELT UP: A sharp advance or increase in financial values. Tends to be used for broader indicators such as market indices or asset classes.

MEMBER: A person eligible to receive, or one currently receiving, benefits from Medicare, an HMO, or other health insurance policy. Includes both those who have enrolled or subscribed and their eligible dependents:

- Member Month (MM): For each member, the recorded count of the months that the member is covered. Per Member per Month (PMPM). *See also* capitation.
- Members Per Year (MPY): The number of members eligible for health plan coverage on a yearly basis.

MEMBER BANK: A bank in the Federal Reserve Bank (FRB) system.

MEMBER FIRM: A brokerage firm with membership on at least one financial stock exchange.

Table 6: Chart of Ten Standardized Medigap Plans A through J

	A	B	C	D	E	F*	G	H	I	J
Basic Benefit	√	√	√	√	√	√	√	√	√	√
Skilled nursing coinsurance			√	√	√	√	√	√	√	√
Part A deductible		√	√	√	√	√	√	√	√	√
Part B deductible			√			√				
Part B excess						√ (100%)	√ (80%)		√ (100%)	√ (100%)
Foreign travel emergency			√	√	√	√	√	√	√	√
At-home recovery				√			√		√	√
Drug benefit								√ (Basic $1,250 Limit)	√ Basic $1,250 Limit)	√ (Extended $2,500 Limit)
Preventive care					√					√

Source: Medicare.gov Web site.

* Plans F and J also have a high-deductible option. This chart is not applicable for all states. Contact your State Insurance Commission for more information.

MEMBER MONTH: The inclusive time frame and economic premium/benefit cost in which a health plan member is included in the plan, including retro additions and deletions.

MERCANTILE AGENCY: A supplier of credit ratings and other financial, accounting, and economic information.

MERGER: The combination of a single firm, from two or more existing companies.

MERGERS AND ACQUISITIONS METHOD: Valuation market approach method that derives pricing multiples from prior transactions relative to similar or same companies in the same health care industry space.

META ANALYSIS: A systematic, typically quantitative method for combining financial information from multiple studies.

MEZZANINE LEVEL: The time period just prior to the initial public offering (IPO) of a health care organization or other company.

MICROECONOMICS: Price theory or the study of choices made by individuals or patients in the health care industrial complex.

MICROHEDGE: A specific transaction aimed at the risk of a clearly identifiable securities trade or position. Generally, these hedges are less efficient than macrohedges for complex investment portfolios.

MID CAP: Companies with a mid-level market capitalization rate (share number outstanding times share price), usually between 1 and 5 billion dollars.

MIDLETON, BLACKFORD: Chairman of the Health Care Information and Management Systems Society in Chicago, Illinois.

MIDYEAR DISCOUNTING: Valuation discounted future earning method that relays economic benefits generated at midyear while estimating the same benefits generated for the remainder of the year.

MIG: The designation used by Moody's Investors Service in rating municipal notes. The term is an acronym for Moody's Investment Grade and, in specific ratings, is followed by the number 1, 2, 3, or 4, denoting successively lower levels of quality.

MILL: One tenth (1/10) of a penny.

MILLER, MARK: Executive Director of the Medical Payment Advisory Commission (MedPAC), in Washington, D.C.

MINIMUM AMOUNT DUE: A loan payment option that covers the minimum amount due monthly. With many adjustable rate loans, payment may not always cover the total interest due. This unpaid portion is called deferred interest and is added to the loan balance. Other loan payment options do not provide for deferred interest.

MINIMUM MAINTENANCE: Lowest amount of equity in a brokerage margin account permissible.

MINIMUM PAYMENT: The minimum amount owed, usually monthly, on a loan or line of credit. In some plans, the minimum payment may be interest only (simple interest). In other plans, the minimum payment may include principal and interest (amortized).

MINIMUM WAGE: Hourly amount paid to workers according to federal statute.

MINORITY DISCOUNT: The dollar amount or percentage deducted from the pro rata share of the value of an entire business to reflect the absence of the power of control.

MINORITY INTEREST: Less than 50% ownership or voting interest in a health care or other business entity.

MINUS TICK: A transaction on the Stock Exchange at a price below the previous transaction in a given security.

MISCELLANEOUS EXPENSE: Ancillary expenses, usually hospital charges other than daily room and board. Examples would be x-rays, drugs, and lab fees. The total amount of such charges that will be reimbursed is limited in most basic hospitalization policies.

MISERY INDEX: Emotional benchmark combining the inflation and unemployment rates.

MIXED COST: A part fixed and part variable cost.

MIXED GOOD: Health care products and services that are a hybrid of private and public benefit.

MOB SPREAD: Yield differential between Federal Treasury and State Municipal bonds.

MODE: A measure of central location, the most frequently occurring value in a set of health data points.

MODE OF PAYMENT: The frequency with which health insurance premiums or other medical bills are paid (e.g., annually, semiannually, monthly, etc.).

MODEL: Mathematical design, reproduction, research and forecast of an economic, financial, or accounting situation.

MODERN PORTFOLIO THEORY: An approach to financial portfolio management that uses statistical measures to develop a portfolio plan. Economic diversification. The theory was developed by Harry Horowitz, PhD, Nobel Laureate in 1990.

MODIFIED ACCELERATED COST RECOVERY SYSTEM (MACRS): Similar to ACRS. Under MACRS the cost of eligible property is recovered over a 3-, 5-, 7-, 10-, 15-, 20-, 27.5-, 31.5-, or 39-year period, depending on the type of property using statutory recovery methods and conventions. It generally applies to most tangible depreciable property placed in service after 1986.

MODIFIED CASH ACCOUNTING: Modification of cash basis accounting in which certain items are included in financial statements (i.e., depreciation).

MODIFIED DURATION: The representation of a bond's weighted cash flow stream. It adjusts the Macaulay Duration by taking into account the yield in the market and the frequency of coupon payments in a year. Modified duration is less than the standard duration. It is computed as: Duration ÷ (1 + yield in market ÷ coupons in year).

MODIFIED FFS: A reduced or discounted fee-for-service medical payment system.

MODIFIER: CPT code suffix acting as a descriptive attachment for reimbursement:

- Level I: descriptive suffix
- Level II: AA–ZZ national carrier code descriptors
- Level III: local and regional code descriptors phased out in 2003
- Pet Scan Modifiers (SCM):

  - N = negative
  - E = equivocal
  - P = positive, not suggestive of ischemia
  - S = positive, suggestive of ischemia

- Ambulance Modifiers (AM):

  - D = other than physician's office
  - E = residence, domicile, or custodial facility
  - G = hospital-based dialysis facility
  - H = hospital
  - I = site of transfer
  - J = non-hospital-based dialysis facility
  - N = skilled nursing facility
  - P = physician's office
  - R = residence
  - S = scene of accident
  - X = intermediate stop

MODIGLIANI-MILLER THEOREM: Suggests that the total value of the bonds and equities issued by a firm is independent or insensitive to the number of bonds outstanding or their interest rate. Nobel Laureates Franco Modigliani and Merton-Miller formed modern thinking on capital structure in 1958, suggesting dividend policy does not matter.

MOLINA, MARIO: Chairman, CEO, and President of Molina Health Care in Long Beach, California.

MOMENTUM: Rate of economic, business, or financial acceleration.

MONETARIST: Belief that money supply is the most important economic factor in the United States.

MONETARY POLICY: Federal Reserve Board (FRB) actions that determine the rate and size of money supply growth and interest rates, through the Federal Open Market Committee (FOMC).

MONETIZATION: A strategy that allows an investor to generate cash from a position without realizing a sale of the underlying position.

MONEY: Physical or electronic medium, and common exchange denominator of value.

MONEY MARKET: Market for cash, ultra short-term debt issues and checks.

MONEY MARKET ACCOUNT (MMA): A checking account that earns interest comparable to money market funds, although the rates paid by any particular bank may be higher or lower.

MONEY MARKET DEPOSIT ACCOUNT (MMDA): An account instrument offered at a banking institution that has features similar to a money market mutual fund. Accounts under $100,000 are insured by the Federal Deposit Insurance Corporation.

MONEY MARKET FUND (MMF): An investment vehicle whose primary objective is to make higher interest securities available to the average investor who wants immediate income and high investment safety. This is accomplished through the purchase of high-yield money market instruments, such as U.S. government securities, bank certificates of deposit, and commercial paper.

MONEY MARKET INSTRUMENTS: Obligations that are commonly traded in the money market. Money market instruments are generally short term and highly liquid.

MONEY MARKET MUTUAL FUND (MMMF): A registered investment company that invests in securities that have short-term maturities (usually from several days to several weeks). It is an investment vehicle whose primary objective is to make higher interest securities available to the average investor who wants immediate income and high investment safety. This is accomplished through the purchase of high-yield money market instruments, such as U.S. government securities, bank certificates of deposit, and commercial paper.

MONEY SUPPLY: The amount of money in circulation. The money supply measures currently (as of 1985) used by the Federal Reserve System are:

- M1—Currency in circulation + demand deposit + other check-type deposits.
- M2—M1 + savings and small denomination time deposits + overnight repurchase agreements at commercial banks + overnight Eurodollars + money market mutual fund shares.

- M3—M2 + large denomination time deposits (Jumbo CDs) + term repurchase agreements.
- M4—M3 + other liquid assets (such as term Eurodollars, bankers acceptances, commercial paper, Treasury securities and U.S. Savings Bonds).

MONGAN, JAMES: Health care economist and President of Partners Health Care Systems in Boston, Massachusetts.

MONOPOLY POWER: The ability of a health care entity to influence its price by making more or less product or service available to patients.

MONOPSONY POWER: A single input purchaser in a health care market without rivals.

MONTE CARLO SIMULATIONS: Financial outcomes data obtained by simulating a statistical model in which all parameters are numerically specified, as in an investment portfolio risk and return model.

MOODY'S INVESTMENT GRADE (MIG): Rating assigned by Moody's Investors Service, Inc. (MIS).

MOODY'S INVESTORS SERVICE, INC. (MIS): An independent service subsidiary of Dun & Bradstreet that provides debt and solvency ratings to various financial services companies of hospital and municipal securities and other financial information to health care sector and other investors.

MORAL BACKING: Nonlegal backing of a debt issue.

MORAL HAZARD: Patients who change their health care behavior in unforeseen ways due to health insurance, money, or lack thereof.

MORAL OBLIGATION BOND: A bond, typically issued by a state agency or authority, that is secured by the revenues from the financed project and, additionally, by a nonbinding undertaking that any deficiency in pledged revenues will be reported to the state legislature which may apportion state monies to make up the shortfall. Legislation authorizing the issuance of moral obligation securities typically grants the state legislature the authority to apportion money to support the debt service payments on any such securities, but does not legally oblige the legislature to do so.

MORAL SUASION: Exhortations to follow suit in the absence of legal enforcement powers.

MORNINGSTAR RATING SYSTEM: System for ranking and rating closed- and open-ended investments (mutual funds) and annuities by Chicago-based Morningstar, Inc.

MORTGAGE: Creditor claim (loan) on real estate assets. *See also* collateral; promissory note.

MORTGAGE BACKED SECURITIES (MBS): A term that encompasses generic and specific securities predicated on real property, such as:

- Accrual or Accretion Bond
- ARMs

- Companion or Support
- Constant Maturity Treasury
- Floaters
- Gnomes
- Gold
- Inverse Floaters or Reverse Floaters
- Interest Only (IO)
- IO-ette or IOette
- Jump Bonds
- Jump Z
- Mega
- PAC PO
- Pass Throughs
- Planned Amortization Class
- Principal Only (PO)
- Reverse TAC
- Scheduled Bonds
- Stripped Mortgage Backed Securities
- Super Floater
- Super PAC
- Super PO
- Support
- Targeted Amortization Class
- VADM
- Z Bond
- Z PAC

MORTGAGE BOND: The most prevalent type of secured corporate bond, as bondholders are protected by the pledge of a corporation's real assets (real estate), evaluated at the time of issuance.

MORTGAGEE: One who is the lending party in a mortgage transaction.

MORTGAGOR: One who is the borrowing party in a mortgage transaction.

MOST ACTIVE LIST: Equities with the most shares traded on a specific day.

MOVING AVERAGE: The omission of the most distant price data (technical analysis), and the inclusion of the most recent price data, when computing the average or mean price securities or markets. It is an oversold or overbought measurement.

MR = MC RULE: Marginal revenue (MR) equals marginal cost (MC) for an economic profit-maximizing health care entity.

MULTINATIONAL FIRM: A firm that makes direct investments in other countries.

MULTIPLE: Inverse of a capitalization rate. The relative multiple is the company's P/E ratio relative to the multiple of the market, usually the S&P 500, but sometimes the price/earnings ratio of an index that more closely mirrors the company's sector.

MULTIPLE PARTY ACCOUNT: Account owned by two or more parties. Parties own the account during the lifetime of all parties in proportion to their net contributions, unless there is clear and convincing evidence of a different intent.

MULTIPLIER EFFECT: Money supply expansion from Federal Reserve member banks who lend money, enhancing its supply.

MULTISERVICE FIRM: A health care company that provides many different products and services.

MULTIYEAR BUDGET: A budget for more than a year, and usually 2 to 5 years.

MUNDELL TOBIN EFFECT: Suggestion that nominal interest rates rise less than one-for-one with inflation because patients and the public hold less in money balances and more in other assets, which would drive interest rates down. Suggested by Robert R. Mundell, 1965.

MUNI: Slang term for municipal (bond) security.

MUNICIPAL BOND FUND: A mutual fund that invests in a broad range of tax-exempt bonds issued by state, city, and other local governments. The interest obtained from these bonds is passed through to share owners free of federal tax. The fund's primary objective is current income, while health care systems, clinics, entities, and hospitals are often included in the fund.

MUNICIPAL BOND INSURANCE ASSOCIATION (MBIA): An association of five insurance companies (The Aetna Casualty & Surety Co., Fireman's Fund Insurance Companies, The Travelers Indemnity Company, CIGNA Corporation, and The Continental Insurance Company) that offers insurance policies on qualified municipal issues under which the payment of principal and interest when due is guaranteed, in the event of issuer default. The two principal rating agencies assign their highest ratings to all municipal issues insured by MBIA Members.

MUNICIPAL BONDS: Municipal bonds issued by state and local governments for building schools, bridges, hospitals, clinics or health care systems, and other municipal facilities. These bonds depend upon their tax base to generate the income to pay the interest and retire the debt. The most important feature of municipal bonds is their tax-exempt status, and although the interest earned is free from federal income tax, state and local governments may levy taxes on that income. Because of the tax advantage, municipalities can borrow at lower rates of interest than can corporations. Investors benefit because the tax advantages associated with the interest, albeit lower than that of corporate or government bonds, may provide a higher rate of return. Municipal bonds are usually sold in increments of $5,000 or more, although municipal bond funds may have lower minimums. Municipal bonds are available in various types, depending upon whether the debt is paid by the issuing authority or by the revenue earned from the facility.

MUNICIPAL SECURITIES RULEMAKING BOARD (MSRB): An independent self-regulatory organization established by the Securities Acts Amendment of 1975, which is charged with primary rulemaking authority over dealers, dealer banks, and brokers in municipal securities. Its 15 members represent three categories—securities firms, bank dealers, and the public—each category having equal representation on the Board.

MUNIFACTS: A private wire communication system originating in the New York editorial offices of The Bond Buyer. Munifacts transmits current bond market information that is printed out on terminals located in the offices of its subscribers.

MURPHY, EDWARD L., MD: President and CEO of the California Health System in San Francisco, California.

MUTATIS MUTANDIS: Substituting new terms for older health care economic and financial assumptions.

MUTILATED CERTIFICATE (NOTE OR BOND): A certificate which has been torn, defaced, or otherwise damaged to such an extent that information needed at the time of its redemption or to assure its validity is no longer ascertainable. A mutilated certificate cannot be used in a delivery until the certificate has been validated. The standards used in evaluating whether a certificate is mutilated are set forth in MSRB Rule G-12(e)(ix).

MUTILATED COUPON: A coupon that has been torn, defaced, or otherwise damaged to such an extent that information needed at the time of its redemption or to assure its validity is no longer ascertainable. A security to which a mutilated coupon is attached cannot be used in a delivery until the coupon has been validated. The standards used in evaluating whether a coupon is mutilated are set forth in MSRB Rule G-12(e)(vii).

MUTUAL COMPANY: A company that has no capital stock or stockholders. Rather, it is owned by its policyowners and managed by a board of directors chosen by the policyowners. Any earnings, in addition to those necessary for the operation of the company and contingency reserves, are returned to the policyowners in the form of policy dividends.

MUTUAL FUND: An open-end company is a financial institution whose business is investing other people's money. By pooling their resources, investors obtain supervision and diversification of their investments. Mutual fund shares are ordinarily redeemable by the holder at any time at net asset value. Most new shares are offered for sale continuously at net asset value plus a fixed percentage as a sales charge. The assets of a mutual fund are the actual securities that it purchases, and its income consists of the dividends and interest on these securities. The earnings of the business are paid out in the form of dividends and capital gains distributions to the shareholders. Mutual funds do not issue bonds, debentures, or preferred stock.

MUTUAL FUND SYMBOL: Five letter exchange symbol ending with an X.

MUTUALIZATION: The process of converting a stock insurance company to a mutual insurance company, accomplished by having the company buy in and retire its own shares.

N

N: Commodity futures symbol for a July delivery month.

NAKED OPTION: An uncovered option position. When the writer (seller) of a call option owns the underlying stock (said to be long the stock), the option position is a covered call. If the writer (seller) of a put option is short the stock, then the position is a covered put. Writing a covered call is the most conservative options strategy, but writing a covered put is the most dangerous because there is no limit to how high the stock can go and thus to how great the loss can be on the short sale.

NAKED OPTION WRITING: Selling of a naked (unowned) option.

NARROW SPREAD: A small difference in asked and bid securities prices.

NASDAQ: National Association of Securities Dealers Automated Quotations (NASDAQ).

NASDAQ COMPOSITE INDEX: A market-value weighted index of the stocks listed on the NASDAQ over-the-counter exchange.

NASDAQ STOCK MARKET: This index is often used as an indicator of the performance of small company stocks.

NASH, DAVID, MD, MBA: The Dr. Raymond C. and Doris N. Grandon Professor of Health Policy and Medicine at Jefferson Medical College of Thomas Jefferson University in Philadelphia, Pennsylvania. He is a board certified internist who directs the Office of Health Policy and Clinical Outcomes, which he founded in 1990. He was named the first Associate Dean for Health Policy at Jefferson Medical College in 1996, and is a graduate of the Wharton School.

NASH EQUILIBRIUM: A competitive market theory that suggests that health care entities operate most efficiently when given the economic, financial, operational, and marketing decision of others.

NATIONAL ASSOCIATION OF SECURITIES DEALERS, INC. (NASD): A voluntary association of broker/dealers in over-the-counter securities organized on a nonprofit, non-stock-issuing basis. The general aim is to protect investors in the OTC market. It is the Self-Regulatory Organization (SRO) for broker/dealers in the OTC market.

NATIONAL ASSOCIATION OF SECURITIES DEALERS AUTOMATED QUOTATIONS (NASDAQ): An electronic data terminal device furnishing subscribers with instant identification of market makers and their current quotations, updated continuously.

NATIONAL CPA HEALTHCARE ADVISORS ASSOCIATION (NCPAHAA): A nonprofit association of accomplished CPA firms committed to providing high-quality financial and consulting services to health care professionals, based in Omaha, Nebraska.

NATIONAL CREDIT UNION ADMINISTRATION: An agency of the U.S. government that insures deposits in health care and other credit unions.

NATIONAL CREDIT UNION SHARE INSURANCE FUND: A program of the National Credit Union Administration that insures shareholders of credit unions.

NATIONAL COVERAGE POLICY: Medicare coverage and payment decisions that apply to all U.S. states.

NATIONAL HEALTH INSURANCE: Financial, access, and delivery systems where all citizens have access to health care services, goods, and products, including drugs.

NATIONAL INCOME AND PRODUCT ACCOUNTS (NIPA): A GDP account for the United States.

NATIONAL MEDIAN CHARGE: The middle amount of all amounts charged for the same medical service. This means that half of the hospitals and community mental health centers charged more than this amount, while the other half charged less than this amount for the same service.

NATIONAL UNIFORM BILLING COMMITTEE (NUBC): An organization chaired and hosted by the American Hospital Association that maintains the UB-92 hardcopy institutional billing form and the data element specifications for both the hardcopy form and the 192-byte UB-92 flat file EMC format. The NUBC has a formal consultative role under HIPAA for all transactions affecting institutional health care services.

NATIONAL UNIFORM CLAIM COMMITTEE (NUCC): An organization chaired and hosted by the American Medical Association that maintains the HCFA-1500 claim form and a set of data element specifications for professional claims submission via the HCFA-1500 claim form, the Professional EMC NSF, and the X12 837. The NUCC also maintains the provider taxonomy codes and has a formal consultative role under HIPAA for all transactions affecting nondental, noninstitutional professional health care services.

NATIONALIZED INDUSTRY: Company or industry owned and operated by a public authority, such as a city charity hospital.

NATURAL MONOPOLY: A single seller in the marketplace due to some competitive advantage or externality.

NATURAL PREMIUM: The premium that is sufficient to pay for a given amount of insurance from one premium date to the next. A policy issued on this basis is called a *yearly renewable term policy,* and the net natural premium rate for it is called a *yearly renewable term rate.* The premium advances each year with the age of the insured. The yearly renewable term plan is usually impracticable because, at the older ages, few persons can afford or are willing to pay the necessary premiums.

NAV MUTUAL FUND: Assets minus Liabilities.

NAV MUTUAL FUND SHARES: Fund Net Asset Value / Number Shares Outstanding; NAV / NSO.

NEAMAN, MARK: President and CEO of Northwestern Health Care in Evanston, Illinois, and chairman of the American College of Health Care Executives in Chicago, Illinois.

NEAR MONEY: Assets that can be quickly converted into cash, such as government bills and notes.

NECESSITY: An economic good or service whose consumption does not vary greatly with changes in personal income and is relatively resistant to the business cycle, as in health care.

NEGATIVE AMORTIZATION: Deficit financing where payments are less than borrowing costs, thereby increasing the principle amount rather than decreasing it.

NEGATIVE ASSURANCE: Accounting report based on limited procedures that states that nothing has come to attention to indicate that the financial information is not fairly presented.

NEGATIVE CARRY: Deficit financing where payments for financial futures positions are less than borrowing costs, thereby increasing the principle amount rather than decreasing it

NEGATIVE EXTERNALITY: Cost not reflected in the price associated with the use of health care resources and inputs.

NEGATIVE LEVERAGE: Opportunity cost loss associated with the purchase of an option on a future. This is due to the fact that futures can be initially margined with certain approved securities whereby the client continues to collect interest.

NEGATIVE PLEDGE: A bond or debt terms and conditions restricting liens on real estate to other creditors, as in a covenant.

NEGATIVE RELATIONSHIP: Two financial, health care, or other economic variables that move opposite one another, for example, smoking and cost containments.

NEGATIVE WORKING CAPITAL: Situation where current liabilities exceed current assets.

NEGATIVE YIELD CURVE: Graphical illustration where long-term interest rates are less than short-term interest rates.

NEGATIVELY CORRELATED: Two financial securities that move in opposite directions.

NEGLECTED FIRM EFFECT: Tendency of smaller or unknown stocks to outperform the market.

NEGLIGENCE: The omission to do something that a reasonable person would do, or the doing of something that a reasonable and prudent person would not do under similar circumstances. It refers only to that legal delinquency that results whenever one fails to exhibit the care that ought be exhibited, whether it be slight, ordinary, or great. It is characterized by inadvertence, thoughtlessness, and inattention, and is founded on reasonable conduct or reasonable care under all circumstances of particular care.

NEGOTIATED SALE: The sale of new municipal securities by an issuer through an exclusive agreement with an underwriter or underwriting syndicate selected by the issuer. A negotiated sale should be distinguished from a competitive sale, which requires public bidding by the underwriters. The primary points of negotiation for an issuer are the interest rate and purchase price on the issue. The sale of a new issue of securities in this manner is also known as a negotiated underwriting.

NEGOTIABILITY: The easy ability to transfer title upon delivery.

NEGOTIABLE CD: A certificate of deposit with rates, terms, and conditions individually determined.

NELSON, JOHN: Health care economist and former President of the American Medical Association in Chicago, Illinois.

NEST EGG: Slang term for one's savings, usually personal.

NET: The amount by which a health care company's total assets exceed its total liabilities, representing the value of the owner's interest, or equity in the company.

NET ACCOUNTS RECEIVABLE (NAR): The amount projected to be received by a payer of health care services.

NET ADDITIONS/WITHDRAWALS: Any capital adjustments made to an investment account or portfolio for the fiscal year to date. Includes investment management fees and income withheld due to distributions from foreign securities.

NET ASSET: Stockholder's equity, net worth, or assets minus liabilities on the balance sheet.

NET ASSET VALUE (NAV): The market worth of a mutual fund's total resources, securities, cash, and any accrued earnings, after deduction of liabilities.

NET ASSET VALUE PER SHARE (NAVPS): The market worth of a mutual fund's total resources, securities, cash, and any accrued earnings after deduction of liabilities, divided by the number of shares outstanding.

NET BENEFIT: The total benefit of a health care product or service purchased minus the dollar sacrifice needed to purchase that health care output. It is total benefits minus total costs.

NET BOOK VALUE: The balance sheet difference between total assets and total liabilities, or stockholder's equity.

NET CHANGE: Change in securities prices from one day to the next.

NET EARNINGS: For the self-employed taxpayer, net earnings represent revenues less expenses (accrual basis) or receipts less disbursements (cash basis). This term is comparable to net income before tax (NIBT) for a corporation.

NET FINANCIAL ASSET: Financial assets minus financial liabilities.

NET INCOME: Excess of total income over total expenses for a health care corporation.

NET INCOME EARNED: The total of all taxable and nontaxable income earned in an account or portfolio. Margin interest charges and credit interest for the fiscal year to date are factored in as well.

NET INCOME STATEMENT (NIS): The Profit and Loss (P&L) statement reflects items such as patient services revenues and money from research grants, educational programs, gift and cafeteria sales, office space and parking lot rental, and investment income. Hospital and medical office expenses include general overhead, nonoperating expenses such as salaries and wages, fringe benefits, supplies, interest, professional fees, bad debts, depreciation, and amortization. But, increases in working capital, current assets, or the retirement of debt and investment in new fixed assets are usually not considered as expenses.

NET INTEREST COST (NIC): A common method of computing the interest expense to the issuer of issuing bonds, which usually serves as the basis of award in a competitive sale. NIC takes into account any premium and discount paid on the issue. NIC represents the dollar amount of coupon interest payable over the life of the serial issue, without taking into account the time value of money (as would be done in other calculation methods, such as the true interest cost method). While the term actually refers to the dollar amount of the issuer's interest cost, it is also used to refer to the overall rate of interest to be paid by the issuer over the life of the bonds.

NET INTEREST MARGIN: Difference between interest revenue and interest expense. A spread.

NET INVESTMENT: Net additions to capital stock. Gross investments minus depreciation.

NET LEASE: In addition to the rental payments, a net lessee assumes all property charges such as taxes, insurance, and maintenance.

NET LOSS: For the self-employed taxpayer, net losses represent a situation where expenses exceed revenues or disbursements exceed receipts.

NET LOSS RATIO: The ratio of health insurance claims and other expenses, over premium revenues. Also referred to as medical loss ratio.

NET PATIENT SERVICE REVENUE: The operating revenue derived from the patient business operations of a health care entity.

NET PAY: Gross pay minus all allowed deductions.

NET POSITION: Difference between longs and comparable shorts or the difference of the combined market values of all long and short positions.

NET PRESENT VALUE (NPV): The difference in amount between initial payment and related future cash inflows after cost of capital adjustments (interest rate), as of a specific date. NPV is the cumulative differential between the revenue and cost stream discounted at the discounted rate minus the investment.

$$NPV = \sum_{t=1} ((R_t - C_t) / (1 + r)^t) - I$$

where t represents time, n represents the number of time periods, R is revenue impacts, C is cost impacts, r is the discount rate, and I is the investment.

NET PROCEEDS FROM A BOND ISSUE: Gross funds received from a debt issue, minus underwriter, marketing, sales printing, advertising, and other fees.

NET PROFIT MARGIN: Percentage of earnings after taxes and interest.

NET PROFITS: A term broadly used to describe only the profits remaining after including all earnings and other income or profit and after deducting all expenses and charges of every character, including interest, depreciation, and taxes.

NET PURCHASES: All purchases less purchase discounts, allowances, and returns.

NET QUICK ASSETS: Cash, accounts receivable, and marketable securities sans current liabilities.

NET SALES: All sales revenues less sales discounts, allowances, and returns.

NET TANGIBLE ASSET VALUE: Tangible assets (excluding nonoperating and excess assets) value minus liabilities value.

NET WORKING CAPITAL (NWC): Difference between current assets and current liabilities. The lower the NWC, the more economically efficient the care provided.

NET WORTH: The surpluses and capital of a health care entity. It may occasionally refer to the common shareholder's position, or assets minus liabilities plus stockholders equity.

NET YIELD: Rate of return on securities minus all costs.

NETWORK CAPITATION: Any global or hospital capitation, or fixed payment arrangement, between a payer and medical provider or facility and its organization or network.

NEUTRAL INCENTIVE: Payment system void of physician enticements or economic motivations that may impact clinical care quality, as with a salaried doctor.

NEW ISSUE: A security (usually stock) offered to the public for the first time, as in an Initial Public Offering (IPO).

NEW ISSUE MARKET: Securities market for private businesses issuing shares to raise money.

NEW YORK STOCK EXCHANGE (NYSE): Auction securities market in lower Manhattan, New York, where bid and ask prices are determined in an open and free manner, with full disclosure, as customers are represented on the trading floor by professionals in order to obtain the best prices.

NEWHOUSE, JOSEPH, PhD: The John D. MacArthur Professor of Health Policy and Management & Director of the Division of Health Policy Research & Education Department of Health Policy and Management at Harvard Medical School in Boston, Massachusetts.

NICHE: Particular specialty or area of expertise, such as the health care industrial complex.

NIELSON, DON: Senior Vice President of the American Hospital Association in Chicago, Illinois.

NIKKEI INDEX: An index of more than 200 blue chip stocks traded on the Tokyo Stock Exchange (TSE).

NINE BOND RULE: All orders for nine listed bonds or less must be sent to an exchange floor for a diligent attempt at execution, unless a better price may be obtained over-the-counter or if the customer specifically directs the trade be done OTC.

NO LOAD (MUTUAL) FUND: Mutual funds offered directly to the public at net asset value, with no sales charge.

NO PAR STOCK: Stock authorized to be issued but for which no worth is set in the articles of incorporation. A stated value is set by the board of directors on the issuance of this type of stock.

NO PAR VALUE: Stock or bond that does not have a specific value indicated.

NOB SPREAD: Slang term for the difference in interest rates between Treasury bonds (long-term) and Treasury notes (short-term).

NOCHOMOVITZ, MICHAEL, MD: President and Chief Medical Officer of University Primary Care Practices in Cleveland, Ohio.

NOISE: Unsubstantiated activity in the financial markets.

NOMINAL: Expressed in current dollars or actual money amounts.

NOMINAL ACCOUNT OWNER: Account owner whose names securities are registered if other than the beneficial owner.

NOMINAL DOLLARS: U.S. dollars adjusted for inflation.

NOMINAL INCOME: Number of dollars received in a specified time period.

NOMINAL QUOTATION: An indication of the approximate market value of a security, provided for informational purposes only. A nominal quotation does not represent an actual bid for or offer of securities and may be referred to as an indication.

NOMINAL RETURN: The return that an investment produces.

NOMINAL VALUE: A measurement of economic amount that is not corrected for change in price over time (inflation). Not expressing a value in terms of constant prices, that is, a relative value.

NOMINAL YIELD: The annual interest rate payable on a bond, specified in the indenture and printed on the face of the certificate itself (if a bearer bond). Also known as the coupon rate.

NOMINEE: A partnership established by a bank, securities firm, or other corporation to be used as the holder of record for registered securities owned by the bank, securities firm, or corporation. These entities register securities in the name of a nominee to avoid the difficulties of registering and transferring securities in a corporate name. Additionally, this form of registration is satisfactory for purposes of delivery on interdealer transactions.

NONACCELERATING INFLATION RATE OF UNEMPLOYMENT (NAIRU): A steady state unemployment rate above which inflation falls and below which inflation rises. It is estimated at 6% in the United States.

NONACCREDITED INVESTOR: One who does not meet the net worth requirements of SEC Regulation D (Rules 505 and 506).

NONCASH CHARGE: Depreciation expense.

NONCASH CREDIT: The opposite of a noncash charge.

NONCONTRIBUTORY: Fee paid by an employer, not the employees, usually regarding health insurance or other fringe employment benefits.

NONCUMULATIVE PREFERRED: Preferred stock that does not accumulate dividends for later possible distribution if missed.

NONCURRENT ASSETS: Assets with a life of more than 1 year.

NONCURRENT LIABILITIES: Liabilities with a life of more than 1 year.

NONDISCRETIONARY: Order that an investor client gives to a stockbroker.

NONDISCRETIONARY ACCOUNT: Securities account where the client makes all the trading decisions. However, one may give very limited discretion in terms of price or time. An order to buy or sell, quantity, and exact financial instrument is still needed.

NONEQUITY OPTIONS: Any option that does not have common stock as its underlying asset. Nonequity options include options on futures, indexes, interest rate composites, and physicals.

NONEXCLUDABLE: One who cannot be economically excluded from consuming a good or service even upon refusal to pay.

NONFONTIER STUDY: Comparison of the relationship of actual health care outputs and costs for two or more health care entities.

NONINVESTMENT GRADE BOND: Bonds considered by rating services such as Moody's or Standard & Poor's to carry a higher risk of default. These bonds are typically given low credit ratings (ranging from BB to D). Also called "junk" bonds, these securities attempt to compensate investors for their higher risk by paying higher yields.

NONOPERATING ASSETS: Those assets not required for ongoing health care or other business operations.

NONOPERATING EXPENSES: Expenses incurred though non-health care related activities, such as marketing, sales, and advertising.

NONOPERATING INCOME: Health care entity income received though non-health care related activities, such as marketing, sales, and advertising.

NONOPERATING REVENUES: Money earned from non-health care related activities.

NONPARTICIPATING PHYSICIAN (PROVIDER): A physician or medical provider who does not sign a participation agreement and, therefore, is not obligated to accept assignment on all Medicare claims.

NONPHYSICIAN PRACTITIONER (PROVIDER): A health care professional who is not a physician but participates in the Medicare program. Examples include advanced practice nurses, and physician assistants.

NONPRICE COMPETITION: Methods that a health care entity uses, other than fee reductions, to increase product or medical services sales revenue, such as value-added Medicare competition.

NONPRICE RATIONING: Free health care or other services on a first come, first served basis.

NONPROFIT: Organization prevented by law to distribute assets or profits to private citizens and that may provide only certain services, such as health care. Not-for-profit. Committed legally not to distribute any profits to individuals with control over it such as members, officers, directors, or trustees, but a nonprofit may pay for services rendered and goods provided.

NONPROFIT INSURANCE COMPANY: Companies exempted from some taxes to provide health or medical expense insurance on a service basis, such as Blue Cross Blue Shield and some dental service corporations.

NONPUBLIC INFORMATION: Material private information (good or bad) about a public company that may affect stock price.

NONQUALIFIED BENEFIT: Any employee benefit that does not meet the qualification standards of the Employee Retirement Income Security Act (ERISA).

NONQUALIFIED DEFERRED COMPENSATION (NQDC): An arrangement deferring the receipt of currently earned compensation that does not comply with the requirements for qualified plans.

NONRECURRING EXPENSES REVENUES: Irregular health care business or other operating expenditures or revenues, the timing of which during a year may not be determined precisely, or expenditures that occur less frequently than monthly.

NONRECOURSE FINANCING: Loans for which partners, both general and limited, have no personal liability. In health care facility real estate programs only the value of such loans, if qualified, is part of the partners' basis in the partnership.

NONREGULAR CASH FLOWS: Irregular cash flows from a project.

NONRESIDENT ALIEN: A citizen that is not a resident or citizen of the United States. Income of such individuals is subject to taxation if it is effectively connected with a U.S. trade or business.

NONRIVAL: One who can consume a good or service without exhausting or depleting it for others.

NONROUTINE TRANSACTIONS: Activities that occur only periodically. The data involved are generally not part of the routine flow of transactions.

NONSUFFICIENT FUNDS (NSF): A bounced check whose maker has insufficient funds to cover the draft.

NONSYSTEMIC RISK: Company or industry specific risk. Risk apart from the markets or economy as a whole (systematic risk).

NONTAX QUALIFIED ANNUITY: An annuity that does not qualify for tax-deductibility of contributions under IRS codes. These annuities are funded with after-tax dollars, but the earnings accrue tax-deferred. Upon payout, all distributions in excess of the cost basis are taxed as ordinary income.

NONTAXABLE DIVIDENDS: Tax-exempt shares of a health care or other company's net profits distributed by the company to its shareholders.

NONTAXABLE INCOME FOR SHORT-TERM SECURITIES: Fiscal year-to-date income from tax-exempt holdings of less than 1 year.

NONTAXABLE MUNICIPAL INTEREST: Fiscal year-to-date income from tax-free municipal securities

NONVALUE ADDED ACTIVITIES: Any activity that does not increase patient value.

NORLING, RICHARD: Chairman and CEO of Premier in San Diego, California.

NORMAL DISTRIBUTION: A popular probability distribution frequently depicted as the bell-shaped curve and often relied upon for financial modeling, because two variables define its location and shape, the mean and the standard deviation. Normal distributions with larger standard deviations (or variances) are wide or flat because greater volatility is dispersed over a wider range. Conversely, smaller standard deviations generate tighter formations that have a pronounced peak appearance. These parameterized regions are crucial to the understanding of value at securities risk programs and many option pricing models. Also, many linear analysis techniques depend on the assumption and stability of normal independent probability functions, while many option pricing models use the annualized standard deviation as the volatility proxy:

- If the mean value of a normal distribution is bounded by one standard deviation (plus or minus) then it is expected that 68.3% of the values will occur in that region.
- If the mean value of a normal distribution is bounded by two standard deviations (plus or minus) then it is expected that 95.5% of the values will occur in that wider region.

- If the mean value of a normal distribution is bounded by three standard deviations (plus or minus) then it is expected that 99.7% of the values will occur in that still wider region.
- If the distribution's mean is bounded by a plus and a minus standard deviation, the design is considered as Two-Tailed because both sides of the distribution are being evaluated.

NORMAL GOOD: A health care good or service that patients purchase more or less of at any price point when their incomes decrease or increase.

NORMAL PROFIT: Minimum payment to medical workers to obtain professional health care ability.

NORMAL TRADING UNITS (NTUS): A round lot of 100 shares.

NORMALIZED EARNINGS: The revised economic benefits of a company adjusted for nonrecurring or unusual items eliminated from financial statements. Company earnings adjusted for cyclic economic ups or downs.

NORMALIZED FINANCIAL STATEMENTS: The revised economic benefits of a firm's financial statements adjusted for nonrecurring or unusual items or nonoperating assets and liabilities.

NORMATIVE ECONOMICS: The health care economics of what a person or organization ought to do, should do, or be.

NORMATIVE STATEMENT: Proclamation about what ought to be done in health care economics and finance.

NOT ELSEWHERE CLASSIFIED: An ill-defined ICD-9-CM term.

NOT-FOR-PROFIT: Ownership group that includes certain health care organizations and all church-related and other facilities that are organized and operated under a policy by which no trustee or other person shares in the profits or losses of the enterprise.

NOT HELD ORDER: An order that does not hold the executing member financially responsible for using his personal judgment in the execution price or time of a transaction.

NOTE: A written, short-term promise of an issuer to repay a specified principal amount on a date certain, together with interest at a stated rate, payable from a defined source of anticipated revenue. Notes usually mature in 1 year or less, although notes of longer maturities are also issued. The following types of notes are common in the municipal hospital–revenue bond market:

- Bond Anticipation Notes (BANs): Notes issued by a governmental unit, usually for capital health care projects, that are paid from the proceeds of the issuance of long-term bonds.
- Construction Loan Notes (CLNs): Notes issued to fund construction of hospital projects. CLNs are repaid by the permanent financing, which may be provided from bond proceeds or some pre-arranged commitment, such as a GNMA takeout.

- Revenue Anticipation Notes (RANs): Notes issued in anticipation of receiving hospital or other revenues at a future date.
- Tax Anticipation Notes (TANs): Notes issued in anticipation of future tax receipts, such as receipts of ad-valorem taxes which are due and payable at a set time of the year.

NOTES PAYABLE (NP): A legal obligation to pay creditors or holders of a valid lien or claim.

NOTES RECEIVABLE (NR): A written promise for the future collection of cash.

NOTICE OF SALE: A publication by an issuer describing the terms of sale of an anticipated new offering of municipal securities. It generally contains the date, time, and place of sale, amount of issue, type of security, amount of good faith deposit, basis of award, name of bond counsel, maturity schedule, method of delivery, time and place of delivery, and bid form.

NOTIONAL: Economic value assigned to liabilities and assets that is not based on cost or market (e.g., the value of a medical service not yet rendered).

NOW ACCOUNT: Negotiable Order of Withdrawal (NOW) checking account that earns interest.

NSF CHECK: Nonsufficient Funds, as in a bounced or dishonored check.

NUMBER OUTSTANDING SHARES: Shares issued minus Treasury shares.

NUMBER SHARES FOR CONVERSION: Par value / Conversion price.

NUMBERED ACCOUNT: A brokerage or other account identified by something other than the customer's name, and usually an identification number.

NUMERAIRE: Macroeconomic model in which there is no actual money or currency, as in a barter exchange system.

NUSSBAUM, SAMUEL, MD: Chief Medical Officer and Executive Vice President for WellPoint, Indianapolis, Indiana.

NYSE COMPOSITE INDEX: An index of all stocks listed on the New York Stock Exchange.

O

OBJECTIVITY: Emphasizing or expressing the nature of economic or fiscal reality as it is apart from personal reflection or feelings. Independence of mind.

OBLIGATION: A legal responsibility as with a debt or loan. Any amount which may require payment by an entity at a future time.

OCCUPATIONAL LICENSURE: Societal, governing, and economic restrictions that increase the difficulty for health care workers to obtain professional standing, as in a medical or nursing license.

ODD COUPON: An interest payment for a period other than the standard 6 months. A payment for a period of less than 6 months is a short coupon, and a payment for a period of more than 6 months is a long coupon. Usually only the first interest payment on an issue would be an odd coupon, but some issues have an odd last coupon. It is an initial interest payment period of other than 6 months on a registered security.

ODD LOT: An amount of stock less than the normal trading unit.

ODD-LOT THEORY: A theory of market activity stating that the small (odd-lot) investor frequently becomes a heavy buyer as the market peaks and sells heavily on balance in a declining market, just prior to a rally. The opposite of conventional wisdom. The supposition that small investors, who tend to buy in smaller units than the standard round lot of 100 shares, are always wrong. To buy when odd-lot investors are selling and sell when they are buying. This is a theory that has not been proven correct.

OFF BALANCE SHEET FINANCING: The acquisition of assets or services with debt that is not recorded on the balance sheet, but may appear as a small footnote.

OFF THE RUN: Previously issued treasury securities that are not generally used for benchmark or pricing purposes. They are less active and liquid than more recent issuances in respect to time remaining to maturity.

OFFER: The price at which a person is ready to sell a security or other asset.

OFFER & ACCEPTANCE: (1) An offer occurs by signing an insurance application for purchase, having a physical examination, and prepaying the first premium. Policy issuance and delivery as applied for constitute acceptance by the company. (2) Offer made by the company and premium payment constitutes acceptance by the applicant.

OFFER CURVE: Graphical representation of how much of a health care good or service an individual patient will offer for trade, barter, or monetary purchase, given income or earnings levels.

OFFER WANTED (OW): Potential buyer notice for a potential seller; of securities.

OFFERING CIRCULAR: A prospectus.

OFFERING MEMORANDUM: Terms and conditions of a private securities placement. A prospectus.

OFFICE OF THE INSPECTOR GENERAL (OIG): The office responsible for auditing, evaluating, and criminal and civil investigating for the Department of Health and Human Services (DHHS), as well as imposing sanctions, when necessary, against health care providers. It is an unconstrained federal unit within the DHHS that performs health care audits, investigates medical fraud and abuse cases, collects data, and performs special monitoring functions.

OFFICE OF THRIFT SUPERVISION (OTS): Bureau of the Treasury Department that was authorized by Congress in the Financial Institutions Reform, Recovery, and Enforcement Act of 1989, to charter, regulate, examine, and supervise savings institutions.

OFFICE OF SUPERVISORY JURISDICTION (OSJ): An office set up by individual member firms in compliance with the NASD Rules of Fair Practice, managed by a registered principal, to administer a firm's supervisory responsibilities in that and other offices.

OFFICIAL STATEMENT: A document published by the issuer that generally discloses material information on a new issue of municipal securities including the purposes of the issue, how the securities will be repaid, and the financial, economic, and social characteristics of the issuing government. Investors use such information to evaluate the credit quality of the securities.

O'KANE, MARGARET: President of the National Committee for Quality Assurance in Washington, D.C.

OKUN, ARTHUR, PhD: Health care economist that suggested transferring wealth or health insurance benefits from one group of people or patients to another, and generated disincentives that discourage productive work or appropriate medical utilization.

O'LEARY, DENNIS, MD: President of the Joint Commission on Accreditation of Health Care Organizations (JCAHO) in Oakbrook Terrace, Illinois.

OLIGOPOLY: A marketplace where a few sellers dominate the sales of a health care product or service.

OLIGOPSONY: The buy-side counterpart of an oligopoly.

OMEGA: A volatility pricing model for derivatives.

OMNIBUS ACCOUNT: Futures account carried on the books by one futures commission merchant (FCM) for another FCM.

ONLINE BANKING: Personal and business account information accessible through a personal computer and the Internet.

ONLINE BILL PAY: Bill payment available by a computer internet service and allows bill payments to several different vendors. Paper checks are issued when payments are not available through bill payment.

ONLINE TRADING: Investment activity that takes place over the Internet without a stockbroker.

ON THE CLOSE; OPEN: A buy or sell securities order to be executed as close as possible to the close or opening of a trading day.

ON THE RUNS: Newly issued treasury securities often used as benchmarks for indices and pricing purposes.

ON THE SIDELINES: Those individuals or institutions not investing in the financial markets.

ONE TAIL TEST: Statistical test that focuses on one side of a probability distribution curve and is related to extraordinary losses and/or extraordinary gains.

OPEN ACCOUNT: A mutual fund account where a shareholder, by virtue of an initial investment in the fund, automatically has reinvestment privileges and the right to make additional purchases without a formal accumulation plan.

OPEN ECONOMY: An economy that imports and exports medical products, goods, or services. Health care industry links with other industries.

OPEN END CREDIT: A consumer line of credit that may be used repeatedly up to an established overall limit. Commonly known as revolving credit or a charge account, in which the customer may pay in full or in installments that include a finance charge. The term does not include negotiated advances under an open -end real estate mortgage or a letter of credit.

OPEN END FUND: A mutual fund formed to continuously issue and buy back shares to meet investor demand. The share price is determined by the market value of the securities held by the fund's portfolio, and it may be higher or lower than the original purchase price. Open -end funds can range from load to no-load.

OPEN END INVESTMENT COMPANY: Mutual funds that buy and sell securities for redemption by shareholders.

OPEN END MANAGEMENT COMPANY: The technical term for a mutual fund.

OPEN END PROVISION: A mortgage bond provision that enables a corporation to use the same real assets for more than one bond issue. In the event of default, creditors on all issues have equal claims.

OPEN INTEREST: Options with a strike price, expiration date, and specific stock.

OPEN MARKET COMMITTEE: Federal Open Market Committee (FOMC).

OPEN MARKET OPERATIONS: The purchase or sale of government securities by the Federal Reserve.

OPEN ORDER: A Good-Till-Canceled (GTC) order to purchase securities.

OPENING INVENTORY: The cost of durable medical equipment (DME) and other supplies and inventory onhand at the beginning of the year.

OPENING PURCHASE: A transaction in which an investor becomes the holder of an option. The position is terminated by entering a closing sale order, known as taking a long position.

OPENING SALE: A transaction in which an investor becomes a writer (seller) of an option. The position is terminated by entering a closing purchase order known as taking a short position.

OPENING TRANSACTION: An addition to or creation of a trading position. An opening purchase transaction adds long options (or long securities) to an investor's total position, and an opening sell transaction adds short options (or short securities).

OPERATING ACTIVITIES: Activities of a health care or other organization directly related to its mission statement.

OPERATING AGREEMENT: Written document that sets out the rules by which a Limited Liability Company (LLC) is to be operated. It is the LLC equivalent of hospital corporate bylaws or a medical practice partnership agreement.

OPERATING BUDGET: The operational inflow and outflow projections of a health care or other entity.

OPERATING CASH FLOW: The cash flows received from the main business activities of a health care or other organization.

OPERATING CYCLE: Period of time between the acquisition of medical goods and services, involved in the manufacturing or medical care delivery process, and the final cash realization resulting from sales and subsequent collections.

OPERATING EXPENSES: The expenses incurred from the main business activities of a health care or other organization. In the securities industry, the costs of running a mutual fund, which are paid out of a fund's assets before earnings are distributed to fund shareholders.

OPERATING INCOME: The income earned from the main business activities of a health care or other organization.

OPERATING LEASE: A short term or cancelable rental agreement.

OPERATING LEVERAGE: The degree to which fixed costs are used in health care or other firms' operations.

OPERATING MARGIN: Income (loss) from health care operations plus mortgage interest expenses plus other interest expenses divided by net patient service revenue. It is a ratio that indicates the percentage of net patient service revenue that remains as income after operating expenses, except interest expense, have been deducted.

OPERATING PROFIT MARGIN: Percentage of services or sales before taxes or interest expense is deducted.

OPERATING RATIO: Any number of so-called financial percentages used to determine how well an organization is using its economic inputs to produce outputs. It is an efficiency measurement.

OPERATING REVENUES: The revenues generated by a health care entity through its operational activities and provision of medical services.

OPERATIONS: The normal activities of a health care entity, company, or agency in the course of conducting its business.

OPERATIONS AND MAINTENANCE FUND: A fund established by the bond contract of a revenue bond issue into which monies to be used for the purposes of meeting the costs of operating and maintaining the financed project are deposited. Under a typical revenue pledge, this fund is the first (under a net revenue pledge) or the second (under a gross revenue pledge) to be funded out of the revenue fund.

OPPORTUNITY COST: The revenue lost by missing another business opportunity.

OPTIMIZING: Balancing health care benefits against health care costs.

OPTION: Contracts to buy (call option) or sell (put option) a security at a stated price within a stated time period. Puts and calls are *types* of options. All the same type options of the same security are said to be of the same *class*. Options of the same class may have different exercise prices (the stated buy or sell price, called the *strike price*) and different dates. All options of the same class with the same strike price and expiration date are called a *series*. The price of an option is called a *premium*. The price of a premium is made up of *intrinsic value* (the difference between the current price and the strike price) and *time value* (the difference between the premium and the intrinsic value). An option is said to be *covered* when the investor has another position that will meet the obligation of the option contract. When option rights are used they are *exercised*; unexercised options are said to *expire* after their set time period is up. A buyer of an option is called a *holder* and a seller is called a *writer*. Companies often offer employees *incentive options* as part of their compensation. These operate more like rights or warrants and allow the employee to purchase stock in the company at a specified price for a certain number of years.

OPTION ADJUSTED DURATION: Measurement of duration targeted for the stated first option (put or call) feature, reducing the duration statistic from its ordinary measurement.

OPTION CLEARING CORPORATION (OCC): The issuer and guarantor of listed option contracts. Also serves as the clearing agency for listed options transactions. It is jointly owned by the participating exchanges.

OPTION MODELS: Mathematical tools to determine the price, premium, or volatility for puts, calls, convertible securities, asset backed securities, warrants, and other derivatives. Option models may be categorized as credit, currency, equity, index, futures, and physical or cash oriented, according to factors such as: market, strike or exercise price, interest rate for discounting purposes, volatility, and time to expiration. Some models require expected dividends, coupons, and foreign exchange considerations. Examples are:

- Binomial Model
- Black Scholes Model
- Cox, Ingersoll, and Ross Model
- Gastineau and Madansky Model
- Heath, Jarrow, and Morton Model
- Ho and Lee Model
- Hull and White Model
- Jamshidian, Rendleman, and Bartter Model
- Vasicek and Whaley Model

OPTION SPREAD: The sales or purchase of options within the same contract class.

OPTION TRADING STRATEGIES: Fundamentals are puts and calls, either American Style or European Style, or ordinary, plain vanilla, and exotic. Can be market directional, volatility directional, market neutral, volatility neutral, time value capture, time value or payment, and so forth. Specific strategies include: Backspreads, Bear, Box, Bull, Butterflies, Condors, Conversion, Credit, Debit, Diagonal, Fence, Guts, Horizontal, Purchased Call, Purchased Put, Ratio, Reverse Conversion, Sold Call, Sold Put, Straddles, Strangles, Synthetic Long Call, Synthetic Long Futures or Underlying, Synthetic Long Put, Synthetic Long Straddle, Synthetic Short Call, Synthetic Short Futures or Underlying, Synthetic Short Put, Synthetic Short Straddle, Vertical, and Volatility. There are also compound and nested options or strategies, such as: a call-on-a-call, a call-on-a-put, a put-on-a-put, and a put-on-a-call.

OPTION WRITER: The seller of an option contract who is obligated to meet the terms of delivery if the option holder exercises his or her right.

ORDER: An order for new issue municipal securities placed with a syndicate by a member of the syndicate, where the securities would be confirmed to that member at syndicate terms (e.g., less the total takedown). It is a set of instructions executing a securities transaction, such as:

- All or None (AON)
- All or Nothing
- Buy on Close
- Buy on Opening
- Contingent
- Discretionary
- Nondiscretionary
- Do Not Reduce (DNR)
- Exchange for Physicals (EFP)
- Fill or Kill (FOK)
- Good Till Canceled (GTC)
- Immediate or Cancel (IOC)
- Limit (LMT)
- Market, Market if Touched (MIT)
- Market on Close (MOC)
- Market on Opening
- Not Held
- One Cancels the Other (OCO)
- Open Order
- Sell on Close
- Sell on Opening
- Stop (STP)

- Stop Limit (STP LMT)
- Other combined spreads, options, and instruments

ORDER PERIOD: The period of time following the competitive sale of a new securities issue during which nonpriority orders submitted by account members are allocated without consideration of time of submission. The length of the order period is usually determined by the manager. In a negotiated sale the order period is the period of time established by the manager during which orders are accepted from account members. The order period generally precedes the sale by the issuer. At times, order periods occur when securities are repriced or market conditions improve dramatically.

ORDERLY: Securities trading or markets that behave in a rational manner.

ORDERLY LIQUIDATION VALUE: The sale of business assets, over time, in a manner to maximize sales proceeds.

ORDINAL UTILITY: Health care or medical care utility as measured by patient satisfaction, and where each unit of health care output is not essential.

ORDINARY ANNUITY: A series of payments received or made at the end of each predetermined payment period.

ORDINARY DIVIDEND: A payment declared or paid by a health care or other corporation. It reflects the recently established or declared amount. It is not expected to be a one-time or special declaration, but regular.

ORDINARY INCOME: Income derived from normal health care business operations, but not the sale of capital assets. It is one of two classes of income and capital gains taxed under the IRC. Usually ordinary income is taxed at a higher rate than capital gains.

ORDINARY REPAIR: Any business repair work that creates revenue expenditure, debited to an expense account.

ORGANIZATION EXPENDITURES: The costs of organizing a trade, medical practice, or for-profit clinic or activity before it begins active business. A taxpayer may elect to amortize such expenses for a term of no less than 60 months; and if the expenses are not deductible, they may only be recovered when the business ceases operation or is sold.

ORIGINAL HOUSE: The investment banking firm that syndicates or sells original securities issues to the marketplace.

ORIGINAL ISSUE DISCOUNT (OID): An amount by which the par value of a security exceeds its public offering price at the time it was originally offered to an investor. The original issue discount is amortized over the life of the security and, on a municipal security, is generally treated as tax-exempt interest. When sold before maturity, any profit realized is figured for tax purposes on the adjusted cost basis, which is calculated for each year the security is outstanding by adding the accretion value to the original offering price. The amount of the accretion value (and the existence and total amount of original issue discount) is determined in accordance with the provisions of the Internal Revenue Code and the rules and regulations of the Internal Revenue Service.

ORPHAN STOCK: Stocks neglected by research analysts.

OTC BULLETIN BOARD: OTC electronic bid and ask stocks not meeting NASDAQ minimum requirements for listing, as in penny stocks.

OTHER COMPREHENSIVE BASIS OF ACCOUNTING (OCBOA): Consistent accounting basis (other than GAAP) used for financial reporting. Examples include cash or income tax basis.

OTHER EXPENSES: Miscellaneous cost or expense category.

OTHER INCOME: Miscellaneous income category.

OTHER POST-RETIREMENT EMPLOYEE BENEFITS (OPREB): All benefits other than pensions, provided by employers to employees.

OTHER REVENUE: Nonreported operating income, included elsewhere in the profit and loss statement.

OUT OF LINE: Securities priced too high or too low, in like-kind comparisons.

OUT OF THE MONEY: An option that has no intrinsic value. A call option is out of the money when the exercise price is higher than the underlying security's price. A put is out of the money when the exercise price is lower than the underlying security's price.

OUT-OF-POCKET COSTS: Total costs paid directly by consumers for insurance co-payment and deductibles, prescription or over-the-counter drugs, and other services.

OUT-OF-POCKET EXPENSE: Cost borne directly by a patient without the benefit of health insurance or additional out-of-pocket expenses, such as deductibles or co-payments.

OUT-OF-POCKET LIMIT: A cap placed on patient out-of-pocket health care costs, after which benefits increase to provide full coverage for the rest of the year.

OUT-OF-POCKET MAXIMUM: The maximum amount of expenses, as set by a health care plan, that a person is obligated to pay directly during each calendar year.

OUTFLOW: Financial disbursements, also known as outlay.

OUTLAY: Financial disbursements, also known as outflow.

OUTLIERS: Statistically economic, financial, medical, or other remote and independent events that differ from a benchmark or normal distribution.

OUTPUT EFFECT: Change in price impact of a health care input or resource, on its ultimate medical output.

OUTSIDE DIRECTORS: Most mutual funds registered with the SEC under the Investment Company Act of 1940 are required to have at least 40% of their Board of Directors made up of persons who are considered to be outside or noninterested. This means that they have no affiliation with the adviser, principal underwriter, or custodian bank.

OUTSOURCING: Buying elsewhere instead of making in-house.

OUTSTANDING CHECKS: A check issued but not yet paid by the bank.

OUTSTANDING STOCK: Stock in the possession of stockholders.

OVERBOUGHT/SOLD: Security that has experienced a rapid rise in price and may be susceptible to a dramatic decline, or, a security that has experienced a rapid drop in price and may be susceptible to a dramatic rise.

OVERDRAFT: Credit extension for a checking account by a banking institution. It is the amount by which account withdrawals exceed deposits.

OVERDRAFT PROTECTION: A service that allows the customer to write checks for an amount over and above the amount in their checking account. Funds are transferred from their line of credit or other designated account to their checking account as needed. This service must be applied for and approved.

OVERHANG: A large volume of securities that would depress prices if released to the markets.

OVERHEAD: Indirect corporate expenses not traced to a specific patient, client, or customer.

OVERHEAT: A too rapidly expanding economy.

OVERLAPPING DEBT: The issuer's proportionate share of the debt of other local governmental units that either overlap it (the issuer is located either wholly or partly within the geographic limits of the other units) or underlie it (the other units are located within the geographic limits of the issuer). The debt is generally apportioned based upon relative assessed values.

OVERUTILIZED CAPACITY: Health care output production that is more than its minimum total average cost.

OVERVALUED: A stock whose current market price is estimated to be too high given the firm's earnings, growth potential, or other criteria. The opposite of undervalued.

OVER-THE-COUNTER (OTC) MARKET: A market for securities made up of securities broker/dealers who may or may not be members of securities exchanges. Over the counter is a market conducted anywhere other than on an exchange.

OVER-THE-COUNTER OPTIONS: Nonlisted put and call options whose expiration dates and exercise prices are not standardized. OTC options are not cleared or guaranteed by the Options Clearing Corporation.

OVER-THE-COUNTER SECURITY: As thousands of companies have insufficient shares outstanding, stockholders, or earnings to warrant application for listing on the New York Stock Exchange, securities of these companies are traded in the over-the-counter market between firms who act either as agents for their customers or as principals (for themselves).

OWNER WITHDRAWALS: Money removed from a medical, health care practice, or other business by the doctor or owners.

P

P2P: (1) Patient to Patient. (2) Patient to Physician. (3) Peer to Peer.

P = MC RULE: Medical product or service price equals marginal cost in a profit-maximizing health care or other business entity.

PAASCHE INDEX: The official method for U.S. price deflators is an algorithm like the Laspeyres index but whose base quantities are chosen from the second, later time period.

PACKAGE: A combination of several different types of health insurance coverage.

PACKAGE(D) PRICING: Combines the fees for the professional and institutional services associated with a medical procedure into a single payment. Package pricing, also known as service bundling or global pricing, sets the price of the bundled procedures and implicitly controls the volume of services provided as part of the global service.

PAID AMOUNT: The portion of a submitted charge that is actually paid by both third-party payers and the insured, including co-payments and balance bills. For Medicare this amount may be less than the allowed charge if the submitted charge is less, or it may be more because of balance billing.

PAID AS BILLED: Medical invoice paid as submitted without change or adjudication.

PAID CLAIMS: Medical reimbursement that meets contracted terms and conditions. A *clean-claim.*

PAID CLAIMS LOSS RATIO (PCLR): Paid medical claims divided by total premiums.

PAID IN CAPITAL: Money received by a corporation from investors, for equity.

PAPER: Very short-term unsecured commercial debt.

PAPER PROFIT/LOSS: An unrealized profit/loss on a security still held. Paper profits are realized only when a security is sold at prices above the cost of acquisition.

PAR: An arbitrary dollar amount assigned to a share of common stock by the corporation's charter. At one time, it reflected the value of the original investment behind each share, but today it has little significance except for bookkeeping purposes. Many corporations do not assign a par value to new issues, assigning a stated value instead. In preferred shares or bonds, it has importance insofar as it signifies the dollar value on which the dividend or interest is figured and the amount to be repaid upon redemption.

PAR OPTION: A redemption provision that permits the issuer to call securities at par.

PAR VALUE: For common stocks, the value on the books of the corporation. It has little to do with market value or even the original price of shares at first issuance. The difference between par and the price at first issuance is carried on the books of a corporation as paid-in capital or capital surplus. Par value for preferred stocks is also liquidating value and the value on which dividends (expressed as a percentage) are paid, generally $100 per share.

PARDES, HERBERT: President and CEO of the New York-Presbyterian Health Care System in New York, New York.

PARENT COMPANY: A company that owns or otherwise controls another company or companies.

PARETO EFFICIENCY (OPTIMUM): The inability to improve health care quality or lower costs, without decreasing the clinical quality, or increasing the costs for another patient.

PARETO ENDOWMENT: An allocation of health care and economic goods to patients is "Pareto Optimal" if no other allocation of the same medical goods or services would be preferred by every patient.

PARITY (BOND): The condition that exists when a convertible security and its underlying stock are equal in value. Bond Market Value / Number of Shares.

PARITY (OPTION): An option trading for its intrinsic value, that is, the premium is equal to the amount the option is in the money. There is no time value when an option is trading at parity.

PARK: To place cash and/or assets in a safe investment haven during volatile markets.

PARKINSON'S LAW: Positive relationship between hospital bed availability and cohort utilization of those space-occupying beds. *See also* Roemer's Law; Say's Law.

PARTIAL CAPITATION: An insurance arrangement where the payment made to a health plan is a combination of a capitated premium and payment based on actual use of services. The proportions specified for these components determine the insurance risk faced by the plan.

PARTIAL RISK CONTRACT: Hybrid reimbursement method combining discounted FFS with discounted fixed payments, per patient group.

PARTICIPATING PREFERRED STOCK: Preferred stock that is entitled to its stated dividend and also to additional dividends on a specified basis, if declared, after payment of dividends on common stock.

PARTICIPATING PROVIDER (PHYSICIAN): A medical provider, physician, or dispenser of health care services or products that agrees to third-party reimbursement terms and conditions in order to access (treat) a cohort of patients.

PARTICIPATION: A medical provider or health care facility that is included in the Medicare compensation health care system in the United States.

PARTICIPATIVE BUDGET: Managerial methodologies where those involved in operations provide cognitive input into the budget construction process.

PARTNERSHIP: There are two basic forms of partnerships:

- A limited partnership has two or more classes of partners. Each partner has certain rights to the partnership's income, distributions, and so forth. The general partners manage the partnership and assume its potential liabilities. The limited partners are not active in the business, and their liability is essentially limited to their initial investment in the partnership. Restrictions as to sale or other disposition of the partnership units are generally placed on the limited partners.
- A general partnership has no limited partners. All partners share the income, expenses, and liabilities in percentages agreed to by them at the time the partnership agreement is prepared. All partners are jointly liable for the partnership's liabilities. Sale or disposition of the partnership positions may or may not be restricted.

PARTNERSHIP CAPITATION: Mutual fixed-payment risk sharing arrangement between providers and hospitals.

PASS THROUGH ENTITY: Individual or organization who receives the profits of an S-corporation or partnership for income tax purposes.

PASSIVE: Investment in which there is no material participation. It is the opposite of aggressive (risky).

PASSIVE ACTIVITY LOSS: Deficit generated from activities involved in the conduct of a trade or business in which the taxpayer does not materially participate.

PASSIVE INCOME: Derived from such sources as dividends, interest, royalties, rents, amounts received from personal service contracts, and income received as a beneficiary of an estate or trust.

PATIENT INCENTIVE: Some motivator to alter or change patient behavior. It is usually a cost containment measure.

PATRIOT ACT: Uniting and Strengthening America by Providing Appropriate Tools Required to Intercept and Obstruct Terrorism (USA Patriot Act) Act of October 26, 2001.

PATRIOT BONDS: Series EE bonds are marked "Patriot Bond," whose proceeds go into the U.S. Treasury General Fund and are not specifically earmarked for the war. Monies for the war and other federal government spending also draw from this general fund, which may contribute to fighting the war on terrorism. They are also known as war bonds.

PAULY, MARK, PhD: Bendheim Professor, and Professor of Health Care Systems, Business, and Public Policy, Insurance and Risk Management, and Economics at Wharton School of the University of Pennsylvania.

PAULY GOODMAN PROPOSAL: Original innovators of tax subsidized MSA and HSA styled high-deductible health insurance policies.

PAULY SATTERTHWAITE INDEX: A patient medical information model that offers an alternative explanation for high health care fees and costs.

PAY-AS-YOU-GO: The tax system employed by the U.S. government (and many states) requiring that estimated amounts of tax be paid as income is earned. Failure to make timely estimated tax payments may result in the imposition of nondeductible interest (penalties) at rates comparable to those available from commercial lenders.

PAYABLE: Financial amount owed.

PAYABLE DATE: The date on which a dividend is paid. Payable date or the day on which a mutual fund pays distributions to its shareholders.

PAYABLES DEFERRAL PERIOD (PDP): Accounts Payable / Daily Credit Purchases.

PAYBACK PERIOD: The time it takes for net health care entity revenues to return the cost of investment.

PAYEE: The person or entity receiving payment, such as a medical professional for services rendered.

PAYER: An entity that assumes the risk of paying for medical treatments. This can be an uninsured patient, a self-insured employer, a health plan, or HMO. Also known as payor or carrier.

PAYER-ID: Centers for Medicare and Medicaid's term for their pre-HIPAA National Payer ID initiative.

PAYER MIX: Allocation of reimbursement sources for a medical facility, clinic, or provider (see Table 7).

PAYING AGENT: The entity responsible for transmitting payments of interest and principal from an issuer of municipal securities to the security holders. The paying agent is usually a bank or trust company, but may be the treasurer or some other officer of the issuer. The paying agent may also provide other services for the issuer such as reconciliation of the securities and coupons paid, destruction of paid securities and coupons, and similar services.

PAYMENT CAP: The maximum amount an ARM payment can increase at a payment change date regardless of the amount of increase in the interest rate.

Table 7: Sample Payer Mix

Sample	2008	2009
Medicare	25.7%	23.9%
Medicaid	16.4%	15.3%
Managed care	39.7%	42.2%
Commercial	2.7%	4.0%
Self pay	15.5%	14.5%

For example, a current loan payment of $1,000, with an 8.5% payment cap, may increase to no more than $1,085 on the next payment change date.

PAYMENT DATE: The date on which interest, or principal and interest, is payable on a debt security. Interest payment dates usually occur semiannually for bonds.

PAYMENT-IN-KIND: Securities that pay interest or dividend payment in additional securities of the same kind.

PAYMENT LEVEL: Amount paid for medical services, per-provider, per-unit by both patient and insurer. *See also* payment rate.

PAYMENT RATE: The total payment that a hospital or community mental health center receives when they give outpatient services to Medicare patients. It is the total amount paid for each unit of service rendered by a health care provider, including both the amount covered by the insurer and the consumer's cost sharing. It is sometimes referred to as payment level. For Medicare payments to physicians, this is the same as the allowed charge. *See also* payment level.

PAYMENT REVIEW PROGRAMS: A program used to discover medical fraud and health care abuse by providers and practitioners.

PAYMENT SAFEGUARDS: Activities to prevent and recover inappropriate Medicare benefit payments including MSP, Medical Review, Utilization Review, provider audits, and fraud and abuse detection.

PAYOR: *See* Payer.

PAYOUT RATIO: The ratio of dividends-to-earning of a company.

PAYROLL: Employee compensation, or the major expense of most health care businesses.

PAYROLL TAX: Employer and employee surcharge equal to a percentage of all wages and salaries received.

PCP CAPITATION: A reimbursement system for health care providers of primary care services that receive a prepayment every month. The payment amount is based on age, sex, and plan of every member assigned to that physician for that month. Specialty capitation plans also exist but are rarely used.

PE RATIO: Price Earnings Ratio or price of a stock in relation to its per share earnings.

PEAK: A high output point relative to inputs.

PECUNIARY EXTERNALITY: An effect of health care production or medical care transactions on outside patients and parties through economic prices but not real allocations.

PEGGING: Market manipulation using a combination of capping and supporting moves in an attempt to fix an underlying security's price at a certain level.

PENNY STOCKS: Stocks selling for under $1. They are usually highly speculative.

PENSION: Salary replacement plan for retirement. Either defined benefit (DB) plan (older type pension plan in which the company assumes risk), or defined contribution (DC) plan (newer type pension plan in which the participant assumes risk). Traditional and Roth IRAs, Traditional, Individual and Roth 401(k)s and 403(b)s, and so forth.

PENSION BENEFIT GUARANTEE CORPORATION (PBGC): Federal corporation established following ERISA in 1974 that insures certain unfunded defined pension benefits up to certain limits.

PEOPLE PILL: The resignation of the entire senior management team in the case of a hostile corporate takeover.

PER CAPITA: Statistical allocation of data to an individual. Also, per patient, per head, *per capitus.*

PER CAPITA DEBT: The amount of an issuing municipality's debt outstanding divided by the population residing in the municipality. It is often used as an indication of the issuer's credit position because it can be used to compare the proportion of debt borne per resident with that borne by the residents of other municipalities.

PER CAPITA HEALTH CARE SPENDING: Annual spending on health care per person.

PER CAUSE DEDUCTIBLE: Requirement that a deductible be made for each separate illness or accident before benefits are paid.

PER DIEM: Total medical reimbursement charges per day, rather than by actual charges and services.

PER DIEM PAYMENTS: Fixed daily payments that do not vary with the level of services used by the patient. This method generally is used to pay institutional providers, such as hospitals and nursing facilities.

PER DIEM RATES: Fixed daily rates that do not vary with the level of services used by the patient. This method generally is used to pay institutional providers, such as hospitals and nursing facilities.

PERCENT (%) OF EQUITY: The percentage of a total portfolio a particular holding comprises. Computed by dividing the current market value of a security type (or total for a security type) by total current market value of the managed portfolio. It factors in short positions and accrued interest and dividends.

PERCENT (%) OF PREMIUM METHOD: The financial proportion or cost of any element (medical, facility, drug, or DME) taken against the premium price of an insurance charge for a specific benefit or service.

PERCENTAGE (%) OF COMPLETION METHOD: An accounting procedure for determining partial payments on a large contract where identifiable portions of the work are completed, invoiced and paid before the entire project is finished and paid in full.

PERCENTAGE (%) OF HOLDINGS: The ratio of holdings represented by a component of an account or portfolio.

PERCENTAGE (%) OF RECEIVABLES METHOD: A method of estimating uncollectible receivables.

PERCENTAGE (%) OF SALES METHOD: A method of estimating sales ratios.

PERFECT COMPETITION: A marketplace where there are many medical providers, health care services are homogenous, each health care business entity has a very small share of the market, no competitive threats exist, information is readily available, and providers may enter and exit easily.

PERFECT ELASTICITY OF DEMAND: A change in health care quantity demanded that needs no change in the price of health care products or services.

PERFECT ELASTICITY OF SUPPLY: A change in health care quantity supplied that needs no change in the price of health care products or services made available by providers.

PERFECT INELASTICITY OF DEMAND: A change in health care prices that results in no change in quantity of health care products or services demanded.

PERFECT INELASTICITY OF SUPPLY: A change in health care prices that results in no change in quantity of health care products or services supplied by providers.

PERFECT PRICE DISCRIMINATION: Charging a different price for each unit of health care output that a patient is able and willing to maximally pay.

PERFORMANCE BASED PAY: Any compensation method used to economically incent or provide a bonus or additional monetary benefits to providers in exchange for cost efficient utilization of rendered medical care or services.

PERFORMANCE BUDGET: Projected performance goals, along with line item projections of inflows and outflows, that measure a health care entity's performance.

PERIOD CERTAIN: Annuity guarantying a minimum number of periodic payments.

PERIOD COSTS: Operational costs expensed in the time period incurred.

PERIOD DIGESTION: The time after a corporate merger when company styles and culture are acclimating.

PERIODIC BALANCING: The act of reshifting capital from asset classes that performed well to those that did not, in order to maintain a set ratio between asset classes.

PERIODIC INTERIM PAYMENT: Medical provider lump sum payment to a health care provider. It is an end of year bonus adjustment.

PERMANENT ACCOUNT: Account not closed at the end of a period, such as assets, liabilities, and capital accounts.

PERMANENT FINANCING: Usually stocks and/or long-term bonds.

PERPETUAL BOND: Corporate debt without a maturity date.

PERPETUAL INVENTORY: A continuing running record of inventory and cost of goods sold.

PERPETUITY: An investment generating an income stream over an extended period of time. The formula is the expected income stream divided by a discount factor or market rate of interest that reflects the expected present value of all payments. For example, if a preferred hospital issue pays a $2.00 quarterly dividend and the annual interest rate is 5%, then one would expect to be willing to pay $2.50/0.0125, or $200 per share. Here, the 5% interest rate was adjusted for a simple quarterly disbursement $(0.05/4 = 0.0125)$.

PERQUISITE: A fringe benefit. An economic perk.

PERSONAL CONSUMPTION EXPENDITURES HEALTH CARE: The expenditures of average households for medical products, goods, and services.

PERSONAL DISTRIBUTION OF HEALTH CARE INCOME: The manner in which one allocates income for health care among different medical products and services.

PERSONAL FINANCE: Income, savings, investments, insurance, taxes, speculations, loans, mortgages, budgets, spending, gifting, and other financial affairs such as retirement, estate, and medical practice succession planning on an individual basis.

PERSONAL FINANCIAL SPECIALIST (PFS): A CPA who specializes in personal financial planning.

PERSONAL HEALTH CARE CONSUMPTION: The personal use of health care products or services.

PERSONAL HEALTH CARE EXPENDITURES: These are outlays for goods and services relating directly to patient care. It is the part of total national or state health expenditures spent on direct health care delivery, including hospital care, physician services, dental services, home health, nursing home care, and prescription drugs.

PERSONAL IDENTIFICATION NUMBER (PIN): An account holder's secret number or code used to authorize transactions or obtain information regarding an account. It is often used in conjunction with a plastic card (ATM or Debit card), online account access, or with a telephone voice response system.

PERSONAL INCOME: Total earnings derived from wages, and passive and active investments.

PETERSON, DIANE: President of D. Peterson & Associates in Houston, Texas, and the immediate past chairman of the American College of Health Care Executives in Chicago, Illinois.

PETTY CASH: Small cash fund for paying minor expenditures.

PHANTOM BILLING: Billing for medical services not actually performed. Fraudulent medical claims submissions versus CPT *code creep.*

PHANTOM INCOME: Income on paper but not in the form of cash.

PHANTOM STOCK PLAN: An arrangement under which an employee is allowed the benefits of owning employer securities even though shares are not actually issued to the employee.

PHARMACEUTICAL INDUSTRY ROI: Among the most consistent industries in the U.S. Fortune 500, and leaders in Return on Revenues (ROR), Return on Assets (ROA) and Return on Stockholders Equity (ROSE).

PHILLIPS CURVE: Relationship between interest rates and unemployment levels.

PHYSICIAN BONUS: Additional lump sum of money given as an incentive to a medical provider for specific behavior.

PHYSICIAN CHANNELING INCENTIVE: Additional medical provider compensation for health care work load or other services to lower cost-of-care providers (i.e., optometrist versus ophthalmology for a routine eye examination) (see Table 8).

PHYSICIAN CONTINGENCY RESERVE (PCR): Financial set-aside or cash account for excessive medical claim losses. A bonus, risk, capitation or economic withhold pool.

PHYSICIAN FISCAL CREDENTIALING: The economic outcomes analysis of one or more procedures in an attempt to gather, allocate, analyze, and interpret meaningful information relative to a medical practitioner or venue of performance. When used to establish comparative norms or, when compared to the appropriate benchmarks, cost and charge reductions are documented without comprising quality. Economic heuristic beliefs are then corroborated or dismissed.

PHYSICIAN PRODUCTION FORMULA: Typically a fee-for-service pro rata share of funds received for patient care under a fixed-rate capital reimbursement model. Capitated FFS percentage.

PHYSICIAN UNIT COST HOSPITAL POOL: A shared economic risk strategy between doctors and hospitals as a financial incentive to doctors to lower inpatient unit costs through the use of outpatient facilities, stepped-down care units, early discharges, and so forth.

PICK-UP: The value or profit gained in a bond swap.

PIGGYBACK: Illegal stockbroker practice of buying or selling securities after a customer does the same.

PIGOU EFFECT: A wealth impression on health care consumption as prices fall. A lower price level leads to a greater existing private wealth of nominal value, leading to a rise in health care consumption.

PINK SHEETS: Slang term for the daily publication of wholesale prices of over-the-counter (OTC) stocks that are generally too small to be listed in newspapers. They are named for the color of paper used. It is a list issued by the National Quotation Bureau (NQB) identifying market makers dealing in corporate equity securities in the over-the-counter market.

Table 8: Physician Compensation

Specialty	All Physicians	Starting	East	West	South	North
Allergy & Immunology	$207,278	$154,080	$193,480	$210,802	$204,870	$206,241
Anesthesiology	$315,300	$250,000	$275,000	$298,000	$334,200	$334,033
Cardiac & Thoracic Surgery	$421,620	$310,000	$387,298	$343,050	$421,240	$469,860
Cardiology	$336,000	$280,000	$264,900	$343,646	$386,957	$369,566
Colon & Rectal Surgery	$327,927	****	$300,000	****	****	$350,798
Critical Care Medicine	$228,740	****	$220,235	****	$227,242	$228,740
Dermatology	$274,014	$200,000	$225,000	$289,409	$322,138	$263,201
Diagnostic Radiology - Interventional	$410,250	$320,000	$345,860	$410,000	$537,942	$410,250
Diagnostic Radiology - Non-Interventional	$364,899	$257,367	$330,000	$350,224	$383,319	$383,256
Emergency Care	$230,930	$175,500	$200,327	$228,814	$225,905	$239,984
Endocrinology	$185,000	$140,000	$166,675	$185,000	$177,665	$201,241
Family Medicine	$164,209	$120,000	$141,225	$166,750	$163,417	$168,488
Family Medicine - with Obstetrics	$163,334	$125,000	$140,643	$162,352	$161,421	$167,222
Gastroenterology	$308,246	$250,000	$263,594	$325,698	$325,033	$306,994

General Surgery	$294,000	$200,000	$250,028	$275,336	$301,761	$330,903
Geriatrics	$159,492	****	$150,000	****	$158,400	$170,278
Gynecological Oncology	$334,009	****	$290,795	$345,355	****	$347,005
Gynecology	$217,283	****	$220,794	****	$224,420	$217,256
Gynecology & Obstetrics	$250,196	$180,000	$232,276	$240,118	$258,756	$275,419
Hematology & Medical Oncology	$255,007	$200,000	$207,300	$261,004	$293,043	$255,007
Hospitalist	$171,991	$150,000	$153,515	$175,084	$183,775	$171,913
Hypertension & Nephrology	$214,751	$165,000	$186,683	$238,750	$253,228	$214,751
Infectious Disease	$185,920	$140,111	$161,206	$179,402	$175,000	$203,640
Intensivist	$231,111	****	****	$230,391	****	****
Internal Medicine	$169,569	$120,000	$158,824	$171,246	$167,740	$170,511
Neonatology	$229,486	$165,000	$242,492	$222,750	$223,312	$232,738
Neurological Surgery	$465,006	$400,000	$352,352	$495,266	$553,500	$465,006
Neurology	$201,241	$151,960	$180,882	$199,614	$204,000	$201,241

(Continued)

Table 8: Physician Compensation

Specialty	All Physicians	Starting	East	West	South	North
Pediatric Gastroenterology	$193,193	****	****	****	****	$190,345
Pediatric Hematology/Oncology	$195,249	****	****	$193,387	$198,940	$196,897
Pediatric Intensive Care	$200,000	****	****	****	$200,000	$200,000
Pediatric Nephrology	****	****	****	****	****	****
Pediatric Neurology	$185,212	****	****	****	****	$192,528
Pediatric Pulmonary Disease	$158,429	****	****	****	****	****
Pediatric Surgery	$326,399	****	****	****	****	$354,871
Pediatrics & Adolescent	$169,267	$115,000	$155,916	$168,301	$191,511	$168,609
Pediatric Infectious Disease	$173,993	****	****	****	****	$173,993
Perinatology	$341,922	****	$246,597	$336,537	****	$399,360
Physical Medicine & Rehabilitation	$193,468	$145,000	****	$183,362	$204,775	$201,993
Plastic & Reconstruction	$328,764	$220,020	$273,000	$344,059	$344,998	$353,983
Psychiatry	$177,000	$135,000	$155,673	$197,021	$168,160	$177,000
Psychiatry - Child	$192,416	****	****	$220,055	****	$183,621

Specialty						
Pulmonary Disease	$222,000	$163,626	$199,831	$249,865	$225,400	$228,359
Radiation Therapy (MD only)	$334,171	****	$285,940	$343,844	$328,350	$368,240
Reproductive Endocrinology	$263,568	****	****	****	****	****
Rheumatologic Disease	$188,260	$150,000	$153,000	$192,026	$181,525	$193,301
Sports Medicine	$193,573	****	****	****	****	****
Surgical Pathology (MD only)	$	$	****	****	****	****
Surgical Sports Medicine	$391,497	****	$485,670	$459,592	****	$389,997
Transplant Surgery - Kidney	$345,000	****	****	****	****	$379,995
Transplant Surgery - Liver	$349,788	****	****	****	****	$379,995
Trauma Surgery	$312,272	****	$265,457	****	$310,385	$352,352
Urgent Care	$176,353	$125,500	$179,300	$179,357	$180,395	$173,683
Urology	$324,690	$219,229	$270,493	$302,600	$351,585	$358,008
Vascular Surgery	$335,642	$221,500	$297,636	$318,388	$337,762	$350,000
Gastroenterology	$308,246	$250,000	$263,594	$325,698	$325,033	$306,994

Source: 2005 AMGA Physician Compensation Survey.

PIPELINE OR CONDUIT THEORY: A theory of investing by which tax liabilities by mutual funds are avoided by passing a certain percentage (currently 98%) of income and profits on to a fund's stockholders as dividends and capital distributions. The fund pays taxes on the 2% retained.

PLACE: To sell or market new securities.

PLACE, REV. MICHAEL: President and CEO of the Catholic Health Association in St. Louis, Missouri.

PLACEMENT RATIO: The amount of bonds sold by underwriting syndicates each week as a percentage of the amount issued that week by issuers selling $1,000,000 par value or more of securities. The placement ratio is compiled weekly and is published in *The Bond Buyer.*

PLATYKURTIC (PLATYKURTOSIS): A relatively flat condition for a probability distribution that is evaluated against the normal distribution and its usual bell-shaped curve.

PLAY OR PAY: Slang term for an economic insurance suggestion for employers to provide health insurance for employees, or pay into a fund that would provide coverage.

PLAYING THE MARKET: The amateurish buying or selling of securities.

PLEDGED RECEIVABLES: Use of anticipated accounts receivable payments as collateral.

PLEDGED REVENUES: The money obligated for the payment of debt service and other deposits required by the bond contract:

- Gross Pledge or Gross Revenue Pledge: A pledge that all revenue received will be used for debt service prior to deductions for any costs or expenses.
- Net Pledge or Net Revenue Pledge: A pledge that all funds remaining after certain operational and maintenance costs and expenses are paid will be used for payment of debt service.

PLOW BACK: Reinvesting profits back into a business, rather than distributing it as dividends or profit to shareholders, investors, or capital suppliers.

PLUS TICK: A transaction on a stock exchange at a price higher than the last transaction.

PMPM: Per Member Per Month.

PMPY: Per Member Per Year.

POINT: In stocks, a point means $1. In bonds, because a bond is quoted as a percentage of $1,000, it means $10. In market averages, it means simply a point, a unit of measurement.

POISON PILL: Slang term for strategies to make stock less attractive in the event of a hostile corporate takeover attempt.

POLITY: A group with organized governance, such as the American Medical Association.

POOLED INCOME FUND: A mutual fund that commingles property gifted by several donors, where each donor designates a noncharitable person to receive income for life and a charity to receive the remaining interest. [Regs. §1.642(c)-5]

POOLING: Combining assets and resources as a strategy for a common economic goal.

POOLING OF INTERESTS: Combining the financial statements of two health care firms that merge. It is the summation of assets on the balance sheet of the new or surviving firm, and voting common stock exchange for the voting common stock of an acquired company when certain criteria are met.

POOLING OF INVENTORY: Combining inventory, equipment, and/or DME as a strategy for a common economic goal.

PORTER, MICHAEL E., PhD: Director of the Institute for Strategy and Competitiveness (ISC) at Harvard Business School. Porter is also Harvard's Bishop William Lawrence University Professor and a leading authority in health care competition.

PORTFOLIO: An aggregation of assets to preserve and increase purchasing power in the future. Holdings of securities by an individual or institution, which may include bonds and preferred and common stocks of various enterprises.

PORTFOLIO ANALYSIS: Quantified systematic (market) and nonsystematic (business) risk for investment holdings developed by Harry Markowitz, PhD, who is considered to be the originator of this theory, and the father of asset allocation or modern portfolio theory.

PORTFOLIO CHOICE: Decision about which assets and liabilities to purchase, trade, and hold.

PORTFOLIO DISCOUNT: The discount for nonrelated or nonintegrated health care business sectors or service lines.

PORTFOLIO INCOME: Investment income including interest income, dividend income, and net gains and losses from the sales of securities and other capital assets.

PORTFOLIO INSURANCE: A form of hedging equity and credit products because it requires quick adjustments in the hedge.

PORTFOLIO MANAGER: A professional who manages a portfolio of securities.

PORTFOLIO RISK: The sum of systematic (market) and nonsystematic (business) risk (see Figure 4).

PORTFOLIO SUMMARY: Statement of account value information for the fiscal year-to-date through prior month end and fiscal year-to-date through prior business date. Provides a snapshot of portfolio or account valuation and fiscal year-to-date income.

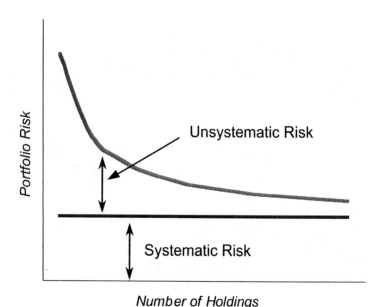

Figure 4: Portfolio Risk.

PORTFOLIO THEORY: Concept that evaluates the reduction of nonsystematic or diversifiable risks through the selection of securities or other instruments into a composite holding or "efficient portfolio." Efficiency means that a portfolio would offer lower risks or more stable returns for a targeted return level. Instruments that have independent returns lower nonsystematic risks. Also, instruments that are inversely related on a return basis reduce the diversifiable risks. A basic theory assumes that returns are independent, investor expectations are homogeneous, and that the normalized probability distributions are stable. *See also* portfolio analysis.

PORTFOLIO TURNOVER: A measure of a mutual fund's trading activity that indicates how much buying and selling of securities has taken place.

POSITION: A stake in a certain set of securities, or the financial condition of a company.

POSITION BUILDING: The gradual acquisition of certain securities to a portfolio.

POSITION LIMITS: The maximum number of open option contracts that an investor can hold in one account or in a group of related accounts. Some exchanges express the limit in terms of option contracts on the same side of the market, and others express it in terms of total long or short delta.

POSITIVE CARRY: The cost of capital to finance securities is lower than the yield on those securities.

POSITIVE ECONOMICS: Health care or other economics testable by appeal to the facts.

POSITIVE EXTERNALITY: Benefit not reflected in price and associated with the use of health care or other resources.

POSITIVE YIELD CURVE: Usual graphical representation when interest rates are higher on long-term debt than they are on short-term debt.

POSITIVELY CORRELATED: Two securities or industries that have market movement in the same direction.

POST: Recording accounting transactions.

POST-CLOSING-TRIAL BALANCE: A list of ledger accounts.

POST HOC, ERGO PROPTER HOC: Fallacious Latin phrase that reasons when one economic act follows another, the first act is the cause of the second.

POSTING: The transferal of amounts from the accounting journal into the ledger of accounts.

POSTING DATE: The actual day a medical service charge or professional fee is noted on a patient ledger or account.

POTENTIAL COMPETITION: The possibility of new medical or health care economic competitors, for example, MD versus DO, hospitals versus ASCs, and so forth.

POVERTY: Personal income thresholds below the Social Security Administration Index of 1964. Indexed annually.

POWERS AND AUTHORITIES DOCUMENT: A formal document similar to an Investment Policy Statement (ISP) that outlines position taking and risk management limits for a hospital, large portfolio or other endowment type fund or portfolio, which lists trading parameters, such as:

- aging limits
- cash limits
- concentration limits
- contract limits
- conversion limits
- counterparty limits
- country limits
- CPV adjusted values
- cross border limits

- currency limits
- day trading limits
- delta adjusted limits
- dollar loss limits
- duration limits
- funding limits
- gross limits
- instruments may or may not be traded
- inventory limits
- investment limits
- long position limits
- margin limits
- market value limits
- maximum individual trade limits
- net position limits
- notional value limits
- overnight exposure limits
- premium and discount limits
- principal or share limits
- regulatory capital limits for the firm, desk, trader, and instrument
- short position limits
- size of market limits
- supervisory limits
- time value decay limits
- VAR limits
- volatility limits
- who is authorized to trade, when, where, and with whom

PPS INPATIENT MARGIN: A measure that compares Prospective Payment System operating and capital payments with Medicare-allowable inpatient operating and capital costs. It is calculated by subtracting total Medicare-allowable inpatient operating and capital costs from total PPS operating and capital payments and dividing by total PPS operating and capital payments.

PPS OPERATING MARGIN: A measure that compares Prospective Payment Systems operating payments with Medicare-allowable inpatient operating costs. This measure excludes Medicare costs and payments for capital, direct medical education, organ acquisition, and other categories not included among Medicare-allowable inpatient operating costs. It is calculated by subtracting total Medicare-allowable inpatient operating costs from total PPS operating payments and dividing by total PPS operating payments.

PRACTICE EXPENSE: The cost of nonphysician resources incurred by the physician to provide services. Examples are salaries and fringe benefits received by the physician's employees and the expenses associated with the purchase and use of medical equipment and supplies in the physician's office. A component of the Medicare Resource Based Relative Value Scale (RBRVS).

PRACTICE EXPENSE RELATIVE VALUE (PERV): A value that reflects the average amount of practice expenses incurred in performing a particular service. All values are expressed relative to the practice expenses for a reference service whose value equals one practice expense unit.

PRECAUTIONARY SAVINGS: Accumulated funds by patients of laymen to prepare for future periods in which income is low.

PREDATORY PRICING: Providing or selling a health care or other service, good, or other product at below variable or incremental costs (less than profitable) in order to gain market share or reduce competition.

PREEMPTIVE RIGHTS: The right to maintain a proportionate share of ownership in a health care or other corporation.

PREFERRED STOCK: Owners of this kind of stock are entitled to a fixed dividend to be paid regularly before dividends can be paid on common stock. They also exercise claims to assets, in the event of liquidation, senior to common stockholders but junior to bondholders. Preferred stockholders normally do not have a voice in management.

PRE-FISC: Slang term meaning prior to considering the government's health care fiscal policy.

PRELIMINARY OFFICIAL STATEMENT (PROSPECTUS) or RED HERRING: A preliminary version of the official statement that is used by an issuer or underwriter to describe the proposed issue of securities prior to the determination of the interest rate(s) and offering price(s). The preliminary official statement may be used by issuers to gauge underwriters' interest in an issue and is often relied upon by potential purchasers in making their investment decisions. Normally, offers for the sale of or acceptance of securities are not made on the basis of the preliminary official statement, and a statement to that effect appears on the face of the document generally in red print, which gives the document its nickname, red herring. The preliminary official statement is technically a draft.

PREMISE OF VALUE: The most reasonable set of circumstances applicable to a valuation project.

PREMIUM: The price of an option agreed upon by the buyer and seller through their representatives on the floor of an exchange. The premium is paid by a buyer, to a seller. The premium is quoted on a per share or per unit basis.

PREMIUM BONDS: Coupon bonds with a higher rate of interest than the prevailing rate and that sell at a higher price than par. Because the yield is higher, premium bonds compensate the investor for the premium paid. Also, this type of bond has less volatility than discounted securities.

PREMIUM CALL: A redemption provision that permits the issuer to call securities at a price above par or, in the case of certain original issue discount or multiplier securities, above the compound accreted value.

PREPAID ASSET: A benefit such as rent, utilities, leases, or insurance that is paid for in advance.

PREPAID CARE: Health care paid for in a fixed-rate installment basis.

PREPAID EXPENSE: An expense paid before due. An asset on the balance sheet.

PREPAID GROUP PRACTICE: Prepayment health care arrangements with selected medical practitioners to provide fixed-rate care for a population of patients.

PREPAID GROUP PRACTICE PLAN: A plan where specified health services are rendered by participating physicians to an enrolled group of persons, with a fixed periodic payment made in advance by (or on behalf of) each person or family. If a health insurance carrier is involved, it is a contract to pay in advance for the full range of health services to which the insured is entitled under the terms of the health insurance contract. *See also* health maintenance organization (HMO).

PREPAID HEALTH PLAN: Health care given to a cohort of patients, by physicians, providers, and facilities, who accept periodic fixed interim payments. It is a prepaid program.

PREPAID HOSPITAL SERVICE PLAN: The common name for a health maintenance organization (HMO). It is a plan that provides comprehensive health care to its members, who pay a flat annual fee for services.

PREPAID PRACTICE: Medical care reimbursement prior to the delivery of health care services. It is an accounting liability.

PREPAID PREMIUM: An insurance or other premium payment paid prior to the due date.

PREPAID PRESCRIPTION PLAN: Drug reimbursement plan that is paid in advance.

PREPAYMENT: Payment made before due, as in prepaid or prospective health care financial arrangements by contract. It is a method providing in advance for the cost of predetermined benefits for a population group, through regular periodic payments in the form of premiums, dues, or contributions including those contributions that are made to a health and welfare fund by employers on behalf of their employees.

PREPAYMENT PENALTY: Cost or surcharge if a debt is paid off prematurely.

PREPAYMENT PLANS: A term referring to health insurance plans that provide medical or hospital benefits in service rather than dollars, such as the plans offered by various health maintenance organizations.

PREPAYMENT PREMIUMS: Advanced payment by an insured of future health care insurance premiums, through paying the present (discounted) value of the future premiums or having interest paid on the deposit.

PREREFUND: A second bond issued to pay off a first bond at its call date. A form of bond payment insurance.

PREREFUNDED (ADVANCE-REFUNDED) BONDS: Securities that are refinanced by the proceeds of a new bond issue. Proceeds are generally invested in either U.S. government securities or federal agency securities. This type of security has an added element of security, high current income, higher yield to maturity, and lower volatility.

PRESALE ORDER: An order given to a syndicate manager prior to the purchase of securities from the issuer, who indicates a prospective investor's intention to purchase the securities at a predetermined price level. Presale orders are normally afforded top priority in allocation of securities from the syndicate.

PRESENT (DISCOUNTED) VALUE (PV OR PDV): The amount of money that, if invested at a specified rate of interest, will, at a given future time, accumulate to a specified sum, calculated by: $PV = $ Future Value $\times$ Present Value Factor. It is the current value of a future payment or income stream discounted at some appropriate interest rate.

PRESENT VALUE ANNUITY: The worth today, for an equal value of streaming income, considering the time value of money.

PRESENT VALUE FACTOR (PVF): The discounting of future cash flow, such as ARs by the formula: $[1 / 1 + i)^n]$.

PRESOLD ISSUE: Municipal securities sold prior to public announcement.

PREVAILING CHARGE: One of the factors determining a physician's payment for a service under Medicare, set at a percentile of customary charges of all physicians in the locality.

PREVENTION COSTS: Costs incurred to prevent or reduce poor quality medical goods or services.

PREVENTIVE CONTROLS: Methods to reduce errors or fraud from occurring that could result in a misstatement of the financial statements.

PRICE: Revenue posted per health care product, good, or service unit rendered. A charge.

PRICE CEILINGS: Legal maximum charges for health products or services resulting in a shortage.

PRICE DISCRIMINATION: The practice of selling certain health care services or products for different prices, to different buyers.

PRICE/EARNINGS RATIO (P/E RATIO): Often called a stock's multiple. Current price per share divided by earnings per share. Earnings can be forward (predicted/projected) or trailing (actual last four quarters). It is a benchmark of earnings growth and prospects.

PRICE EFFECT: A result in the change in price based on the quantity of health care services consumed.

PRICE ELASTICITY OF DEMAND: The percentage change in quantity demanded of a health care good resulting from each 1% change in the price of the service.

PRICE ELASTICITY OF SUPPLY: The percentage change in quantity supplied of a health care good resulting from each 1% change in the price of the service.

PRICE FIXING: Conspiracy among participants to establish market prices for health care services. It is illegal and collusionary.

PRICE FLOOR: Legal minimum charges for health care or other services resulting in a glut for market flood.

PRICE INDEX: A measurement of health care product or service value, set at 100 in the base year.

PRICE LEADERSHIP: A dominant company in the health care industry that sets its price to maximize profits, after which other firms follow suit at the same price level.

PRICE LEVEL: Weighted average of health care prices in a given area.

PRICE LEVEL SURPRISE: Unanticipated change in the price point of health care products, goods, and services.

PRICE MAKER: A buyer or seller of health care products, goods, and/or services that is able to affect the sales price point by altering the quantity it buys or sells, according to the CMS fee schedule.

PRICE SUPPORT: Floors imposed on certain goods or services.

PRICE SYSTEM: Model by which health care resource use is guided by their price.

PRICE TAKER: A seller or buyer of health care products or services that is unable to affect a price point change by altering the amount it sells or buys. *See also* Medicare fee schedule.

PRICE VARIANCE: A measure, benchmark, or spread of standardized costs for an industry.

PRICE WAR: The continual erosion of prices by rival companies in the same marketplace or space, such as ambulatory or outpatient surgery centers (ASCs or OSCs).

PRICER REPRICER: A person, organization, software package, or subscription electronic application that reviews procedures, diagnoses, fee schedules, and other data and determines the eligible amount for a given health care service or supply. Additional criteria can then be applied to determine the actual allowance, or payment, amount.

PRICEY: An unusually high or low bid for securities.

PRIMARY CARE CAPITATION: Prospective medical payment system that provides a fixed amount of reimbursement to a gatekeeper or primary care physicians for medical care, regardless of quantity delivered in the aggregate, to patient population cohorts.

PRIMARY DISTRIBUTION (OFFERING): The original sale of a security. All further trades are in the secondary market.

PRIMARY PAYER: The insurer who pays the first medical claim. Medicare or other private health insurance.

PRIME COSTS: The sum of direct material and labor costs.

PRIME MARKET: Market for new issue securities. Initial Public Offerings.

PRIME PAPER: High quality commercial paper. Short-term unsecured corporate debt.

PRIME RATE: The cost of capital or interest rate a bank charges its most creditworthy customers or institutions.

PRINCIPAL: (1) A lump sum or corpus of money or funds. (2) The role of a broker/dealer firm when it buys and sells for its own account. In a typical transaction, it buys from a market maker or contrabroker and sells to a customer at a fair and reasonable markup. If it buys from a customer and sells to the market maker at a higher price, it is called a markdown.

PRINCIPAL OF PAYMENT: Advanced monthly funds given to HMOs as an economic equivalent per capita, of each enrolled member of a group of Medicare beneficiaries.

PRINCIPAL REGISTRATION: A form of registration with the National Association of Securities Dealers, entitling the registrant to participate in all supervisory phases of the member organization except preparation and approval of the financial statements and net capital computations.

PRINCIPLE OF MINIMUM DIFFERENTIATION: The tendency of health care industry competitors to make themselves almost identical in order to appeal to the largest possible market.

PRIOR DEDUCTIBLE CREDIT: A provision that allows a member or family to apply any health insurance deductible credit.

PRIOR PERIOD ADJUSTMENT: A correction to retained earnings for a mistake of a prior accounting period.

PRIOR PREFERRED (PREFERENCE) STOCK: A kind of preferred stock entitling the owner to prior claim to forthcoming dividends or claim to assets in liquidation proceedings.

PRIORITY: Order of creditors in a liquidation action (secured to unsecured).

PRIORITY PROVISIONS: The rules adopted by an underwriting syndicate specifying the priority to be given different types of orders received by the syndicate. The most common priority provision gives presale orders top priority, followed by group net orders, designated orders, and member orders. MSRB rules require syndicates to adopt priority provisions in writing and to make them available to all interested parties.

PRIVATE COSTS: Price paid by individuals for the use of a good or service such as health care.

PRIVATE EXPENDITURES: These are outlays for medical services provided or paid for by nongovernmental sources: consumers, insurance companies, private industry, and philanthropic and other nonpatient care sources.

PRIVATE FOUNDATION: A tax-exempt organization, such as a hospital or other designated health care entity, under IRC §501(c)(3) that does not enjoy a broad base of public support. [IRC §§508, 509]

PRIVATE INUREMENT: The payment for medical goods, services, and equipment, at above market rates, at the expense of tax-exempt health care entities (501[c]3 charitable or community health care facilities and hospitals).

PRIVATE PLACEMENT: The distribution of unregistered securities to a limited number of purchasers without the filing of a registration statement with the SEC. Such offerings generally require submission of an investment letter to the seller by all purchasers.

PRIVATE SECURITIES TRANSACTIONS: The practice described in the National Association of Securities Dealers (NASD) Rules of Fair Practice, under which an associated person of a member firm engages in a securities related transaction without his firm's knowledge. This is prohibited. An associated person is required to inform his firm of any securities type activity and must have its permission in order to engage in same. If the associated person is to receive compensation for this transaction, the firm is required to run it through its books and records and has ultimate supervisory responsibility.

PRIVATIZATION: The conversion of a public company into a privately held one. This is usually through a leveraged buy out with extreme debt.

PRO FORMA FINANCIAL STATEMENTS: Estimates or projections of the four consolidated financial statements: (1) Balance Sheet, (2) Cash-Flow Statement, (3) Net Income Statement, and (4) Statement of Operations.

PRO RATA: According to a calculated share or portion. In proportion.

PRO RATA CANCELLATION: The termination of a health insurance or other contract or bond, with the premium charge being adjusted in proportion to the exact time the protection has been in force. When the policy is terminated midterm by the insurance company, the earned premium is calculated only for the period coverage was provided. For example: an annual policy with premium of $1,000 is cancelled after 41 days of coverage at the company's election. The earned premium would be calculated as follows: $40 / 365 \text{ days} \times \$1,000 = 0.109 \times \$1,000 = \$109$.

PRO RATA PREMIUM: A fractional or percentage premium.

PRO RATA RATE: A short-term rate proportionate to the rate for a longer term.

PRO RATA UNEARNED PREMIUM RESERVE: A health insurance reserve calculated to represent the unearned portion of the liability to policy owners to be discharged in the future with future protection, by return to the policy owner in event of cancellation, or by reinsuring the business with another insurer.

PROBABILITY DISTRIBUTION: A statistical tool used to show the dispersion around an expected result. A normal distribution with a "bell-shaped curve." Other distributions have bell-shaped curve appearances but do not necessarily behave in a normal manner, such as:

- Bernoulli
- Beta
- Binomial
- Cauchy
- Chi Square
- Exponential
- F
- Gamma
- Geometric
- Lognormal
- Negative Binomial
- Normal
- Pascal
- Poisson
- t
- Uniform

PROBLEM ORIENTED V-CODE: ICD-9-CM code that notates potential situations that might affect a patient in the future but are not a current injury or illness.

PROCEEDS SALE: A transaction where a customer sells a security and uses the proceeds to purchase another security.

PROCESS: A cost and quality assessment of delivered health care.

PRODUCER PRICE INDEX (PPI): Monthly measure wholesale price changes in industry segments.

PRODUCER SURPLUS: The difference between health care revenue and the opportunity cost of production.

PRODUCT MARGIN: Total contribution margin minus avoidable fixed costs.

PRODUCTION: The conversion of health care or other inputs, to outputs. *See also* productivity.

PRODUCTION COST: The operations expenditures of a processing department.

PRODUCTION COST REPORT: Summary of the operations of a processing department for a specific period.

PRODUCTION FUNCTION: Relationship between varied health care outputs and inputs. It is the greatest number of health care outputs that a health care entity can produce or serve from various quantities of inputs.

PRODUCTIVE: The amount of health care economic output, per unit of input.

PRODUCTIVE EFFICIENCY: Occurs when the maximum output of health care goods and services is derived from the output of other goods or services.

PRODUCTIVITY: A measure of health care work output per unit of input.

PROFESSIONAL FEES: Monies paid to contracted medical providers, while nursing compensation is usually a line-item labor item.

PROFESSIONAL LIABILITY INSURANCE: Medical malpractice insurance.

PROFIT: The difference between revenues taken in by a health care or other business entity and the costs incurred for operations and the receipt of those revenues.

PROFIT AND LOSS (P&L) STATEMENT: *See* Net Income Statement (NIS).

PROFIT CENTER: Health care organizational units responsible for earning revenues and controlling their own costs, such as the emergency room or a cardiac care center. Health care entities include traditional, capitation, and administrative subunit profit centers.

PROFIT MARGIN: Earnings expressed as a percentage of revenues (i.e., the percentage of sales a company has left over as profit after paying all expenses).

PROFIT MARGIN ON SALES (PMOS): Net income to share (stock) holders / Sales.

PROFIT SHARING PLAN: Corporation-employer agreement to share in company profits or losses by purchasing stock.

PROFIT TAKING: To sell appreciated securities for gain and/or profit.

PROFITABILITY RATIOS: A financial success measurement of a health care or other organization (i.e., Return on Assets, Return on Equity, Return on Investment, etc.).

PROGRAMMED TRADING: Integrated sales or purchase of securities triggered by computers.

PROGRESSIVE TAX: A tax rate that increases with the tax base.

PROJECT COMPLETION CLAUSE: A protective covenant found in many municipal and hospital revenue bonds. The contractor(s) building the revenue producing project have an obligation to complete the work (and have the facility ready to produce revenue by a certain, specified date). If the facility is not completed as scheduled, the issuer is entitled to collect a monetary penalty from the contractor. The contractor is protected with a project completion bond from a casualty insurance company.

PROJECTED COSTS: Claims and/or retention costs projected for a given patient population for a specific time period.

PROJECTION: Economic estimate of future financial or business performance in a particular sector such as health care, or the nation as a whole.

PROMISE TO PAY: As specified in a policy or contract, a company's stated agreement to make payment of all stipulated sums to designated beneficiaries in the event of certain, specified occurrences.

PROMISSORY NOTE: Written promise to pay back a sum of money over specific time period and noted interest rate.

PROPORTIONATE SHARE OF ASSETS IN LIQUIDATION: A common stockholder's right to assets in proportion to his interest, upon liquidation, after all liabilities have been satisfied.

PROPORTIONATE TAX: A fixed tax rate in the face of a variable tax base.

PROPRIETORSHIP: A medical practice or health care entity owned and operated by a single individual or doctor.

PRORATE: Adjustment of health care or other policy benefits for any reason of change in occupation or significant or existence of other coverage.

PRORATION: Percentage formula allocation of assets.

PROSPECTIVE PAYMENT: The reimbursement or payment in advance for medical services rendered.

PROSPECTIVE PAYMENT SYSTEM (PPS): A system used by Medicare to pay medical providers, hospitals, and clinics a set amount of money per diagnostic related group (DRG).

PROSPECTUS: A document stating material information for an impending offering of securities (containing most of the information included in the registration statement) that is used for solicitation purposes by the issuer and underwriters.

PROTECTIVE COVENANTS: Agreements in the bond contract that impose duties upon the issuer, in order to protect the interests of the bondholders. Typical protective covenants relate to such items as maintenance of rates adequate to cover debt service, segregation of funds, proper project maintenance, and insurance, maintenance of specified books and records, and tests for the issuance of additional parity bonds.

PROVIDER DISCOUNTS: The amount of money contracting health care providers deduct from their charge because of contracts between themselves and a health plan.

PROVISION FOR BAD DEBTS: A health care entity operations account that estimates the portion of write-offs, nonpayments, and bad debts expenses in a cumulative account on the balance sheet.

PROXY: A short-term voting authorization issued by a corporation to its stockholders.

PROXY FIGHT: The persuasion and arguments used by a takeover artist to convince corporate shareholders to sell stock, with or without a premium or discount.

PRUDENT BUYER: The efficient purchaser of market balance between value and cost.

PRUDENT INVESTOR RULE: Rule suggesting that one in a fiduciary capacity (a trustee, executor, custodian, etc.) is required to conduct himself faithfully and exercise sound judgment when investing monies under his care and taking measured and reasonable investment risks in return for the anticipation of future rewards. Allows for investments into mutual funds, stocks, bonds, and variable annuities, and believes in asset allocation and Modern Portfolio Theory (MPT).

PRUDENT MAN RULE: Named after a court case decided in 1830, providing that operating in a fiduciary capacity (a trustee, executor, custodian, etc.) is required to conduct himself faithfully and exercise sound judgment when investing monies under his care. "He is to observe how men of prudence, discretion and intelligence manage their own affairs, not in regard to speculation, but in regard to the permanent distribution of their funds, considering the probable income as well as the probable safety of the capital to be invested" (*Harvard College v. Armory, 9 Pick.* [26 Mass.] 446, 461; 1830). In most cases, this rule may allow investments into mutual funds and variable annuities.

PRYOR, DAVID: Senior Vice President of Ascension Health in St. Louis, Missouri.

PSYCHIATRIC HOSPITAL (BEHAVIORAL HEALTH/MENTAL HOSPITAL/ ASYLUM): A hospital specializing in treatment of patients with mental illness or drug related illness or dependencies. Psychiatric wards differ only in that they are a unit of a larger hospital.

PUBLIC CHARITY: A tax-exempt organization, such as a hospital, clinic, or other designated entity, under IRC §501(c)(3) that enjoys a broad base of public support. [IRC §509(a)(2)]

PUBLIC COMPANY ACCOUNTING OVERSIGHT BOARD (PCAOB): A private sector, nonprofit corporation created by the Sarbanes-Oxley Act of 2002, to oversee the auditors of public companies in order to protect the interest of investors and further the public interest in the preparation of informative, fair, and independent audit reports.

PUBLIC GOOD: A product or service such as safety, health care, or national defense that can be consumed by one person or patient, without depleting it for another.

PUBLIC LAW 107–56 [H.R. 3162].: An Act to deter and punish terrorist acts in the United States and around the world, to enhance law enforcement investigatory tools. It is applicable to medical offices, clinics, health care, and hospital facilities who perform research and development related to bioterrorism countermeasures.

PUBLIC OFFERING: Securities sold to the public through an underwriter or investment bank.

PUBLIC OFFERING PRICE: Shares priced at the initial public offering (IPO); NAV per Share / (100% – Sales Charge Percentage).

PUBLIC OVERSIGHT BOARD (POB): Independent committee composed of public members who monitor and evaluate peer reviews conducted by the

SEC Practice Section (SECPS) of the AICPA's Division for CPA Firms as well as other activities of the SECPS.

PUBLICLY HELD: Company whose shares are traded and held by public investors.

PULL BACK: Retreat in an upward securities price trend.

PUMP AND DUMP: Slang term for the illegal actions by stockbrokers to attract new buyers with an illusion of high trading volume by inflating or pumping up the market for a specific security. This engineers a brief period of inflated prices that may dupe investors to purchase the securities only to have the broker dump many shares on the market place at the momentarily higher prices, thereby triggering a rapid decline in values that impacts the most recent investors.

PUNT: Closing a securities or other market position.

PURCHASE ACCOUNT: A listing of all purchases.

PURCHASE JOURNAL: Journal used to record all purchases of DME, inventory, and related items.

PURCHASE METHOD OF ACCOUNTING: Financial and economic corporation merger method by adding the acquired company's assets at the price paid for them to the acquiring company's assets.

PURCHASE ORDER: Ticker or invoice authorization to buy an asset.

PURCHASED CALL: A bullish investment strategy that confers the right, but not the obligation, to exercise an options contract into a long-position in underlying securities. The risk is limited to the premium paid, and the reward is theoretically considered to be unlimited.

PURCHASED PUT: A bearish investment strategy that confers the right, but not the obligation, to exercise an options contract into a short position in the underlying securities instrument. The risk is limited to the premium paid, and the reward is theoretically considered to be limited to the difference between the strike price less a zero market price.

PURCHASER'S REPRESENTATIVE: Under SEC Rule 506 of Reg. D, a purchaser's representative is required for any nonaccredited investor who does not have sufficient knowledge or experience to personally analyze the risks and merits of an investment.

PURCHASING POWER RISK: Potential of inflation to erode purchasing power or value of future income and assets.

PURE INDEMNITY: Traditional fee-for-service medical payment reimbursement.

PURE INFLATION: Occurs when the price of all goods and services rise over a time period.

PURE MONOPOLY: Environment where there is a single seller of a health care product or service without an alternate and without similar substitutes.

PURE MONOPSONY: Environment where a single company buys the entire market supply of a health care input, with few alternative employment opportunities.

PURE PLAY: A single line of business, especially in a company or firm without diversified products, goods, or services (i.e., an MRI imaging center).

PUSH DOWN ACCOUNTING: Method in which the values that arise from an acquisition are transferred or "pushed down" to the accounts of an acquired company.

PUT BONDS: Put bonds allow bondholders to give bonds (put) back to the issuer at par on specified dates prior to maturity. Put bonds have either a fixed or variable interest rate and may have single or multiple tender dates. They may be either mandatory (in which case the investor has a specified period of time to keep the bonds at the new rate) or optional (in which case the investor has a specified time period to tender the bonds).

PUT OPTION: An instrument that grants the holder the right to sell a stated number of shares (typically 100) of the underlying security within a stated period of time at the exercise price.

PUT WRITER: One who receives a financial premium and accepts, for a time period, the obligation to buy an underlying security for a specific price at the put buyer's discretion.

PUTTY-PUTTY: An attribute of health care capital in some economic models. It is capital transformed into durable health care goods or services, and then transformed back into general capital.

PY: Per Year.

PYRAMIDING: Credit abuse of a loan taken for recurring purposes and not fully paid when needed again for a new loan.

Q

Q: Commodity futures symbol for an August delivery month.

Q-RATIO: Ratio of a health care or other firm's market assets value to their replacement cost. It is also known as Tobin's Ratio.

QUALIFIED ANNUITY: An annuity that qualifies for tax deductibility under the IRS code. These annuities will be funded with pretax dollars and the earnings received into the account will accrue tax deferred. When the annuitant begins payout, the entire distribution, whether in monthly installments or in a lump sum, will be taxed as ordinary income. Examples of these annuities would be 403(b) plans for public education employees, doctors, nurses, hospitals, and clinics and 501(c)(3) plans for private nonprofit organizations.

QUALIFIED APPRECIATED STOCK: Stock for which a market price quotation is readily available and that would generate a capital gain if sold. [IRC §170(e)(5)]

QUALIFIED CHARITY: An organization described in IRC §170(c) that includes hospitals and health care organizations. Gifts to these entities can be deducted by donors for income, gift, or estate tax purposes.

QUALIFIED DEFERRED COMPENSATION PLAN: Pension plan contributions that are deductible to an employer and have no current tax implications for employees, according to IRS code. These plans are especially for hospital and health care personnel.

QUALIFIED DOMESTIC RELATIONS ORDER (QDRO): Decree issued by a judge as part of a property settlement, usually in divorce, that allows an individual transfer of retirement plan assets into a separating spouse's account and still retains tax-deferred status for the new spousal owner, as with a divorced physician.

QUALIFIED LEGAL OPINION: Conditional affirmation of the legality of financial securities, before or after they are sold. An unqualified or clean legal opinion, on the other hand, is an unconditional affirmation of the legality of securities.

QUALIFIED MEDICAL EXPENSE: Defined by IRS Code 213(d) as an expense used to alleviate or prevent mental defects, illnesses, or physical defects.

QUALIFIED OPINION: An author's opinion that appears on financial statements which calls attention to exceptional items of interest. It is an accounting or audit opinion that states, except for the effect of a matter to which a qualification relates, that financial statements are fairly presented in accordance with GAAP. Reviewers are required to qualify when there is a scope limitation.

QUALIFIED PLAN: A deferred compensation plan (DCP) that receives favorable tax benefits but is subject to the extensive regulatory requirements of the Internal Revenue Code (IRC) and the Employee Retirement Income Security Act (ERISA).

QUALIFIED RETIREMENT PLAN: A private retirement plan that meets the rules and regulations of the Internal Revenue Service. Contributions to a qualified retirement plan are, in almost all cases, tax deductible, and earnings on such contributions are always tax sheltered until retirement. These plans include 401(k) plans, 403(b) plans, or Keogh plans, which allow individuals to contribute both pre- and after-tax money for a tax-deferred investment. These plans are usually funded by contributions from employee wages, which may be enhanced by employer contributions.

QUALIFYING RATIOS: Comparisons of a borrower's debts and gross monthly income.

QUANGO: Slang term for a quasi-nongovernmental organization, such as the U.S. Federal Reserve.

QUANT: One who is mathematically inclined to apply various numerical approaches in analyzing or trading securities or markets, such as a statistician or mathematician.

QUANTISE: Slang term meaning to denominate a liability or asset in a nonregular (non-USD) currency trade.

QUANTITATIVE ANALYSIS: Financial analysis, based on measurable mathematical actualities that ignore considerations of quality of management.

QUANTITY DECREASING EFFECT: The result of a demand or supply decrease on the equilibrium price point for health care products or services.

QUANTITY DEMANDED: The amount of health care products or services a patient-buyer or insurance company is willing and able to purchase, at a certain price, over time.

QUANTITY DISCOUNT: Price reductions for goods or services according to volume.

QUANTITY INCREASING EFFECT: The result of a demand or supply increase on the equilibrium price point for health care products or services.

QUANTITY SUPPLIED: The amount of health care products or services a medical provider or supplier is willing to make or provide at a certain price, over time.

QUANTO OPTION: An option that pays out in an interest or current rate, in a denomination other than issued.

QUARTERLY REPORT: A report of securities performance sent every 3 months to stockholders.

QUASI-REORGANIZATION: Shareholder approval that allows management to revalue assets and eliminate deficits by charging it to other equity accounts without the creation of a new corporate entity or without court intervention.

QUASI-RENTS: Investment returns in excess of the short-run opportunity cost of the resources devoted to the health care economic activity.

QUINIAN, PATRICK, MD: CEO of Ochsner Clinic Foundation in New Orleans, Louisiana.

QUBES (QQQQ): NASD technology-laden tracking exchange traded fund (ETF) index on the American Stock Exchange (Amex).

QUICK ASSETS: Cash, or those assets that can quickly be converted into cash.

QUICK ASSETS RATIO: The ratio of cash, accounts receivable, and marketable securities to current liabilities.

QUICK RATIO: A measure of health care entity financial liquidity: cash + marketable securities + ARs / current liabilities. *See also* acid test.

QUICK TURN: A security traded quickly, as in a day trade.

QUINN, JOHN: CTO of Capgemini's provider health practice in New York City.

QUI-TAM: The method in the Federal False Claims Act that allows lawsuits against the health care fraud and abuse wrongdoers, in "the name of the king, as for himself, who sues in this matter" (Latin phrase).

QUID PRO QUO: The expectation by a donor that he or she will receive a bargained-for benefit in exchange for a gift to a charity [Rev. Rul. 76–185] (Latin phrase).

QUOTA: Restrictions on health care input quantity. An imposed limit on the amount of inputs or outputs.

QUOTE: Current buy and sell prices of a security. The lowest price any seller will accept at a given time is *asked,* and the highest price any buyer has offered for a stock at a given time is the *bid.* The difference between bid and asked is the *spread.*

R

R-SQUARED: Mutual fund performance percentage explained by variations in its compared benchmark index.

RABBI TRUST: An arrangement used to provide informal funding for a non-qualified deferred compensation agreement. Assets of the trust must be forfeitable by the employee who is a party to the agreement. Generally, this is achieved by making the trust assets subject to claims by the employer's creditors.

RACKETEER INFLUENCED AND CORRUPT ORGANIZATION ACT (RICO): Federal legislation used against individuals accused of insider trading activities.

RAIDER: One who buys controlling stock in a company and instills new senior management.

RALLY: A rise in a stock market or individual security.

RAMSEY EQUILIBRIUM: A government's choice in certain kinds of economic or health care business models. The government's choice in a Ramsey problem and its solution is called a Ramsey outcome.

RANDOM: A condition in finance or economics where changes occur on a probabilistic basis while the underlying probability function may be known or unknown.

RANDOM SELECTION OF HEALTH CARE CLAIMS: CMS has an internal policy that states that a percentage of particular claims must be reviewed. Depending on the area of concern or incidents of fraudulent activities, the carriers will allocate resources to investigate the concerns. They are also mandated to review a certain percentage of claims on a regular basis to ensure program integrity. The HHS Office of Inspector General's 2005 Work Plan focuses on a wide variety of compliance issues. Some of the areas include:

- Postacute Care Transfer: OIG will be looking at the payments for services provided in acute care hospitals and admitted to post-acute care settings.
- Diagnosis-Related Group Coding: OIG will be evaluating codes that have a history of aberrant coding patterns that have led to overpayment to hospitals.
- Improper Medicare Payments: For inpatient psychiatric stays due to medical necessity or coverage issues.

- Appropriateness of coronary artery stents and cardiac rehabilitation services.
- Outlier payments to home health agencies.
- Imaging and laboratory services in nursing homes will be evaluated for overpayment and to ensure that medical necessity criteria are met.
- Continued monitoring of coding of evaluation and management services and use of modifiers in physician reimbursements.

RANDOM WALK THEORY: A direct refutation of technical analysis that posits that financial markets cannot be predicted because they move in a random manner like the walking pattern of a drunkard.

RANGE: A set of data or securities prices consisting of the opening sale, high sale, low sale, and the last sale of the day for a given security.

RATCHET EFFECT: The trend for rising health care price levels when aggregate demand increases, but not for decline when aggregate health care demand declines.

RATE REGULATIONS (RRs): State or locally administered hospital reimbursement scales.

RATE OF RETURN: The percentage amount of income, loss, or change in value anticipated or realized on an investment, over time.

RATE OF RETURN REGULATION: A rule to set health care prices at a level that enables the entity to earn a specific target profit on its capital.

RATINGS: Evaluations of the credit quality of notes and bonds usually made by independent rating services. Ratings are intended to measure the probability of the timely repayment of principal and interest on debt securities. Ratings are initially made before issuance and are periodically reviewed and may be amended to reflect changes in the issuer's credit position. The information required by the rating agencies varies with each issue, but generally includes information regarding the issuer's demographics, debt burden, economic base, finances, and management structure. Many financial institutions also assign their own individual ratings to securities.

RATIO ANALYSIS: A method of analyzing a health care or other entity's financial condition calculated from line items in the financial statements. There are four major categories:

- Liquidity;
- Profitability;
- Capitalization; and
- Activity.

RATIO OF CHARGES (COSTS) TO CHARGES (RCC): Percentage ratio of initial patient charges to total patient charges. Percentage ratio of initial or total patient costs to total patient charges.

RATIO OF CHARGES TO CHARGES (OR COSTS TO CHARGES) APPLIED TO COSTS (CHARGES): Retrospective medical payment formula that multiples RCC by allowable costs, or by patient charges.

RATIONAL BEHAVIOR: Actions, especially economic and financial, that seek to achieve a gain by undertaking and understanding the psychological processes for which the extra benefit exceeds the extra cost.

RATIONAL CHOICE: Best financial selection out of all possibilities.

RATIONAL EXPECTATIONS: The use of all available information to produce an economic forecast.

RATIONAL IGNORANCE: Option of a patient not to acquire or process health care information about some medical condition, illness, or treatment.

RATIONALIZE: To take an observed health care economics behavior and find a model financial environment in which that behavior is an optimal solution to a medical care optimization problem.

RATIONED HEALTH CARE: Artificial constraints on either the demand side or the supply side of the free health care marketplace.

RAWLSIAN FAIRNESS: Distributive health care economic justice that suggests giving the largest income to the leasts well-off, and most needy.

REACTION: A precipitous drop in securities prices after a long rising bull market.

READY TRANSFERABILITY OF SHARES: A shareholder's right to give away or sell shares without prior consultation with corporate directors.

REAL: Expressed in constant dollars. Inflation adjusted.

REAL ASSET: Tangible, fixed asset.

REAL ESTATE INVESTMENT TRUST (REIT): A company that manages a portfolio of real estate holdings for capital appreciation, income, or both. It is a type of mutual fund. REITs are required to distribute to investors at least 95% of their net earnings annually.

REAL ESTATE MORTGAGE INVESTMENT CONDUIT (REMIC): An investment vehicle to minimize double taxation of income from a pooling of mortgages.

REAL GNP: Gross National Product calculated from a base, nominal, or reference year. Nominal GDP / GDP deflator.

REAL GROWTH: Increased demand or supply for health care or other goods or services, with corresponding unit (not price) increase.

REAL INCOME: Income purchasing calculated from a base, nominal, or reference year.

REAL RATE OF RETURN: The actual rate of investment return after factors such as inflation, commissions, fees and expenses, and taxes are taken into consideration.

REAL VALUE: A measurement of economic worth, or amount corrected for changes in price over time (inflation), or expressing a value in terms of constant dollar prices for health care services and products.

REAL WAGES: Constant nominal wages adjusted for inflation and purchasing power loss.

REAL YIELD: Nominal yield of an asset or investment minus a percentage change in the Consumer Price Index (CPI) or rate of inflation.

REALIZED GAINS OR LOSS: The increase or decrease in securities value from the time of purchase to the time of sale.

REASONABLE ASSURANCE: Management assessment of the effectiveness of internal controls over financial reporting as expressed at a level of reasonable assurance. It includes the understanding that there is a remote likelihood that material misstatements will not be prevented or detected on a timely basis. It is a high level of assurance.

REASONABLE AND CUSTOMARY CHARGE (RCC): The medical or health care charges or fees common within a geographic area. These fees are reasonable if they are within the average charge for service parameters for that area, and if the charges for participating providers are what have been contracted with the health plan.

REASONABLE CHARGES (RC): Under Medicare or a major medical health insurance policy, the customary charges for similar services made by physicians. The range of prevailing charges for physicians engaged in specialty practices may be different from one locale to another.

REBALANCE: To sell or buy securities in a portfolio in order to return to a prescribed set allocation or proportional constraints.

REBATE: A controversial health or other insurance practice where a portion of an agent's commission or anything of value is given to the prospective patient or insured as an inducement to buy. Rebates are considered unethical and illegal in most states.

REBATING: Granting any form of inducement, favor, or advantage to the purchaser of a health insurance or other policy, good, or service that is not available to all under the standard policy terms. Rebating in some states is a penal offense for which both the agent and the person accepting the rebate can be punished by fine or imprisonment, and in virtually all states the agent is subject to revocation of license. It is unethical or illegal behavior.

REBILL: To bill again for noncovered or nonpaid health care services.

RECAPITALIZATION: An alteration or change in a health care or other firm's sources of finance. It is the internal reorganization of a corporation including a rearrangement of the capital structure by changing the kind of stock or the number of shares outstanding or issuing stock instead of bonds. It is distinguished from most other types of reorganization because it involves only one corporation and is usually accomplished by the surrender by shareholders of their securities for other stock or securities of a different type.

RECEIPT: A written acknowledgment of a payment.

RECEIPTS OF ACCRUAL ON MUNICIPAL SECURITIES: Receipts of Accrual on Municipal Securities (RAMS) are stripped municipals. Similar to government CATS, RAMS have the added tax-exempt feature common to municipal securities. RAMS come in three types: coupon RAMS represent the claim to future coupon interest; corpus RAMS are claims to the principal, due either at maturity or upon the date the bond is refunded; converting RAMS have the coupons stripped up to the call date, and then the certificates convert to a tax-free interest-bearing security at the underlying bond's coupon rate.

RECEIVABLES: Monetary claims against a business entity or individual. Average Day Sales / Days Sales Outstanding.

RECEIVABLES COLLECTION PERIOD (RCP): Receivables / Sales / 360; DSO (Days Sales Outstanding); or the time it take to convert health care or medical receivables into cash.

RECEIVABLES TURNOVER: Speed of accounts receivable (AR) collections.

RECEIVER IN BANKRUPTCY: An impartial, court-appointed administrator of a corporation that has sought protection from its creditors' claims under federal bankruptcy laws. The receiver is appointed to help the court decide between liquidation and reorganization and is paid out of the remaining assets of the corporation.

RECESSION: A decline in real GNP for two consecutive, 3-month reporting periods.

RECLAMATION: If good securities delivery is not made between broker/dealers and such is determined after physical delivery was made, either party (buyer or seller) may commence reclamation procedures.

RECONCILIATION: Comparison of two financial, economics, or accounting numbers and related data to demonstrate the basis for the difference between them.

RECONVEYANCE: A method of releasing a lien against real property.

RECORD DATE: The date set by the corporate board of directors for the transfer agent and registrar to close their financial books to further changes in registration of stock and identify the recipients of the distribution.

RECOUPMENT: The recovery by Medicare of any Medicare debt by reducing present or future Medicare payments and applying the amount withheld to the indebtedness.

RECOURSE: The legal ability to hold the original creditor responsible in a failed financial deal. An action taken to recover a debt.

RECOURSE FINANCING: Loans for which partners have personal liability, such as a medical practice partnership. The value of such loans is part of a partners' basis in a partnership, by providing the ability to return assets for full or partial pre-arranged value.

RECOVERY: Economic expansion after a period of contraction.

RECURRING EXPENSES: Regular health care or other entity's operating expenditures that occur every month.

RED HERRING: Slang term for a preliminary prospectus for securities to be offered publicly by a corporation or underwriter. It is the only form of written communication allowed between a broker/dealer and a potential purchaser before the effective date. The Securities Act of 1933 requires a red-lettered caveat on the front page, hence the derivation of the name.

REDEMPTION: Return of investment principle in a security transaction. A shareholder redeems mutual fund shares at net asset value (NAV). It is a transaction in which one issuer returns the principal amount represented by an outstanding security (plus, in certain cases, an additional amount).

REDEMPTION FEE: A premium charge for a redemption.

REDEMPTION PRICE: The amount per share a mutual fund shareholder receives when he cashes in his shares (also known as bid price). The value of the shares depends upon the market value of the fund's portfolio securities at the time.

REDEMPTION PROVISIONS: The terms of a bond contract giving the issuer the right, or requiring the issuer, to redeem or "call" all or a portion of an outstanding issue of bonds prior to their stated dates of maturity at a specified price, usually at or above par. Common types of redemption provisions include:

- Optional Redemption: The issuer has the right to redeem bonds, usually after a stated date and at a premium, but is not required to do so.
- Mandatory Redemption: The issuer is required to call outstanding bonds based on a predetermined schedule or as otherwise provided in the bond contract. Frequently, the issuer is allowed to make open market purchases in lieu of calling the bonds.
- Extraordinary Mandatory Redemption: The issuer is required to call or redeem all or part of an issue of bonds upon the occurrence of certain events.

REDUCTION RULES: Exceptions to the general rule that gifts to a qualified hospital or charity are deductible to the extent of the fair market value of the donated property. [IRC §170(e)(1)(A)]

REECE, RICHARD L., MD: Pathologist and health industry speaker based in Old Saybrook, Connecticut, who is editor of *Physician Practice Options,* a national monthly health care economics, business, and finance newsletter.

REFLATION: The reverse of deflation through government Federal Open Market Committee (FOMC) interaction.

REFUNDING: The act of issuing new debt and using prior proceeds from old debt to retire existing debt:

REFUNDING (REFINANCING): The issuance of a new debt security (bond) using the proceeds to redeem old bonds at maturity or outstanding bonds issued under less favorable terms and conditions to replace one debt with another, as interest rates have declined.

REGIONAL EXCHANGE: The stock exchange of a particular region of the country.

REGISTERED BONDS: Outstanding debt whose holder name is recorded by the issuing health care or other corporation. Legal title may be transferred only when endorsed by the registered owner.

REGISTERED CHECK: A bank-issued check guaranteed by bank funds.

REGISTERED REPRESENTATIVE: A broker who sells and buys securities for a customer. A securities salesperson.

REGISTERED COMPANY: Securities Exchange Commission mandated disclosure prior to an initial public offering (IPO).

REGISTERED INVESTMENT ADVISOR (RIA): One who is registered with the Securities Exchange Commission (SEC) to sell financial products.

REGISTERED SECONDARY DISTRIBUTIONS: Offering of securities by affiliated persons (insiders) or the issuer (of treasury stock) that requires an effective registration statement on file with the SEC before distribution may be attempted.

REGISTRAR: Usually a trust company or bank charged with the responsibility of preventing the issuance of more stock than authorized by the company.

REGISTRATION: The process of filing with the SEC in order to sell securities to the public.

REGISTRATION STATEMENT: A document filed with the SEC by the issuer of securities before a public offering may be attempted. The Securities Act of 1933 mandates that it contain all material information. Such a statement is also required of an affiliated person's intent upon offering sizable amounts of securities in the secondary market. The SEC examines the statement for a 20-day period (minimum), seeking obvious omissions or misrepresentations of fact, but specifically does not approve the issue.

REGRESSION ANALYSIS: A statistical tool used to measure the relationship between two or more variables, usually securities prices or data points.

REGRESSIVE TAX: A tax rate that declines as the tax base increases.

REGULAR WAY CONTRACT: The most frequently used securities delivery contract. For stock and corporate and municipal bonds, this type of contract calls for delivery on the first business day after the trade. For U.S. government bonds and listed options, delivery must be made on the next business day after the trade.

REGULATED INVESTMENT COMPANIES (RIC): Investment companies that meet certain criteria for eligibility and are exempted by the IRS from paying taxes on investment income and capital gains paid to shareholders as long as at least 98% is distributed. In order to be a RIC, a corporation must make an irrevocable tax election in order to be treated as one.

REGULATION A: An exemption from standard SEC registration for a security, the total offering price of which does not exceed $5,000,000 in a 12-month period.

REGULATION D: The part of the Securities Act of 1933 that deals with private securities placements. The major provisions deal with accredited investors and both dollar limits (aggregation) and investor limits (integration). Under this regulation, private placements meeting the stipulations are exempt from registration with the SEC.

REGULATION G: Federal Reserve Bank (FRB) rules for those lenders who extend credit to purchase or carry securities.

REGULATION Q: Federal Reserve Bank (FRB) ceiling ruling for pass-book and checking account interest rates.

REGULATION T: Federal Reserve Bank (FRB) regulation that explains the conduct and operation of general and cash accounts within the offices of a securities broker/dealer firm, prescribing a code of conduct for the effective use and supervision of credit. According to Regulation T, one may borrow up to 50% of the purchase price of securities that can be purchased on margin. This is known as the initial margin. Also, it dictates that payment must be received no later than 1 business day after the trade and states what happens if you do not pay on time.

REGULATION U: Federal Reserve Bank (FRB) regulation that directs banks to secure a statement of purpose signed by a borrower who uses securities as collateral in order to determine the reason for the loan.

REGULATION Z: Federal Reserve Bank (FRB) regulation covering Truth in Lending (TIL) and Consumer Credit Protection Act (CCPA) of 1968.

REGULATORY CAPITAL: The amount of capital available for trading or position taking purposes by health care, financial, or other institutions. The total capital base is adjusted for memberships, various fixed assets, DME, type and/or maturity of securities, as well as other factors.

REHNQUIST, JANET: Inspector general of the Department of Health and Human Services (DHHS) in Washington, D.C.

REHYPOTHECATION: Stocker-Broker-Dealer pledge of securities in a margin account as collateral for a loan.

REIMBURSABLE COSTS: Allowable expenses for health care services according to Medicare or Medicare schedules, commercial insurance companies, HMOs, or other similar contracts.

REIMBURSEMENT: Repaying out-of-pocket expenses, or the payment of actual charges for health care goods or medical services.

REINHARDT, EWE, PhD: James Madison Professor of Political Economics at Princeton University in New Jersey, an expert on the costs of managed medical care and other social systems, and an opponent of managed care liability. He was the predictor of a three tiered system of patients and medical care reimbursement in the United States: (1) uninsured and uninsurable patients, (2) managed care payments and health maintenance organization care, and (3) fee-for-service payments, traditional reimbursement, and concierge medicine models.

REINVESTMENT PRIVILEGE: A service provided by most mutual funds for the automatic reinvestment of a shareholder's income dividends and capital gains distributions in additional shares.

REINVESTMENT RISK: The risk that a purchaser of a fixed income security incurs that interest rates will be lower when the purchaser seeks to reinvest income received from the security.

REJECTION: The privilege of the purchaser in a transaction to refuse a delivery not deemed acceptable.

RELATED PARTY TRANSACTION: Business between entities or persons who do not have an arm's length relationship, especially between family members or controlled entities. For HIPAA, Stark I, Stark II, and tax purposes, these types of transactions are generally subject to a greater level of scrutiny.

RELATED PORTFOLIO: A portfolio of municipal securities that is operated in some way with a municipal securities dealer (e.g., a dealer bank's portfolio). Certain disclosure requirements under Municipal Securities Rulemaking Board (MSRB) rules are applicable to orders for new issue municipal securities from related portfolios.

RELATIVE EFFICIENCY: The belief that the market reflects current information in its securities prices.

RELATIVE PRICE: The ratio of one health care price to another.

RELATIVE STRENGTH: Individual price performance of a security relative to a related index. It is a relative price performance benchmark.

RELATIVE VALUE SCALE (RVS): A compiled table of relative value units (RVUs) that is given to each medical procedure or unit of health care service. As payment systems, RVS is used to determine a formula that multiplies the RVU by a dollar amount, called a converter.

RELATIVE VALUE STUDY: A guide for the relationships of time, resources, experience, skill, instruments and equipment, venue, and other factors to perform medical procedures or services.

RELATIVE VALUE UNIT (RVU): The unit of measure for a relative value scale. RVUs must be multiplied by a dollar conversion factor to become payment amounts.

RELATIVE VALUE WEIGHT (RVW): Percentages or ratios to reflect consumption associated with a specific DRG.

RELEVANT ASSERTIONS: Assertions that have a meaningful bearing on whether a financial account is fairly stated.

RELEVANT COST: Avoidable expense charge as a result of choosing one alternative over another within a set domain. All costs are considered avoidable, except sunk costs and future costs that do not differ between the germane alternatives at hand.

RELEVANT INFORMATION: Expected information that differs among alternative courses of action.

RELEVANT RANGE: Span where total fixed costs and variable costs per unit remain stable and do not change.

REMAINDER INTERESTS: Property, financial or other rights that can be enjoyed only after prior rights have terminated.

REMAINDERMAN: The person (entity) that receives a trust's principal after the income beneficiary's interest ends.

REMARGIN: The addition of eligible securities or cash for a brokerage account deficiency.

REMITTANCE: Payment of an invoice.

RENEWAL AND REPLACEMENT FUND: A fund established by the bond contract of a revenue bond issue into which monies are deposited to cover anticipated expenses for major repairs of the project or its equipment or for replacement of equipment. Under a typical revenue pledge, this fund is the fifth to be funded out of the revenue fund.

REOFFERING SCALE: The prices and/or yields listed by maturity for securities offered to the public by underwriters.

REORDER POINT: A preset quantity limit for inventory holdings indicating the time to order additional DME or inventory, so as to avoid stock-outs.

REORGANIZATION: The restatement of assets to reflect current market value, whereby a financially troubled health care firm may continue operations, as opposed to liquidation where assets are sold and the entity no longer exists.

REPLACEMENT COST: Charge to replace a similar or like-kind asset at current replacement prices. The present cost of similar property or equipment with the closest utility to the replaced item.

REPO: Repurchase agreements. The purchases of securities under a stipulation that the seller will repurchase the securities within a certain time period at a certain price.

REPORT (8-K): A report that public firms must file with the SEC detailing changes that may affect the value of its securities.

REPORT (10-K): A report that public firms must file annually with the SEC.

REPORT (10-Q): A report that public firms must file quarterly with the SEC.

REPORT (13-D): A report that an individual who acquires 5% of a public company must file with the SEC.

REPORT DATE: The final date that economic, accounting, and/or financial conclusions are relayed to the patient, customer, or client.

REPRESENTATIVE REGISTRATION: The minimum NASD qualification for solicitors of investment banking or securities business, traders, assistant officers of member firms, and training directors and assistants.

REPURCHASE AGREEMENT: Repurchase agreements (repos) are the primary tool used by dealers in government (sometimes municipal) securities to finance the carrying of inventory. It is an agreement between the buyer (the dealer) and seller (the issuer) to reverse a trade at a specified time at a specified yield.

REQUIRED RATE OF RETURN: The lowest acceptable rate of return required from investors for a given level of risk.

REQUISITION: A formal written order for assets.

RESERVATION WAGE: A salary below which a health care laborer will not work.

RESERVE: Monies earmarked by health plans to cover anticipated claims and operating expenses. It is part of a fiscal method of withholding a certain percentage of premium to provide a fund for committed but undelivered health care and such uncertainties as: longer hospital utilization levels than expected, overutilization of referrals, accidental catastrophes, and so forth. A percentage of the premiums support this fund. Businesses other than health plans also manage reserves. For example, hospitals document reserves as that portion of the ARs they hope to collect but have some doubt about collectibility. Rather than book these amounts as income, hospitals will reserve these amounts until paid. It is a common European term.

RESERVES: A fiscal method of withholding a certain percentage of premiums to provide a fund for committed but undelivered health care and such uncertainties as: longer hospital utilization levels than expected, overutilization of referrals, accidental catastrophes, and the like.

RESERVES REQUIREMENT: The money a banking institution must hold against deposit liabilities.

RESET BOND: A bond debt whose coupon interest rate payments are periodically reset.

RESIDUAL VALUE: Remaining value at the end of a time period within a discounting future earnings valuation model.

RESOURCE-BASED RELATIVE VALUE SCALE (RBRVS): A schedule of values assigned to health care services that give weight to medical procedures based upon resources needed by the provider to effectively deliver the service or perform that procedure. Unlike other relative value scales, RBRVSs ignore historical charges and include factors such as time, effort, technical skill, practice cost, and training cost. Established as part of the Omnibus Reconciliation Act of 1989, Medicare payment rules for physician services were altered by establishing an RBRVS fee schedule. This payment methodology has three components: a relative value for each procedure, a geographic adjustment factor, and a dollar conversion factor. It is a Medicare weighting system to assign units of value to each CPT code (procedure) performed by physicians and other providers.

RESPONSIBILITY ACCOUNTING: The evaluation of each individual accountability center of a health care or other organization.

RESTRICTED ACCOUNT: A margin-securities brokerage account, where the equity is less than the current federal requirement (Regulation T).

RESTRICTED ASSETS: Resources limited by legal or contractual agreements.

RESTRICTED COVENANT: A formal written noncompete order.

RESTRICTED DONATIONS: Donated funds with restrictions on use.

RESTRICTED FUND: Account established for assets whose income must be used for purposes established by donors or grantors of such assets.

RESTRICTED SECURITY: A portfolio security not available to the public at large, which requires registration with the Securities and Exchange Commission before it may be sold publicly. A "private placement" frequently referred to as a "letter stock."

RESTRUCTURE: To adapt corporate financial, business, marketing, or other strategies to better compete in changing markets.

RETAIL: One who buys securities, or medical care, products, goods, or services for a personal account, and usually in small quantities.

RETAIL HMO: A small regional or local HMO formed and/or purchased under state insurance rules and regulations to provide health care services in limited quantities. It is a HMO with a license.

RETAIL PRICE: Price for financial products and services charged to individuals without benefit of discounted price breaks.

RETAINED EARNINGS: Profits that a health care business entity keeps to further its mission statement, goals, and objections. It is that part of a company's profits that is not paid out in dividends but used by the company to reinvest in the business.

RETAINER: An ongoing fee paid to a professional person to engage his or her services.

RETENTION DEDUCTIBLE: A health or other insurance clause that stipulates a deductible will apply in the absence of underlying coverage.

RETENTION REQUIREMENT: The amount of money necessary to be retained in an account after sale of a security, presently 50% of the proceeds of the sale. This is only used in a restricted margin account.

RETIREMENT PLAN: 2006 retirement plan limits listed in Table 9, indexed thereafter.

In addition to the statutory limits in Table 9, one must consider whether any hospital or health care employer-sponsored plan has imposed limits. For example, if participating in a hospital 401(k) plan under which salary deferrals are limited to 10% of compensation and compensation is $50,000, the maximum amount that can be deferred to the plan is $5,000 ($50,000 × 10%) instead of the statutory limit of $15,000. After age 50, by December 31, 2006, one can defer an additional $5,000 as catch-up contributions, if the plan allows it.

RETIREMENT PLAN LIMITS (MULTIPLE PLANS):

IRA Contributions: IRA contribution limits for the year are $4,000, or $5,000 if at least age 50 by December 31, 2006. This limit applies regardless of the number of IRAs for the year. Therefore, if one contributes to a Roth and a Traditional IRA, or multiple Traditional and/or Roth IRAs, the $4,000/$5,000 can be allocated among these IRAs, provided the aggregate contribution does not exceed $4,000/$5,000 (see Table 9).

IRA Salary Deferral Contributions: If in multiple retirement plans with deferral features (i.e., SIMPLE IRAs, SIMPLE 401(k), 401(k) and 403-(b) plans), the aggregate deferrals cannot exceed $15,000, plus an additional $5,000 if at least age 50 by December 31, 2006. If in a 457 plan, an additional $15,000, plus $5,000 catch-up, can be deferred to the 457 account.

IRA Deductibility: Amounts contributed to a Traditional IRA are fully deductible, unless an active participant, who must therefore factor in Modified Adjusted Gross Income (MAGI) and marital status in order to determine if a contribution is deductible, as listed in Table 10.

If unable to deduct a Traditional IRA contribution, one may either make a nondeductible contribution or contribute to a Roth IRA, with income limitations.

- 401(k) Plan: An employee benefit plan that allows employees to defer income taxes on a portion of compensation that is paid into a savings trust that meets certain qualifications under the Employee Retirement Income Security Act (ERISA).
- §403(b) Plan: A tax-deferred savings arrangement, similar to a 401(k) plan, that is available to employees of nonprofit hospitals, clinics, schools, and health care, and educational organizations.
- 12b-1 Plan: Named after a section of the Investment Company Act of 1940, which permits mutual funds to levy an asset-based sales charge to cover advertising and distribution costs. The NASD Rules of Fair Practice limit these charges to .75% of assets and do not permit a fund to refer to itself as "no-load" if the charge is higher than 25 basis points. These charges

Table 9: Retirement Plan Limits for 2006

	2005	2006
Traditional and Roth IRA regular contribution	$4,000	$4,000
Traditional and Roth IRA catch-up contribution	$500	$1,000
Regular elective deferrals to SIMPLE IRA and SIMPLE 401(k) plans	$10,000	$ 10,000
Catch-up elective deferrals to SIMPLE IRA and SIMPLE 401(k) plans	$2,000	$2,500
Regular deferrals to 401(k), 403(b) and 457 plans	$14,000	$15,000
Catch-up deferrals to 401(k), 403(b) and 457 plans	$4,000	$5,000
Annual dollar limitation	$42,000	$44,000
Compensation cap	$210,000	$220,000
Minimum compensation for SEP plans	$450	$450
Definition of highly-compensated employee	$95,000	$100,000
Definition of key	$135,000	$140,000

Source: Internal Revenue Service.

must be reviewed by the fund's Board of Directors quarterly and approved annually. The plan may be discontinued by a majority vote of the fund's shareholders OR that part of the Board represented by outside directors.

- 12b-1 Plan Fees: The fees of no load mutual funds for markets and advertising.

RETIREMENT PROTECTION ACT (RPA): 1994 legislation to strengthen the Pension Benefit Guarantee Corporation (PBGC) and assist under- or over-funded legacy company-defined benefit plans (DBPs) such as seen in older hospitals, VAs, and other health care systems.

RETRO ADD: After-the-fact patient-member additions in a capitated medical reimbursement payment model, often requiring payments corrections.

RETRO DELETE: After-the-fact patient-member deletions in a capitated medical reimbursement payment model, often requiring payments corrections.

RETROSPECTIVE PAYMENT: Health care reimbursement determined after the medical care has been rendered.

Table 10: IRA Deductability for 2006

Tax Filing Status	2005 MAGI Range	2006 MAGI Range	Comments – 2006
– Single – Married filing separately, but did not live with spouse during the year	$50,000 to $60,000	$50,000 to $60,000	– Contribution is fully deductible if MAGI is $50,000 or less. –Deductibility amount is phased out for MAGI range, and formula is used to determine deductibility amount. – No deduction is allowed if MAGI is $60,000 or greater.
Married filing jointly – range for active spouse	$70,000 to $80,000	$75,000 to $85,000	– Contribution is fully deductible if MAGI is $75,000 or less. – Deductibility amount is phased out for MAGI range, and formula is used to determine deductibility amount. – No deduction is allowed if MAGI is $85,000 or greater.
Married filing jointly — this range is for a spouse who is not active, but is married to an active spouse.	$150,000 to $160,000	$150,000 to $160,000	– Contribution is fully deductible if MAGI is $150,000 or less. – Deductibility amount is phased out for MAGI range, and formula is used to determine deductibility amount. – No deduction is allowed if MAGI is $160,000 or greater.
Married filing separately and lived with spouse during the year. Applies to both spouses, even if only one spouse is active.	$0 to $10,000	$0 to $10,000	– Deductibility amount is phased out for MAGI range, and formula is used to determine deductibility amount. – No deduction is allowed if MAGI is $10,000 or greater.

Source: Internal Revenue Service.

RETROSPECTIVE PREMIUM: An insurance premium-establishing method in which current costs are adjusted to reflect the prior year's loss or health claim experience.

RETROSPECTIVE RATE: An insurance rating method in which current rates are adjusted to reflect the prior year's aggregate or individual rating experience.

RETROSPECTIVE RATE DERIVATION (RETRO): A rating system whereby the employer becomes responsible for a portion of the group's health care costs. If health care costs are less than the portion the employer agrees to assume, the insurance company may be required to refund a portion of the premium.

RETROSPECTIVE REIMBURSEMENT: The payment to a health care provider or entity prior to the deliverance of medical services.

RETURN: Income, interest, and/or capital gains earned on an asset.

RETURN ON ASSETS (ROA): Net income expressed as an average of total assets.

RETURN ON DEBT (ROD) : Principal payments; interest, or usury payments.

RETURN ON EQUITY (ROE): Liquidating dividends. Net income expressed as a percentage of total equity.

RETURN ON INVESTMENT (ROI): The percentage of loss or gain from an investment.

RETURN ON NET ASSETS (RONA): Excess over revenues, over expenses/net assets.

RETURN ON NET WORTH (RONW): Excess of corporate insurance company end-of-year net worth.

RETURN ON TOTAL ASSETS (ROTA): Excess over revenues, over expenses/total assets.

RETURN TO CAPITAL: Compromised or reduced payment on capital, to capital suppliers.

RETURN TO DEBT: Interest or principal payments to debt suppliers.

RETURN TO EQUITY: Return on equity realized by capital suppliers.

RETURN TO SCALE: Increase in health care outputs that results from increasing all inputs by the same percentage.

REVALUATION: An increase of the value of one currency over another.

REVENUE: Money earned by rendering health care goods and products or by providing services, such as health insurance premium proceeds.

REVENUE ATTAINMENT: Achieving the amount of revenues budgeted.

REVENUE BONDS: Debt loans payable from the earnings of a revenue-generating facility, such as water, sewers, or utility systems, hospitals or clinics. The risk, however, is that the facility will not generate income sufficient to pay the interest, and therefore the yield is somewhat higher than for a general-obligation bond. Revenue bonds are supported only by the revenue earned, so if the project, such as a hospital, does not produce revenues sufficient to pay the interest on the bonds, then the bonds go into default. Therefore, it is important to properly evaluate the municipality's ability to tax and/or the assumptions used to project the facility's revenue.

REVENUE BUDGET: An operating and/or nonoperating revenue forecast.

REVENUE CENTER: Health care or other business unit that produces income.

REVENUE CODE: Payment codes for services or items in FL 42 of the UB-92 found in Medicare and/or NUBC (National Uniform Billing Committee) manuals (42X, 43X, etc.).

REVENUE ENHANCEMENT: Augmenting traditional revenue sources of the enterprise with new sources, products, or health care services.

REVENUE EXPENDITURES: Expensed costs that maintain an asset or restore it to functional working order.

REVENUE FUND: A fund established by the bond contract of an income generating bond issue into which all gross revenues from the financed project are initially placed and from which the monies for all other funds are drawn.

REVENUE PRINCIPLE: The basis for recording the time and amount of revenues.

REVENUE RECOGNITION: Method of determining whether or not income has met the conditions of being earned and realized or is realizable.

REVENUE SHARE: The proportion of a practice's total revenue devoted to a particular type of expense. For example, the medical practice expense revenue share is that proportion of revenue used to pay for practice expenses.

REVENUE VOLUME VARIANCE: (Actual volume − budget volume) × actual volume.

REVERSAL: The often sharp economic change in a financial market, company, or individual, usually in a negative direction.

REVERSE CAPITATION: A health care payment method that capitates or fixes payment to medical specialists by contract, but pays primary care physicians at some fee-for-service rate.

REVERSE ENTRIES: An accounting entry that changes the credit and debit of a prior adjusting entry.

REVERSE LEVERAGE: Condition when interest payments or dividends exceed the cost of borrowed money.

REVERSE SPLIT: A corporate reduction in the number of shares outstanding, thereby increasing the value of each remaining share.

REVERSE SWAP: The exchange of bonds in a portfolio to restore it to its original aggregate position.

REVOCABLE TRUST: An *inter-vivos* trust that may be changed or canceled at the direction of the settlor (creator/grantor). Revocable trusts are called living trusts when the settlor is also the primary beneficiary.

REVOLVING CREDIT LINE: A continuous line of credit up to a pre-negotiated limit.

REVOLVING DEBT/CREDIT: Revolving credit is credit that is repeatedly available up to a specified amount as periodic repayments are made. Revolving debt is the total amount of the credit that has actually been used and is outstanding at any given point in time. Examples of consumer credit plans that provide revolving credit include major bank cards, such as American Express, Visa, MasterCard, and Discover, and department store and gas cards.

REVOLVING FUND: An account where (money) funds are continuously received and disbursed.

REX-WALLER, JOHN: President of National Surgical Hospitals Inc., in Chicago, Illinois.

RHO: Interest rate sensitivity of an option relative to a change in the interest rate option pricing variable that measures its change in value for a given change in the interest rate. Part of the Greek alphabet.

RICARDIAN PROPOSITION: The suggestion that tax financing and bond financing of a given stream of government expenditures, such as for municipal clinics or hospitals, leads to equivalent economic allocations. It's the Modigliani-Miller theorem applied to the government.

RICE, JAMES: Vice Chairman of the Governance Institute in La Jolla, California.

RICH: Cash flow characteristics that suggest an over-valued security.

RIGGED: Illegal securities or other market price manipulations.

RIGHT TO RESCISSION: The legal right to void or cancel a contract in such a way as to treat the contract as if it never existed.

RIGHT TO SETOFF: A debtor's ability to discharge all or a portion of the amount owed to another party by applying against the debt an amount that the other party owes to the debtor.

RIGHTS: Granted to existing shareholders when a company issues more shares in a new issue. Usually the rights last for only a short time and the shares are offered at a lower price than they will be offered to the public. "Preemptive rights" are sometimes mandated by state laws to allow existing shareholders to maintain a proportionate share of ownership, thus preventing "dilution" of their existing shares.

RIGHTS OF ACCUMULATION: A privilege offered by some investment companies that allows the investor to include the total market value of shares already owned in calculating sales charges when a new investment is made in additional shares.

RIGHTS OFFERING: The sale of new securities to existing stockholders.

RISK: Uncertainty. The assignment of outcomes and their associated probabilities. (1) Market risk—the uncertainty that a particular security may fluctuate in price solely due to investor sentiment in the "market," sometimes called systematic risk. This is best observed when bad news hits Wall

Street and almost all stocks go down regardless of their earnings strength. (2) Business or financial risk—the risk that the business in which you have invested money will not do well. If the company's products don't sell and earnings plummet, you can expect the stock price to do so as well. (3) Credit risk—a risk that applies with debt securities (bonds). The investor has extended credit to the issuer when he buys their bonds. Just as in our personal lives, if we loan money to someone, there is always the chance that they will not be able to pay us back. Lower rated bonds, called junk bonds, carry a great deal of credit risk. (4) Liquidity risk—refers to how marketable the investment you're holding is. Some investments, such as real estate, are not easily sold quickly, and therefore, we say that they don't have great liquidity. There is no liquidity risk with mutual funds or variable annuities as Federal Law requires redemption by the issuer after tender of a redemption request. (5) Money rate or interest rate risk—as interest rates go UP, the prices of securities sold primarily for their fixed income (such as bonds and preferred stock) go DOWN. Because the investor has no control over interest rate movements, this is a real risk. (6) Purchasing power or inflation risk—the uncertainty that a dollar will not purchase as much in the future as it does now. This risk is found in all FIXED dollar securities such as bonds and fixed annuities. It was primarily due to this risk that variable annuities and variable life insurance were developed as their portfolios, consisting largely of common stock, provide a hedge against inflation.

RISK ADJUSTED CAPITATION: A method of payment to either a health care organization or individual medical provider that takes the form of a fixed amount per person per period and that is varied to reflect the health characteristics of individuals or groups of individuals.

RISK ADJUSTED RETURN ON CAPITAL (RAROC): Same as Return on Equity (ROE) with the net income numerator, and denominator (capital) adjusted for financial risk.

RISK ADJUSTED RETURN ON EQUITY (RAROE): Same as Return on Equity (ROE) with the net income numerator, and denominator (equity) adjusted for financial risk.

RISK ADJUSTER: A method used to modify health care spending costs for a particular cohort of Medicare patients that are estimated to be above or below expected costs.

RISK ARBITRAGE: A purchase and/or short sale of the same or potentially equal securities at prices that do not immediately guarantee a profit. Alternatively, it is to play one security against another to take advantage of a disparity in price. It is usually used during corporate takeover attempts.

RISK AVERSION: Satisfaction with lower investment returns, all things being equal.

RISK CONTRACT: An arrangement between a managed health care plan and HCFA (now the Centers for Medicare and Medicaid Services) under 1876 of the Social Security Act. Under this contract, enrolled Medicare beneficiaries generally must use the plans' provider network. Capitation payments to plans are set at 95% of the adjusted average per capita cost.

RISK CORRIDOR: A financial arrangement between a payer of health care services, such as a state Medicaid agency, and a provider, such as a managed care organization that spreads the risk for providing health care services. Risk corridors protect the provider from excessive care costs for individual beneficiaries by instituting stop-loss protections, and they protect the payer by limiting the profits that the provider may earn.

RISK EXPERIENCE LOSS RATIO: The frequency and distribution of a health or other insurance company's health care claims or losses.

RISK FACTOR: The amount of economic or financial uncertainty in a pool of patient or managed contracts.

RISK FACTOR REDUCTION: Diminution of economic or financial uncertainty in a pool of patient or managed contracts.

RISK FREE RATE: The rate of return (interest rate) available on a default-free government bond investment (see Figure 5).

RISK INDEX: The present value function factor for riskless cash flow, divided by the present value interest factor for a risky asset.

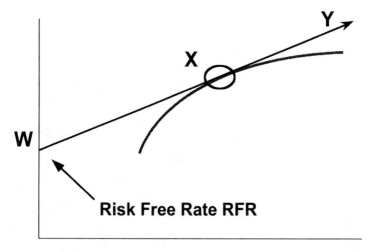

Figure 5: Risk Free Rate RFR.

RISK MANAGEMENT: Adjusting exposures for a portfolio in order to stabilize variability of returns while trimming dominant exposures. Investment policy statements and/or powers and authorities documents.

RISK PREMIUM: The interest rate difference between what investors require for a certain security and the risk-free rate of return.

RISK SELECTION: Health plan or insurance enrollment choices based on premium costs and other financial incentives, such as medical or health savings accounts.

RISK TOLERANCE: The ability of an investor to tolerate the chance of loss on an investment. Risk measurement attempts to quantify these chances, which can result from inflation, interest rates, market fluctuations, political factors, foreign exchange, and so forth.

RISK TYPES: Include the following:

- agency
- bankruptcy
- basis
- capital restrictions
- commodity
- compliance
- concentration
- conversion
- convexity
- corporate
- counterparty
- country
- coupon
- credit
- credit rating
- currency
- default
- dilution
- disaster
- duration
- environmental
- event
- exercise
- force majeure
- funding
- hazards
- legal
- liquidity
- market
- nonsystematic
- obsolescence
- operational
- option
- pin
- political
- prepayment
- price level
- reinvestment
- residual
- roll
- rule change
- software and financial assumptions
- spread
- systematic
- technological
- time value decay
- timing
- volatility
- weather
- yield curves

RISKLESS TRANSACTION: A simultaneous buy-sell transaction with neutral output and no uncertainty.

RIZZO-ZECKHAUSER MODEL: A health care economic theory that relates the importance of personal income targets to physicians and medical practitioners. *See also* supplier induced demand (SID).

ROAD SHOW: Presentation of a company to potential investors, especially in an Initial Public Offering.

ROEMER'S LAW: Positive relationship between hospital bed availability and cohort utilization of those space occupying beds. *See also* Parkinson's Law; Say's Law.

ROGUE TRADER: One who operates outside the limits of his authority, often to hide losses but in the process incurs even greater ones.

ROLL DOWN: Movement out of a higher coupon or option strike price into a lower coupon or option strike price. It is the movement down a yield curve from a relatively longer maturity security into a relatively shorter maturity security.

ROLL UP: Progression from one option to another with a larger exercise price.

ROLLING BUDGET: Continual upgrade of a budget for a given time period, in advance.

ROLLOVER: Transfer of a securities option position into a different delivery month.

ROLLOVER IRA: An individual retirement account established to accept assets from a qualified plan. As long as the assets aren't mixed with other contributions, they may later be moved into another qualified plan. *See also* Conduit IRA.

ROMNEY, MITT: Governor of Massachusetts and proponent of a "personally responsible" and "individually mandated," modified universal health care system in the United States (*Boston Herald,* April 21 2006).

ROTH IRA: Personal retirement account created by the Taxpayer Relief Act of 1997 allowing continued after-tax capital to accumulate tax free under certain conditions. It is a type of individual retirement account in which the investor (subject to income limits) contributes after-tax dollars to the account, which can then grow free of any further taxes on appreciation or income.

ROTH 401(K): Personal retirement account created in 2001 allowing continued after-tax capital to accumulate tax free under certain conditions.

ROTHER, JOHN: Policy director of AARP in Washington, D.C.

ROTHSTEIN, RUTH: Chief of the Bureau of Health Services, in Cook County, Illinois.

ROUND LOT: A unit of trading or a multiple thereof. On the New York Stock Exchange stocks are traded in round lots of 100 shares for active stocks and 10 shares for inactive ones. Bonds are traded as percentages of $1,000, with municipal bonds traded in minimum blocks of five bonds ($5,000 worth).

ROUND TRIP: Sale and purchase of a security within a short period of time.

ROUTINE TRANSACTIONS: Recurring sales and accounting activities reflected in financial statements and recorded in the normal course of business.

ROWE, JOHN, MD: Chairman and CEO of Aetna in Hartford, Connecticut.

ROYER, THOMAS, MD: President and CEO of Christus Health in Irving, Texas.

ROZELL, BILLIE, RN, DSN: Executive committee member for the International Society for Research in Healthcare Financial Management, Towson, Maryland.

RUBBER CHECK: A bounced check with insufficient funds.

RULE OF 72: Divide 72 by an interest rate factor to equal the time period, in years, for a doubling of a principle sum.

RULE OF 78: A formula used to determine interest for installment loans by the sum of the year's digits. $1 + 2 + \ldots + 12 = 78$, so 1/78th of the interest is owed after the first month, 3/78ths after the second month, and so forth. It is more expensive than simple interest payments.

RULE OF 108: Divide 108 by an interest rate factor to equal the time period, in years, for tripling a principle sum.

RULE 144: An SEC rule permitting the occasional sale of restricted ("letter") securities or insider holdings in modest amounts, without registration with the SEC.

RULE 147: Rule dealing with exemption from SEC registration under the 1933 Act for securities offerings limited to residents of one state or territory. It implements and provides standards for the intrastate exemption.

RULE 405: The stockbroker's rule to know each customer.

RULES OF FAIR PRACTICE: A set of rules established and maintained by the NASD Board of Governors regulating the ethics employed by members in the conduct of their business.

RULES OF THUMB: Industry specific mathematical equations for business entity valuation based on several variables such as overhead expenses, revenues, and industry specific risk and combined with hearsay, experiences, or heuristics.

RUN: A sudden demand at a bank for money by its depositors.

RUN AHEAD: Illegal practice of purchasing securities for a stockbroker's account, prior to client order executions.

RURAL HOSPITAL: This category of hospital is determined based on distance and defined as a hospital serving a geographic area 10 or more miles from the nexus of a population center of 30,000 or more. More specifically, a rural hospital means an entity characterized by one of the following:

- *Type A:* Rural Hospitals: small and remote, have fewer than 50 beds, and are more than 30 miles from the nearest hospital.
- *Type B:* Rural Hospitals: small and rural, have fewer than 50 beds, and are 30 miles or less from the nearest hospital.
- *Type C:* Rural Hospitals: considered rural and have 50 or more beds.

RUSH CHARGE: An additional fee imposed for expeditious results, tests, health care goods, products, or medical services.

RUSSELL, THOMAS, MD: Executive Director of the American College of Surgeons in Chicago, Illinois.

RUSSELL 1000 INDEX: Measures the performance of the 1,000 largest U.S. companies based on total market capitalization.

RUSSELL 1000 GROWTH INDEX: Measures the performance of those Russell 1000 companies with higher price-to-book ratios and higher forecasted growth values.

RUSSELL 1000 VALUE INDEX: Measures the performance of those Russell 1000 companies with lower price-to-book ratios and lower forecasted growth values.

RUSSELL 2000 INDEX: Measures the performance of the 2,000 largest U.S. companies having the smallest capitalization in the Russell 3000 Index.

RUSSELL 2000 GROWTH INDEX: Measures the performance of those Russell 2000 Index companies with higher price-to-book ratios and higher forecasted growth values.

RUSSELL 2000 VALUE INDEX: Measures the performance of those Russell 2000 Index companies with lower price-to-book ratios and lower forecasted growth values.

RUSSELL 3000 INDEX: Measures the performance of the 3,000 largest U.S. companies based on total market capitalization.

RUSSELL MIDCAP INDEX: Measures the performance of the 800 smallest companies in the Russell 1000 Index.

RUSSELL MIDCAP GROWTH INDEX: Measures the performance of those Russell Midcap Index companies with higher price-to-book ratios and higher forecasted growth values.

RUSSELL MIDCAP VALUE INDEX: Measures the performance of those Russell Midcap Index companies with lower price-to-book ratios and lower forecasted growth values.

S

S CORPORATION: A corporation that chooses to be generally exempt from federal income tax. Its shareholders, who all must consent to this tax treatment, include in their incomes their share of the corporation's separately stated items of income, deduction, loss and credit, and nonseparately stated income or loss.

SACRED COW: Slang term for a philosophy asset, position, or project considered protected by management. Often this investment is presented as off-limits or nonnegotiable.

SAFE HARBOR: Prudent steps that avoid illegal tax, financial accounting, health care management, or business accusations and charges. Safe harbors may be used where a legal requirement is somewhat ambiguous and carries a risk of punishment for an unintended violation.

SALARIED PROFESSIONALS: Highly trained individuals who work as employees of corporations, hospitals, or other medical facilities, government agencies, scientific and educational institutions, or other organizations, such as employed physicians and nurses.

SALARY CONTINUATION PLAN: A nonqualified deferred compensation plan that provides a stated benefit at retirement or other future event without a stated reduction in the employee's current compensation.

SALARY PAYABLE: Wages owed to employees.

SALARY REDUCTION PLAN: A nonqualified deferred compensation plan under which an employee agrees to reduce currently payable compensation by a stated amount (or according to a specified formula), with the accumulated reduction amount payable at retirement or other future event.

SALES ALLOWANCE: Sales discounts, write-offs, deductions, or expenses.

SALES CHARGE: An amount charged to purchase an asset or shares in most mutual funds. The maximum charge is 8.5% of the initial investment. The charge is added to the net asset value per share in the determination of the offering price. It is an expensive sales commission.

SALES CHARGE PERCENTAGE: Public Offering Price; Net Asset Value / POP.

SALES DISCOUNT: A reduction in the amount receivable to induce a purchase.

SALES JOURNAL: A special journal to record credit sales.

SALES MIX: A combination of products or services that make up total sales, such as a medical payer service mix.

SALES REVENUE: The amount earned by providing health care products or services.

SALVAGE VALUE: Amount received for the sale of a fixed asset at the end of a project or its useful life.

SANTA CLAUSE RALLY: Slang term for the historic rise in stock market prices between New Year's Day and Christmas Day.

SARBANES-OXLEY ACT (SARBOX): 2002 Corporate Responsibility Act (CRA) covering financial, accounting, certification, and new protections governing securities fraud.

SATTERTHWAITE, MARK A., PhD: AC Buehler Professor in Hospital and Health Services Management, Professor of Managerial Economics, and Professor of Strategic Management from the Kellog School of Management at Northwestern University in Evanston Illinois. He is a co-originator of high-deductible health insurance plans.

SAVINGS: Income not consumed in a given time period. Money deferred.

SAY'S LAW: A (defunct) macroeconomic theory that the production of a certain amount of goods and services results in the generation of an amount of income sufficient to buy that output.

SCALPER: One who engages in quasi-legal financial transaction for a quick profit.

SCARCITY: Inequilibrium or unbalance between wants and needs, desires and satisfaction, especially in health care.

SCENARIOS: Economic hypothetical "what-if" outcomes analysis.

SCHAEFFER, LEONARD: Chairman and CEO of WellPoint Health Networks in Thousand Oaks, California.

SCHEDULE: List of amounts payable for medical goods, products, or health care services.

SCHEDULE A: The schedule used to summarize a taxpayer's itemized deductions. Itemized deductions include medical and dental expenses (in excess of 7.5% of the taxpayer's AGI), state and local taxes, deductible interest, charitable contributions, miscellaneous deductions (in excess of 2% of the taxpayer's AGI), and so forth.

SCHEDULE C: The schedule used to summarize revenues and expenses (accrual basis) or receipts and disbursements (cash basis) for the self-employed taxpayer. Profits or earnings from self-employment result in the imposition of the self-employment tax at a rate of 15.3%. It is used to report profits or losses for sole proprietorships.

SCHEDULE D: The tax schedule used to report gains and losses.

SCHEDULE 13D: SEC disclosure rule to document 5% beneficial ownership in a public company.

SCHEDULE E: The tax schedule used to report profits or losses from royalty and rental income properties. It is also used to report most of the information from Schedule K-1.

SCHEDULE K-1: A form issued by partnerships and S Corporations to their partners and shareholders, respectively. This schedule retains the character of the partnership or S Corporation's income and expense items for pass-through to the individual's Form 1040. It is the schedule provided to each partner in a partnership (or shareholder in an S Corporation), and also supplied to the Internal Revenue Service as an attachment to the partnership (or S Corporation) tax return—Form 1065 (Form 1120S), showing the partner's (shareholder's) distributive share of partnership (shareholder's) profits and losses. (Though not attached to the individual taxpayer's/partner's/shareholder's individual tax return—Form 1040—the Schedule K-1 is very similar to a Form W-2 that an employee would receive from an employer at year-end.)

SCHROEDER, STEVEN, MD: President of the Robert Wood Johnson Foundation in Princeton, New Jersey.

SCRAP VALUE: Salvage value of an asset.

SCRIPOPHILY: Hobby of collecting securities certificates for scarcity, rather than investment value.

SCRUSHY, RICHARD: Chairman and CEO of HealthSouth Corp. in Birmingham, Alabama.

SCULLY, THOMAS: Administrator of the Centers for Medicare and Medicaid Services (CMS) in Washington, D.C.

SEARCH GOOD: Any product or service whose worth or value can be fully evaluated upon inspection, unlike health care services.

SEASONAL VARIATION: Annual decrease or increase in health care product or service consumption due to co-payments, end-of-year deductibles, coinsurance, and so forth.

SEASONED ISSUE: Mature securities traded for a length of time with good second market liquidity.

SEAT: Membership on a stock exchange, purchased or leased.

SECONDARY MARKET: (1) The aftermarket for securities, or the resale of outstanding securities. (2) A public offering by selling stockholders. If listed on the NYSE, a member firm may be employed to facilitate such an offering in an over-the-counter net transaction for a purchaser, with prior approval of the Exchange. Both member and nonmember broker/dealers can participate in this distribution.

SECONDARY OFFERING: A sale of a large block of securities already issued by a corporation and held by a third party. Because the block is so large, the sale is usually handled by investment bankers who may form a syndicate and peg the price of the shares close to current market value.

SECTION 1244 STOCK: Stock issued (generally the first $1 million of common or preferred) by a corporation that obtains greater than 50% of its annual gross income receipts from the conduct of an active business. The subsequent dispossession of the stock by a stockholder receives favorable tax treatment.

SECTION 501 (c)(3): IRS Code for a nonprofit organization.

SECTOR: A group of stocks in one industry, such as drug stocks, durable medical equipment, and health care.

SECTOR ROTATION INVESTING: A style of investing in which the goal is to outperform the market by investing more heavily in the sectors that are forecasted to perform better than the market in expected economic scenarios.

SECULAR ANNUITY: An arrangement for funding a deferred compensation agreement that involves the purchase of a commercial annuity by an employer for the benefit of an employee. Amounts paid to the insurance company by the employer are recognized as taxable income by the employee in the year they are paid. Earnings on the annuity are taxed to the employee as they are withdrawn.

SECULAR TRUST: An irrevocable trust for the exclusive benefit of an employee that provides benefit security but not deferral of taxation on amounts transferred to the trust by an employer as compensation.

SECURED BOND: Loan backed by pledged assets, such as more federal bonds, as collateral. It is an insured bond as to payment and principle.

SECURED CLAIM: Receipt backed by assets of the issuing company.

SECURED DEBT: Loan, note, certificate, or bond backed by assets of the issuing company.

SECURED LOAN: Loan backed by specifically pledged assets as collateral.

SECURITIES: Any note, stock, bond, evidence of debt, interest, or participation in a profit-sharing agreement, investment contract, voting trust certificate, fractional undivided interest in oil, gas, or other mineral rights, or any warrant, pre-emptive right or option to subscribe to, or purchase, any of the foregoing. Also includes variable annuities and various other insurance products. A capital claim.

SECURITIES ACT OF 1933: Legislation that protects the public against the issuance and distribution of fraudulent securities by requiring the filing of a revealing registration statement with the Securities Exchange Commission.

SECURITIES EXCHANGE ACT OF 1934: Federal law that covers stockbrokers and dealers (B/Ds) and secondary market activities. This compares to the Securities Act of 1933 which focuses on new issues.

SECURITIES EXCHANGE COMMISSION (SEC): Established by Congress to protect investor interest, the commission administers compliance with the Securities Act of 1933, the Securities and Exchange Act of 1934, the Trust Indenture Act (TIA), the Investment Company Act (ICA), the Investment Advisers Act (IAA), and the Public Utility Holding Company Act (PUHCA).

SECURITIES INVESTOR PROTECTION CORPORATION (SIPC): A government-sponsored, private corporation that guarantees repayment of money and securities in customer accounts valued at up to $500,000 per separate customer ($100,000 cash), in the event of a broker/dealer bankruptcy.

SECURITIES MARKET LINE (SML): Security return-risk relationship using beta as a systemic risk measure (see Figure 6).

SECURITIES REGISTRATION: Compliance procedure where an individual or firm is registered, according to function, supervisory level, and type of customer contact, with the State or SEC. Registration is not a sign of approval by any agency but rather a notification by the corporation to the agent/agency of its intent to sell securities.

SECURITIZATION: The act of aggregating debt or companies in a risk pool, as with Physician Practice Management Corporations (PPMCs), and then floating new securities with reduced risk backed by the pool.

SEED: Initial capital contribution (money) to a start-up company or emerging health care organization.

SEGMENTATION: The separate divisions of a company or business.

SELECTED MEDICAL CONTRACT: Negotiated payment agreement with medical providers and health care facilities to contain and control costs.

SELF DIRECTED: Management by the account or asset holder.

SELF-DIRECTED IRA: A retirement account offered through an investment dealer that allows the owner to actively manage his or her securities portfolio.

SELF-EMPLOYMENT TAX: The self-employment tax of 15.3% represents an amount equivalent to both employee (7.65%) and employer (7.65%)

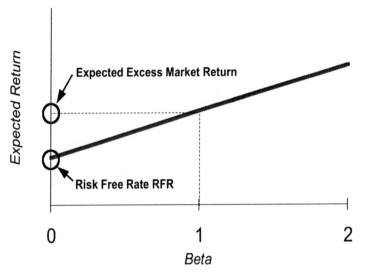

Figure 6: Security Market Line.

contributions to Social Security and Medicare. The self-employment tax rate of 15.3% is a combination of a 12.4% Old Age, Survivors, and Disability Insurance (OASDI) tax plus a 2.9% Medicare tax. The OASDI component is subject to a wage base or ceiling that is inflation-indexed and increases each year. Alternatively, the Medicare tax is computed on all self-employment income and is not subject to a ceiling.

SELF FUNDING: The practice of an employer or organization assuming responsibility for health care losses of its employees. This usually includes setting up a fund against which claim payments are drawn, and processing is often handled through an administrative services contract with an independent organization.

SELF INSURANCE: An individual or organization that assumes the financial risk of paying for health care, life, disability, or other insurable risks and perils.

SELF-INSURED: An individual or organization that assumes the financial risk of paying for health care, life, disability or other insurable risks, hazards, and perils.

SELF PAY: The individual responsible for health insurance claims, sans a health insurance policy contract (private pay).

SELF-REGULATORY ORGANIZATION (SRO): One of eight organizations account-able to the SEC for the enforcement of securities laws within an assigned field of jurisdiction.

SELL: To cover ownership of an asset or security for value or money.

SELL DISCIPLINE: An investor's criteria for selling a security or stock. A value investor, for instance, may sell when the price/earnings ratio of the security is a certain percentage higher than its historical level.

SELL OFF: Pressured securities sales due to unfavorable economic conditions.

SELL ON CLOSE: Order to sell securities at the market's close, at the market or at a limit.

SELL ON OPENING: Order to sell securities at the opening, at the market or at a limit.

SELL ORDER: Stockbroker instructions to sell a securities position or other asset.

SELL OUT: Upon failure of a purchasing firm to accept delivery of a security, and lacking a rejection form, the seller can without notice, dispose of that security in the marketplace at the best available price and hold the buyer responsible for any financial loss resulting from the default.

SELL STOP ORDER: A securities order that becomes a market order to sell if and when someone trades a round lot at or below the stop price used to protect a long position.

SELLER FINANCING: One who provides cash, credit, or securities for an economic transaction.

SELLER'S MARKET: Situation when there is more demand for a health care good, product, or service than available supply.

SELLER'S OPTION: A stock or bond or other settlement contract in which the certificates are due at the purchaser's office on a specific date stated in the contract at the time of purchase.

SELLING CONCESSION: A fraction of a securities underwriter's spread, grant-ed to a selling group member by agreement. It is payment for services as a sales agent for the underwriters.

SELLING COSTS: Expenses incurred by a health care or other entity to influence the sale of products, goods, or services.

SELLING DIVIDENDS: The unfair and unethical practice of soliciting purchase orders for mutual fund shares solely on the basis of an impending distribu-tion by that fund.

SELLING EXPENSE: A fraction of the sales spread on certain securities, granted for associated sales costs. It is payment for sales expenses.

SELLING GROUP: Selected brokers/dealers who contract to act as selling agents for underwriters and who are compensated by a portion of the spread called selling concession on newly issued stocks. They assume no personal responsibility or financial liability to the issuer, as opposed to a syndicate member.

SEMIANNUAL COMPOUNDING: Bi-annual or twice-per-year interest payments.

SEMIFIXED COST: Stepped or incremental cost. Also called semivariable cost.

SEMIVARIABLE COST: Stepped or incremental cost. Also called semifixed cost.

SENIOR SECURITIES: Bonds, debentures, debt, or preferred stocks. These issues have a prior claim, usually in the order named, to assets, earnings, and the proceeds of dissolution. Mutual funds do not issue senior securities, but they may purchase them for their portfolio.

SENSITIVE MARKET: A financial and volatile marketplace easily influenced by bad or good news.

SENTIMENT: The amount of good or bad feelings about a particular financial market, to be either bullish or bearish. Economic emotions.

SEPARATE ACCOUNT: A specialized legal entity created by an insurance company to incorporate contracts offered by the company under a variable annuity insurance plan.

SEPARATE CUSTOMER: As defined by Securities Investment Protection Corporation, the accounts of a given customer at a single brokerage firm. Different types of accounts held by the same person do not constitute separate customers.

SEPARATE PROCEDURES: Procedures that do not have a specific CPT code assigned to them and are usually an integral part of the total health care procedure or medical service rendered. No increase in reimbursement is allowed.

SERIAL BOND: A debt issue that matures in relatively small amounts at periodic stated intervals, as opposed to term or balloon bonds.

SERIAL ISSUE: An issue of bonds or debt having maturities scheduled over several years, thereby allowing the issuer to amortize principal over a period of years. Maturity schedules for serial bonds often provide for level debt service or level principal payments.

SERIES 3: Sales license for commodities futures.

SERIES 4: Registered Options Principal Examination License. Registered Options Principal, Compliance Registered Options Principal, and/or Senior Registered Options Principal.

SERIES 5: Interest Rate Options Examination License.

SERIES 6: Sales license for mutual funds and variable annuities.

SERIES 7: Sales license for all types of securities products, with the exception of commodities futures.

SERIES 8: Trading Supervisor Examination License.

SERIES 15: Foreign Currency Options Examination License.

SERIES 16: Supervisory Analyst Examination License.

SERIES 24: General Securities Principal Examination License.

SERIES 26: Supervisory license for investment company and variable annuity insurance products.

SERIES 27: Financial and Operations Principal Examination License.

SERIES 28: Introducing Broker/Dealer Financial and Operations Principal Examination License.

SERIES 52: Municipal Securities Representative Examination License.

SERIES 53: Municipal Securities Principal Examination License.

SERIES 62: Corporate Securities Representative Examination License.

SERIES 63: License to sell securities and render investment advice.

SERIES 65: Uniform Securities Agent State License.

SERIES E AND EE BONDS: Debt issued by the U.S. Treasury in denominations of as little as $50 and purchased at a discount from their face value. For example, a bond of $50 with a 5-year maturity is sold for $37.36. If it is redeemed at maturity, the bondholder receives the entire $50, thereby earning a 6% annual yield. The rate is a variable rate, 85% of the average rate on 5-year treasury securities. The rate fluctuates every 6 months, thereby giving the investor the opportunity to enjoy higher yields should interest rates rise. The investor who chooses to redeem the bond before maturity would earn a lesser return, reflecting the early redemption. Both purchase and redemption are transacted through a commercial bank. The interest earned on these bonds is exempt from taxation until the bonds are redeemed, thereby giving even those with modest-sized investments the benefit of tax shelter. Also, Series EE bonds provide investors with a way to fund future tuition requirements through the accumulation of tax-free interest.

SERIES H AND HH BONDS: Series HH bonds are sold in larger denominations (with a minimum face value of $500), and have a maturity of 10 years. Unlike that of Series EE bonds, the interest on Series HH bonds does not accrue, so it is subject to federal income taxation annually. These bonds are also purchased and redeemed at commercial banks.

SERIES OF OPTIONS: Options of the same class having the same exercise price and expiration month.

SERVICE COMPANY: A firm that provides intangible services such as medical and health care, rather than merchandise or tangible physical products.

SERVICE DATE: The specific date a charge is incurred, or cost assigned, to a medical procedure, good, or service.

SERVICE LIFE: An asset's period of usefulness.

SERVICE INDUSTRY: Industry that provides intangible services such as medical and health care, rather than tangible or manufactured physical products.

SERVICE V-CODE: ICD-9-CM code for medical examinations, aftercare, or reimbursable ancillary health care services.

SERVICING A LOAN: The ongoing process of collecting loan payments, including accounting for and payment of related taxes, if any.

SETTLEMENT: To complete and pay for a securities transaction.

SETTLEMENT DATE: The date of a financial satisfaction for a securities transaction.

SETTLEMENT METHOD: Accounting for securities as transactions are recorded on the date the securities settle by the delivery or receipt of securities and the receipt or payment of cash.

SETTLEMENT PRICE: The official price at the end of a trading session. This price is established by the Option Clearing Corporation, and it is used to determine changes in account equity or margin requirements, and for other purposes.

SETTLOR: The person who creates and funds a trust. They may also be called a donor, grantor, or creator.

SHADOW PRICES: Slang term for imputed or estimated health insurance costs not valued accurately in the marketplace. Shadow prices also are used when market prices are inappropriate due to regulation or externalities.

SHAM: An unethical or illegal transaction; usually groundless to avoid taxation.

SHAPIRO SNYDER, LYNN: Partner of Epstein, Becker & Green in Washington, D.C.

SHARE: A single unit of a stock security.

SHARE AVERAGING: The periodic purchase of the same number of securities shares to reduce their mean cost basis.

SHARE OF COST: Medicaid initiative for recipients to pay a portion of expenses for medical services.

SHARE PRICE: The net asset value of an individual share of a mutual fund.

SHAREHOLDER: Owner of financial market products or assets such as stocks, bonds, mutual funds, REITs, ETFs, and so forth.

SHAREHOLDERS' EQUITY: Total assets minus total liabilities of a company divided by the number of common shares outstanding. Theoretically, this is the value of the company to the shareholder at liquidation.

SHARPE, WILLIAM, INDEX: A risk adjusted ratio measure of financial performance that correlates the return-in-excess of the risk-free rate of return, by a portfolio's standard deviation.

SHARPE, WILLIAM, PhD, RATIO: Originally formulated by substituting the standard deviation of a securities' portfolio returns (i.e., systematic plus unsystematic risk) in the place of the beta of the Treynor ratio. Thus, a fully diversified portfolio with no unsystematic risk will have a Sharpe ratio equal to its Treynor ratio, while a less diversified portfolio may have significantly different Sharpe and Treynor ratios.

SHELF REGISTRATION: Corporate ability to sell pre-SEC registered shares under favorable economic climates with a minimum of paperwork.

SHELTON, DENNIS: Chairman and CEO of Triad Hospitals in Dallas, Texas.

SHILLER, ROBERT J., PhD: Stanley B. Resor Professor of Economics, Department of Economics and Cowles Foundation for Research in Economics, Yale University, and fellow at the International Center for Finance, Yale School of Management. He coined the term "irrational exuberance" about speculative financial and stock market bubbles, and proposed a variety of risk-management techniques covering the expanding role of public finance, health, and other insurance.

SHORT: Selling a security not owned.

SHORT AGAINST THE BOX: A short sale made when the investor owns securities identical to those sold short. The purpose is to defer, for tax purposes, recognition of gain or loss with respect to the sale of securities in the box.

SHORT COVER: Long (owned) purchase of securities by a short seller investor to replace those borrowed short (unowned) sale.

SHORT INTEREST: Stocks sold short and not repurchased to close out a short position.

SHORT INTEREST THEORY: When short interest positions in a stock are high (see short sale), although it is an indication that many investors feel the stock price will drop, the theory is that the phenomenon is bullish for the stock because the short sellers will all have to purchase the stock in the near future to cover their short positions.

SHORT OPTION: An option that has been written.

SHORT OPTION POSITION: The position of an option writer that represents an obligation to meet the terms of the option if it is assigned.

SHORT POSITION: Any open position that is expected to benefit from a decline in the price of the underlying stock such as long put, short call, or short stock.

SHORT RUN: Period or length of time where some business inputs cannot be varied.

SHORT RUN DEMAND FOR LABOR: Ratio of health care labor wage-rate and quantity of labor demanded when a health care entity has fixed capital, while labor costs are variable.

SHORT RUN DEMAND ELASTICITY FOR LABOR: The percentage change in the quantity of health care demanded divided by the percentage change in the health care labor wage rate when labor is the only variable input.

SHORT SALE: The sale of a security (i.e., stocks and bonds) before it has been acquired. An investor anticipates that the price of a stock will fall, so he sells securities borrowed from the brokerage firm. The securities must be delivered to the firm at a certain date (the delivery date), at which time the investor expects to be able to buy the shares at a lower price to cover his position.

SHORT SALE RULE: SEC regulation that mandates short sales be made only in rising or bull market, on a plus tick.

SHORT SQUEEZE: Sharp upward movement of a futures contract inducing investors to buy in order to prevent loss by covering positions.

SHORT TERM: A less than 1 year investment horizon in the accounting industry. It is a service production time where medical providers can change some, but not all, of the goods or medical services they supply.

SHORT TERM AGGREGATE SUPPLY CURVE: Graphical representation of a time period in which health care input prices remain constant, but price levels fluctuate.

SHORT TERM CAPITAL GAIN OR LOSS: A capital gain or loss that is not long term.

SHORT TERM COMPETITIVE EQUILIBRIUM: Price point at which the total quantity of health care products or services supplied in a short time period and the total quantity of health care outputs demanded are equal, and which is equal or greater to the average variable costs of the health care products or services.

SHORT TERM FINANCING: Borrowing that is paid back in less than a year.

SHORT TERM INVESTMENTS: Financial investments or other assets liquidated in less than a year.

SHORT TERM LIQUIDITY: Ability to meet bills as they come due.

SHORT TERM REALIZED CAPITAL GAINS: Amount by which the net proceeds from the sale of a security that is held for less than 12 months exceeds its cost of acquisition.

SHORT TERM REALIZED CAPITAL LOSSES: Amount by which the acquisition cost of a security that is held for less than 12 months exceeds the net proceeds from its sale.

SHORTAGE: Occurs when the health care quantity demanded exceeds the quantity supplied.

SHRINKAGE: Inventory or Durable Medical Equipment (DME) reduction. It's the difference between recorded and actual inventory, including lost or unaccounted for inventory.

SHUBIK MODEL: A theoretical economic model designed to study the behavior of money. It was created by Martin Shubik, Seymour Knox Professor of Mathematical Institutional Economics at Yale University in New Haven, Connecticut.

SHUT DOWN POINT: Occurs when prices have fallen to a level below that which just allows a physician, clinic, hospital, health care provider, or other entity to cover its minimum average variable costs.

SIGMA: Option term sometimes used as a synonym for vega, lambda, or kappa. It's a letter of the Greek alphabet.

SIGNATURE CARD: A contractual form, executed by an account holder, establishing account ownership and setting forth some of the basic terms of the account and provisions of the deposit contract.

SIGNATURE GUARANTEE: Assurance by a financial institution or other entity that a particular signature is valid. Typical guarantors include commercial banks, trust companies, savings and loan associations, or member firms of a national securities exchange.

SIGNIFICANT ACCOUNTS: Occurs with the likelihood that an account could contain misstatements that individually, or when aggregated with others, could have a material effect on the financial statements, considering the risks of both overstatement and understatement.

SIGNIFICANT DEFICIENCY: A combination of control deficiencies that adversely affects a company's ability to initiate, authorize, record, process, or report external financial data reliably in accordance with GAAP, such that there is a likelihood that a misstatement on annual or interim financial statements that is more than inconsequential will not be prevented or detected.

SIGNIFICANT FINDINGS OR ISSUES: Substantive matters important to auditing procedures performed, evidence obtained, or conclusions reached, including but not limited to:

- significant matters,
- auditing procedures indicating a need for modification of auditing procedures,
- audit adjustments and disagreements among members of an engagement team,
- circumstances that cause difficulty in applying auditing procedures,
- significant changes in the assessed level of audit risk, and
- matters that could result in modification of an auditor's report.

SIMPLE INTEREST: Interest earned on the principal sum only, with no interest computed on interest or interest past due, as in compound interest.

SIMPLE IRA: A form of salary reduction plan.

SIMPLE PLANS (SAVINGS INCENTIVE MATCH PLAN FOR EMPLOYEES): May be adopted if a health care or other company has fewer than 100 employees that received at least $5,000 in compensation in the preceding year.

SIMPLE TRUST: Required to distribute all its income currently, whether or not the trustee actually does so, and it has no provision in the trust instrument for charitable contributions.

SIMPLIFIED ARBITRATION: A method of arbitration to be used when there is a small amount in dispute, no more than $10,000. This method can be used for disputes between members (Simplified Industry Arbitration) and for disputes between a customer and a member (Simplified Arbitration). Two very important points to remember about arbitration are: (1) that decisions and rulings are always final and binding, and (2) A customer will be involved in arbitration only at the insistence of said customer.

This insistence may be done at time of the dispute or the customer may sign a predispute arbitration agreement, in which he is stating in advance that any dispute that may arise will be settled under arbitration.

SIMPLIFIED EMPLOYEE PLAN (SEP): An IRA plan that is simplified and easy to administer for self-employed people. It is a plan that establishes IRAs for employees and independent contractors, providing for the deduction of the lesser of $30,000 or 15% of the employees' taxable compensation (indexed periodically).

SIMULATIONS: A statistical framework for what-if conditions that in a probabilistic sense, suggest expected behavior over an economic, mathematical, or financial time series.

SIMULTANEOUS (RISKLESS) TRANSACTION: A transaction in which the broker/dealer takes a position in security only after receipt of an order from a customer, for the purpose of acting as principal. This is the one dealer transaction that requires disclosure of markup.

SINGLE AUDIT ACT (SAA): Established requirements for audits of states, local governments, and nonprofit organizations that administer federal financial assistance programs above a certain threshold.

SINGLE DRUG PRICER (SDP): Drug-pricing file containing the allowable price for each drug-covered incident to a physician's service, drugs furnished by independent dialysis facilities that are separately billable from the composite rate, and clotting factors to inpatients. The SDP is in effect, a fee schedule similar to other CMS fee schedules.

SINGLE PREMIUM DEFERRED ANNUITY (SPDA): Lump sum tax deferred investment with insurance annuity payout.

SINGLE STEP INCOME STATEMENT: Income statement format that groups all revenues together and then lists and deducts all expenses together without producing subtotals.

SINKER: Debt repaid with a sinking bond fund used to redeem debt and loaned or preferred stock securities.

SINKING FUND: (1) A fund established by the bond contract of an issue into which the issuer makes periodic deposits to assure the timely availability of sufficient monies for the payment of debt service requirements. The amounts of the revenues to be deposited into the sinking fund and the payments are determined by the terms of the bond contract. Under a typical revenue pledge this fund is the first (under a gross revenue pledge) or the second (under a net revenue pledge) to be funded out of the revenue fund. This fund is sometimes referred to as a Debt Service Fund. (2) A separate account in the overall sinking fund into which monies are placed to be used to redeem securities, by open-market purchase, request for tenders or call, in accordance with a redemption schedule in the bond contract.

SITUS: Location of a trust, but it need not be located in the state in which the creator or the trust beneficiaries reside.

SKEWNESS: Exists when a distribution is not symmetrical about its mean. A distribution is symmetrical when its median, mean, and mode are equal. A positively skewed distribution occurs when the mean exceeds the median. A negatively skewed distribution occurs when the mean is less than the median; calculated as $E[(x - mu)^3]/s^3$ where mu is the mean and s is the standard deviation.

SKIMMING: The practice in health programs paid on a prepayment or capitation basis, and in health insurance, of seeking to enroll only the healthiest people as a way of controlling program costs.

SKIMPING: Slang term for providing less than appropriate, optimal, or quality health care services.

SLEEPER: Security with little investor interest but with great potential.

SLIDING PRICE SCALE: Ranges of health care service prices available in exchange for volume discounts preferred provider or facility status or some other concession.

SLIDING SCALE COMMISSION: A health or other insurance commission adjustment on earned premiums under a formula whereby the actual commission (paid by a reinsurer to a ceding insurer) varies inversely with the loss ratio, subject to a maximum and minimum.

SLIDING SCALE DEDUCTIBLE: A health insurance or other deductible that is not set at a fixed amount, but rather varies according to income.

SLIDING SCALE MODEL: A discounted medical fee schedule based on the patients' ability to pay.

SLIPPAGE: The commissions, fees and other costs of executing a securities or other transaction. The other dominant cost is the spread between the bid and offer and price adjustments for size. Sometimes, there are additional expenses in trading odd lots or very large blocks.

SLUGS: Slang term for state and local government series securities used for escrow for advanced refunding, especially with hospital debt issues.

SLUMP: Short-term financial, business, or economic depression.

SMALL AREA VARIATION: Large variations in per capita medical care utilization rates across small or homogenous patient populations.

SMALL BUSINESS STOCK: Stock from a corporation with gross assets of $50 million or less at the time the stock was issued and held by the original owner for more than 5 years prior to the sale of the stock. A sale may receive favorable tax treatment. Unincorporated investors may exclude up to 50% of any gain they realize on the disposition of qualified small business stock issued after August 10, 1993, and held for more than 5 years. The amount of gain eligible for the 50% exclusion is subject to per-issuer limits. In order to qualify for the exclusion, the corporation issuing the stock must be a C Corporation (but excluding certain investment corporations), and it must use at least 80% of its assets in active conduct of one or more qualified trades or businesses.

SMALL CAPITALIZATION STOCKS: Publicly traded company with a market capitalization of $500 million or less.

SMALL FIRM EFFECT: The tendency of securities of smaller corporations to outperform larger ones.

SMITH, THOMAS C.: President and CEO of VHA in Irving, Texas.

SMITH, VERNON L., PhD: George Mason University behavioral economist and psychologist who shared the 2002 Nobel Prize in Economics (formally known as the Bank of Sweden Prize in Economic Sciences in Memory of Alfred Nobel) with Daniel Kahneman, PhD, of Princeton University in New Jersey.

SMITH, WAYNE: President and CEO of Community Health Systems in Brentwood, Tennessee.

SOCIAL SECURITY TAX: The Federal Insurance Contributions Act (FICA) tax.

SOFT DOLLAR: Higher commission sales charge than might be individually negotiated for additional services, such as research, advice, technology connectivity, and so forth.

SOLE PROPRIETORSHIP: An unincorporated business, such as a small medical practice, having a single owner. Although many small businesses are sole proprietorships, this business form is not recommended because of the unlimited liability accruing to the owner. Incorporation serves to shield the owner from liability.

SOLOVIAN GROWTH: Economic growth brought about by investments and increases in capital stock.

SOLOW RESIDUAL: A measure of change in total health care factor productivity, with growth accounting empirically either for an industry, such as health care, or for a macroeconomy. The term was coined by Robert Solow, 1924, a major figure who formed the core of the post-WWII economics department at MIT and contributed to capital theory (1956) development and the Phillip Curve (1960) concepts.

SOLVENCY: Ability to meet financial obligations as they are due.

SORKIN, ALAN L., PhD: Executive committee member for the International Society for Research in Healthcare Financial Management, Towson, Maryland.

SOUR BOND: A bond or other debt obligation in default.

SOURCE DOCUMENT: Original hardcopy of a business, financial, accounting, purchase/sale, or other transaction.

SPECIAL ASSESSMENT BOND: An obligation payable from special assessment revenues.

SPECIAL CASH ACCOUNT: Older reference to a SEC Regulation T account in which the customer is required to make full payment on the first business day after the trade date.

SPECIAL DEALS INTERPRETATION: A mutual fund underwriter's improper practice of disbursing anything of material value (more than $100) in addition to normal discounts or concessions associated with the sale or distribution of investment company shares.

SPECIAL INTEREST PURCHASE: Purchase of a health care or other business interest in order to enjoy economies of scale, market advantages, synergies, or other strategic competitive enhancements.

SPECIAL JOURNAL: Accounting journal to record a specific type of unusual transaction.

SPECIAL TAX BOND: A bond secured by one or more designated taxes other than ad-valorem taxes. For example, bonds for a particular purpose might be supported by sales, cigarette, fuel, or PET scan, or Certificate-of-Need (CON) business license taxes. The designated tax does not have to be directly related to the project purpose, and such debt is not considered self-supporting debt.

SPECIAL US EVALUATION: Pursuant to Code Section 2032A, special-use valuation provides that the highest and best use value may be reduced in the gross estate by up to $750,000 based on special-use valuation for real property used in a farming operation or a trade or medical business that meets certain requirements, and where certain pre-death qualifications are met and post-death commitments are made.

SPECIALIST: A member of a securities exchange with the essential function of maintaining an orderly market, insofar as reasonably practicable, in the stocks in which he is registered as a specialist. To do this, he must buy and sell for his own account and risk, to a reasonable degree, when there is a temporary disparity between supply and demand. In order to equalize trends, he must buy or sell counter to the direction of the market. At all times the specialist must put his customer's interests before his own. All specialists are registered with the exchange, but are not employees of that exchange.

SPECIALIST CAPITATION: Fixed payment, PMPM, accepted by a medical specialist or provider. Specialty department capitation.

SPECIALIST'S BOOK: The notebook a New York Stock Exchange specialist in a given security uses to keep a record of the buy and sell orders he receives for execution at specified prices. He maintains them in chronological sequence of receipt and only limit and stop orders are in the Specialist's Book.

SPECIALIZATION: The production of only one or a few health care products or medical services, as in a single focused, or specialized, physician.

SPECIALIZED INVESTMENT COMPANIES: Investment companies that concentrate their investments in one industry, group of related industries, or a single geographic area for the purpose of reaching their objectives.

SPECIALTY HOSPITAL: This type of health care organization has limited focus to provide treatment for only certain illnesses, such as cardiac care, orthopedic or plastic surgery, elder care, radiology/oncology services, neurological care, or pain management cases. These organizations are often owned by physicians who refer patients to them. In recent years, single-specialty hospitals have emerged in various locations in the United States. Instead of offering a full range of inpatient services, these hospitals focus on providing services relating to a single medical specialty or cluster of specialties.

SPECIFIC IDENTIFICATION METHOD: Inventory costing method used for larger pieces of medical equipment as it traces actual costs to an identifiable unit of product and is usually applied with an identification tag, serial plate, bar code, or RFID scanner. It does not involve flow of cost analysis. But, it does permit the manipulation of income, because health care entities state their cost of goods sold, and ending inventory, at the actual cost of specific units sold.

SPECULATION: A very risky investment with a potential large return.

SPECULATIVE BONDS: High-yield, high-risk, junk bonds.

SPECULATIVE DEMAND: Money needs inversely related to the interest rate.

SPECULATOR: One who accepts large financial risks in return for potential large rewards.

SPIDERS: Shares in a trust that owns stocks in the same proportion as that represented by the S&P 500 stock index. Due to the acronym SPDR, Standard & Poor's Depository Receipts are commonly known as spiders. Each share of a Spider contains one-tenth of the S&P 500 index, and trades at one-tenth the level of the S&P 500, on the AMEX under the symbol SPY. SPDRs are ETFs, and trade like ordinary shares on the stock market with continuous liquidity, and can be short sold, provide regular dividend payments, and incur regular brokerage commissions when traded. Spiders compete directly with S&P 500 index funds.

SPILLOVER BENEFIT: A benefit associated with the production of a health care good or service, obtained without compensation by a third party or someone other than the provider or patient.

SPILLOVER CASH FLOW: Indirect cash-in or cash-outflows that occur elsewhere in a health care organization.

SPILLOVER COST: A consumption expense associated with the production of a health care good or service, obtained without compensation on someone other than the buyer (patient) or seller (medical provider).

SPIN OFF: A distribution of stock in a company that is owned by another corporation and that is being allocated to the holders of the latter institution.

SPLIT: A division of the outstanding shares of a corporation into a larger number of shares, entitling each owner to a fixed number of new shares. The shareholder's overall equity remains the same, though he owns more stock, because the total value of the shares remains the same. For example, the owner of 100 shares, each worth $100, would be given 200 shares, each worth $50, in a two-for-one split.

SPLIT COUPON BOND: A low or zero initial coupon bond that is followed by a higher coupon rate of interest.

SPOT PRICE: The currency price of a commodity.

SPREAD: (1) The difference in value between a bid and offer securities price. (2) The difference between the public offering price and the amount received by the issuer. It is a position in securities consisting of two parts, each of which alone would profit from opposite securities price moves. These opposite parts are entered simultaneously in the hope of limiting risk or benefiting from change or price relationship between the two.

SPREAD (OPTION): Purchase and sale of option contracts of the same class with different expiration dates and/or strike prices.

STABILIZATION: A securities underwriter/syndicate manager is empowered by the members of his group to maintain a bid in the aftermarket at or slightly below the public offering price, thus "stabilizing" the market and giving the syndicate and selling-group members a reasonable chance of successfully disposing of their allocations. This practice is a legal exception to the manipulation practices outlawed by the Securities and Exchange Act of 1934.

STAFFING: Recruiting, interviewing, and hiring health care or other workers.

STAG: One who gets in and out of stocks or a fast profit. *See also* speculator.

STAGFLATION: Slang term for a time of inflation without GNP growth, or a period of high inflation and high unemployment.

STANDARD & POOR'S 500 INDEX (S&P 500): A daily measure of stock market performance that is based on a selected group of 500 companies, and a benchmark for measuring large-cap U.S. stock market performance. The S&P 500 is often used as a general indicator of the equity market, and it includes a representative sample of leading companies in leading industries.

STANDARD & POOR'S CORPORATION: An independent financial service company, a subsidiary of McGraw-Hill Company, that provides ratings for municipal debt securities and other financial information to investors, such as Moody's Investor's Service (see Table 11).

STANDARD COST: A per unit express predetermined cost.

STANDARD DEDUCTION: Individual taxpayers who do not itemize deductions are entitled to an amount by which to reduce adjusted gross income (AGI) in arriving at taxable income which varies by type of taxpayer and is indexed annually. Certain taxpayers may not be entitled to use the standard deduction, such as a married person filing separately, or high income medical practitioners, such as doctors and nurses.

STANDARD DEVIATION: A measure of volatility, risk, or statistical dispersion. It is the positive square root of the variance, calculated by:

- computing the (average) mean of the series,
- then taking the deviation by subtracting the mean from each observation,
- squaring the differences or deviations for each observation,
- dividing the sum of the squared deviations by the number of observations, and
- calculating the positive square root of the sum of squared deviations.

Related terms include:

- *Standard Normal Distribution* or *Standardized Normal Distribution*—Situation that occurs when the underlying normal distribution is converted by changing its scale. The importance of this is that different normal distributions can now be compared to one another. Otherwise, separate tables of values would have to be generated for each pairing of mean and standard deviation values. This standardized variant term is often expressed as Z is N (0,1), or Z is a normal distribution with a mean value of zero and variance equal to one.
- *Static Analysis*—An approach to study market conditions at a moment in time. It is also a "snapshot view" of the market, corporate financial condition, or other economic time series. It reflects one moment, such as the end-of-the-day, end-of-the-month, end-of-the-year, the opening, or any other chronologically defined point.
- *Stationary*—A time series which has a natural mean or tendency toward one. Over time and given larger samples, some economic time series tend to converge toward a natural level with stable volatilities.
- *Statistical Analysis*—A mathematical approach that quantifies securities market action. In its general form, it is reliant on large sample statistics and linear analysis. It assumes independence. Its popular subterms are: mean, variance, standard deviation, alpha, and beta.
- *Stochastic*—A condition in finance or economics whereby changes occur on a more abrupt basis than those expected to be normally encountered. In some ways, stochastic have infinite variance and/or nonconverging means implications.

STANDARD OF VALUE: The exact type of value sought in a valuation engagement, or fair market value, liquidation value, investment value, and so forth.

STANDBY UNDERWRITING AGREEMENT: An agreement between an investment banker and a corporation, whereby the banker agrees, for a negotiated fee, to purchase any or all shares offered as a subscription privilege that are not bought by the rights holders by the time the offer expires.

STANFORD, KATHLEEN, MBA, DBA, FACHE: Vice President of Nursing at Harrison Memorial Hospital in Bremerton, Washington. She is also Commander of her Washington Army National Guard unit.

Table 11: Standard & Poor's Corporation versus Moody's Investment Services

Standard & Poor's		Moody's	
AAA	The obligor's capacity to meet its financial commitment on the obligation is extremely strong.	Aaa	Obligations are judged to be of the highest quality, with minimal credit risk.
AA	The obligor's capacity to meet its financial commitment on the obligation is very strong.	Aa	Obligations are judged to be of high quality and are subject to very low credit risk.
A	The obligor's capacity to meet its financial commitment on the obligation is strong.	A	Obligations are considered upper-medium grade and are subject to low credit risk.
BBB	Obligation exhibits adequate protection parameters. However, adverse economic conditions or changing circumstances are more likely to lead to a weakened capacity of the obligor to meet its financial commitment on the obligation.	Baa	Obligations are subject to moderate credit risk. They are considered medium-grade and as such may possess certain speculative characteristics.
BB	The obligor faces major ongoing uncertainties or exposure to adverse business, financial, or economic conditions, which could lead to the obligor's inadequate capacity to meet its financial commitment on the obligation.	Ba	Obligations are judged to have speculative elements and are subject to substantial credit risk.
B	The obligor currently has the capacity to meet its financial commitment on the obligation. Adverse business, financial, or economic conditions will likely impair the obligor's capacity or willingness to meet its financial commitment on the obligation.	B	Obligations are considered speculative and are subject to high credit risk.

(Continued)

Table 11: Continued

Standard & Poor's		Moody's	
CCC	The obligor is currently vulnerable to nonpayment and is dependent upon favorable business, financial, and economic conditions for the obligor to meet its financial commitment on the obligation. In the event of adverse business, financial, or economic conditions, the obligor is not likely to have the capacity to meet its financial commitment on the obligation.	Caa	Obligations are judged to be of poor standing and are subject to very high credit risk.
CC	The obligation is currently highly vulnerable to nonpayment.	Ca	Obligations are highly speculative and are likely in, or very near, default, with some prospect of recovery of principal and interest.
C	A bankruptcy petition has been filed or similar action has been taken, but payments on this obligation are being continued.	C	Obligations are the lowest rated class of bonds and are typically in default, with little prospect for recovery of principal or interest.
D	The obligation is in payment default.		
+, −	The ratings from 'AA' to 'CCC' may be modified by the addition of a plus or minus sign to show relative standing within the major rating categories.	1, 2, 3	Moody's appends numerical modifiers 1, 2, and 3 to each generic rating classification from Aa through Caa. The modifier 1 indicates that the obligation ranks in the higher end of its generic rating category; the modifier 2 indicates a mid-range ranking; and the modifier 3 indicates a ranking in the lower end of that generic rating category.

Source: Internal Revenue Service.

STARK, FORTNEY "PETE": U.S. Representative (D-Calif.) and ranking member of the Ways and Means health subcommittee.

STARK I: January 1992, from 1989 OBRA (42-USC 1395nn), precludes patient self referrals by a physician or medical provider to another health care entity of interest. It was formerly the Patient in Ethics Referral Act.

STARK II: August 1993, strengthens Stark I and further precludes patient referrals to an expanded list of medical services and physician/providers and family members having a financial interest in the entity.

STARK SELF-REFERRAL PROHIBITION: The Stark Amendment to the Omnibus Budget Reconciliation Act of 1989 (OBRA) was a step by the federal government to prohibit physicians from referring patients to entities in which they have a financial interest. Originally, the Stark Amendment only applied to the referral of Medicare patients to clinical laboratories in which the physician had a financial interest. It was later amended to include many other services called designated health services. The Stark Amendment provides that if a physician (including a family member) has a financial interest in a clinical laboratory, then he or she may not make a referral for clinical laboratory services if payment may be made under Medicare. There are certain exceptions to the Stark Amendment, such as if a physician personally provides a service or if a physician or employee of a group provides the services. Like the safe-harbor regulations, the Stark Amendment permits physician investment in large entities and provides an exception for rural providers. Under Stark, large entities are defined as publicly traded entities with assets greater than $100 million. There are certain other exceptions that are similar to the safe-harbor regulations. They include items such as provision for rental of office space, employment and service arrangements with hospitals, and certain service arrangements. These arrangements must be at arms' length and at fair market value. Stark II was passed in 1993 to modify and expand the Stark amendment. In particular, it acts to bring numerous other entities, besides clinical laboratories, within the prohibitions of the Stark Amendment. The list of designated health services include:

- clinical laboratory services;
- physical therapy services;
- radiology services, including magnetic resonance imaging, computerized axial tomography scans, and ultrasound services;
- radiation therapy services including supplies;
- parenteral and enteral nutrients, equipment, and supplies;
- prosthetics, orthotics, and prosthetic devices and supplies;
- home health services;
- outpatient prescription drugs; and
- inpatient and outpatient hospital services.

The list of current procedural terminology (CPT) codes that relate to the Stark Amendment is updated at least annually, and is published in the Federal Register.

STARRED PROCEDURE: Specific surgical procedures listed in a CPT code book. It's a slang term for an asterisk-term indicating a special denotation.

START UP: A new business venture, such as a medical practice or emerging health care organization (EHO).

STATE TAXATION OF INSURANCE: Authority of the individual states to tax insurance companies in the range of 2%–4% of premiums.

STATED VALUE: Similar to par value, it's an accounting value for stock which is not fair market value or current price.

STATEMENT OF ADDITIONAL INFORMATION (SAI): A supplement to information contained in a mutual fund's prospectus. It provides more detailed information about fund policies, operations, and risks, among other things.

STATEMENT OF CASH FLOWS (SCFs): One of four main financial statements that document where cash went in an organization, for a specific time period. It is a report of cash receipts and disbursements classified according to three major activities: financing, operations, and investments:

- Operating activities include cash inflows (ARs, receipts, donations, and accrued expenses, interest and dividends) and outflows (inventory, pre-paids, supplies, and loans).
- Investing activities include the disposal or acquisition of noncurrent assets, such as equipment, loans, or marketable securities.
- Financial activities generally include the cash inflow or outflow effects of transactions and other events, such as issuing capital stock or notes involving creditors, owners, or shareholders.

Prior to 1988 the formal SCFs was known as a Statement of Changes in Financial Position and projected estimated cash flows by month, quarter, and year, along with the anticipated timing of cash receipts and disbursements.

STATEMENT OF CHANGE IN NET ASSETS: Documents the changes of net assets from one period to another.

STATEMENT OF FINANCIAL CONDITION: A basic financial disclosure statement as of a specified date, listing assets, liabilities, and equity balance.

STATEMENT OF FINANCIAL POSITION: A corporate balance sheet.

STATEMENT OF OPERATIONS: Newer fourth financial statement that documents an entity's revenues and expenses during an accounting period.

STATEMENT OF OWNER'S EQUITY (CAPITAL): Summary of changes in an accounting entry, for owner's equity, during a specific period in time.

STATEMENT OF RETAINED EARNINGS: That part of a health care or other company's profits that is not paid out in dividends but used by the company to reinvest in the business.

STATEMENT OF REVENUES AND EXPENSES: Corporate income statement.

STATEMENT OF STOCKHOLDER'S EQUITY (CAPITAL): Summary of changes in an accounting entry, for stockholder's equity, during a specific period in time.

STATIC BUDGET: A budget prepared for only one level of production volume for goods or services. It is an estimate for a single level of activity.

STATUTE OF LIMITATIONS: The period when legal actions may be brought upon claims or within which rights may be enforced.

STATUTORY MERGER: Acquisition of more than 51% ownership in a corporation.

STATUTORY UNDERWRITER: An individual or corporation that purchases an unregistered security and offers it in a public distribution without an effective registration statement. Such parties are subject to fine and/or imprisonment.

STATUTORY VOTING: A means by which a stockholder is given the right to cast one vote for each share owned in favor or against each of a number of proposals of director/nominees at a formal meeting convened by the corporation.

STEENTH: Slang term for 1/16th of a point.

STEER: Funneling patients to selected medical providers.

STEERAGE DISCOUNT: Volumes of patients sent to selected providers in return for step discounts.

STEP COSTS: Expenses that contain both fixed and variable cost elements.

STEP DOWN COST: A primary cost center that provides resources to other cost centers, such as human resources or nursing. The costs from the primary center are allocated to the other centers, and the primary step down cost center is closed and no other costs are allocated to it.

STEP FIXED COSTS: Fixed costs that increase in total at certain points as the level of activity increases.

STEP UP BASIS: The basis of property acquired by inheritance, bequest, or from a decedent is the FMV of such property on the date of the decedent's death. If the fair market value is more than the decedent's basis, a taxpayer's basis in the property received is increased.

STOCHASTIC: A synonym for financial or economic randomness.

STOCHASTIC INDEX: Technical tool to determine a financial market's oversold or over-bought condition. It is a randomness risk reduction dampening method.

STOCK: Certificate representing ownership in a corporation. They may yield dividends and can appreciate or decline in value. An equity.

STOCK AHEAD: An expression used on the floor of the New York Stock Exchange to signify that one or more brokers had made a prior bid (or offer) at the same price as an order you had entered, so the order was ahead of yours on the Specialist's Book.

STOCK BUYBACK: A corporation may repurchase shares outstanding on the open market and retire them as "treasury shares." This antidilutive action increases earnings per share, which consequently raises the price of the outstanding shares. Companies often announce a share repurchase plan when insiders feel the company is undervalued. The action strengthens the company and helps preclude a takeover.

STOCK COMPANY: Any company that is owned and controlled by a group of stockholders whose investment in the company provides the capital necessary for the issuance of guaranteed, fixed premium, and nonparticipating policies. The stockholders share in the profits and losses of the company. Some stock companies also issue participating policies.

STOCK DIVIDEND: Payment of a dividend in stock rather than cash, usually as a percentage of existing shares held. It may be stock in the original company or that of a subsidiary. A stock dividend is a way for a corporation to maintain its cash position without being subject to the accumulated earnings tax, because it reduces retained earnings and increases capital stock on a company's books. A stock dividend also carries a tax advantage for the shareholder, because a dividend would be subject to ordinary income tax, but the tax on capital gains is not payable until the shares are sold.

STOCK DIVIDEND DISTRIBUTION: A distribution to shareholders made upon declaration of a corporation's board of directors. This distribution differs from the usual disbursement in that it is given in the form of additional shares of stock instead of money.

STOCK INDEX FUTURES: A futures contract that has as its underlying entity a stock market index. Such futures contracts are generally subject to cash settlement.

STOCK INDEX OPTIONS: The right to sell and buy option contracts based on an average of stock prices.

STOCK JOCKEY: Slang term for a stockbroker who sells and buys frequently.

STOCK OPTION: A right to purchase a security at a specified price at some time in the future.

STOCK OUT: Depletion of inventory.

STOCK (OR BOND) POWER: A legal document either on the back of registered stocks and bonds or attached to them, by which the owner assigns his interest in the corporation to a third party, allowing that party the right to substitute another name on the company records in place of the original owner's.

STOCK REPURCHASE: The purchasing and retiring of equity by the issuing corporation.

STOCK REVERSE SPLIT: The reduction of outstanding shares of a company into a fewer number of shares with a higher price, while the overall equity in the company remains the same.

STOCK SCREENING: A computerized method of stock picking according to preselected criteria.

STOCK SPLIT: The division of the outstanding shares of a company into a larger number of shares, with a lower price but while the overall equity in the company remains the same. Shareholders have more shares but the same proportionate interest in the company. Unlike a stock dividend, a stock split does not affect the books of the company. After a split, the shares will immediately fall to a proportionate market value (that is, in a 2-for-1 split, $30 shares will fall to $15 each). A split makes the stock cheaper and helps to broaden ownership in the company. A "reverse split" (1-for-10) allows a company with low share value to be noticed by institutional investors who may be restricted from considering low-priced stocks.

STOCK SYMBOL: Letters used to identify companies on listed stock exchanges. They are also referred to as trader symbols.

STOCK WARRANT: Usually issued along with a stock, bond, or preferred stock, entitling the owner to purchase a specific amount of securities at a specific price, usually above the current market price at the time of issuance, for an extended period, anywhere from a few years to forever. In the case that the price of the security rises to above that of the warrant's exercise price, then the owner can buy the security at the warrant's exercise price and resell it for a profit. Otherwise, the warrant will simply expire or remain unused. Warrants are listed on options exchanges and trade independently of the security with which it was issued.

STOCKBROKER: One who is licensed to perform transactions (usually buy or sell) in financial instruments on a stock market as an agent of his/her/its clients who are unable or unwilling to trade for themselves. A Registered Representative (RR) of a wire house or brokerage firm.

STOCKHOLDER: A person who owns stock in a corporation; equity holder; share holder.

STOCKHOLDER'S (OWNER'S) EQUITY: The owner's equity of a corporation.

STOP ORDER: A securities sale or purchase in order to preserve gains or limit securities losses.

STOP LIMIT ORDER: A securities order that becomes a limit order to sell when someone creates a round lot transaction at, or below, the stop price.

STOP LOSS LIMIT: A way medical providers limit economic risks in cases where costs are greater than reimbursement amounts.

STOP LOSS ORDER: Insuring with a third party against a risk that an MCO cannot financially and totally manage. For example, a comprehensive prepaid health plan can self-insure hospitalization costs with one or more insurance carriers.

STOP LOSS REINSURANCE: Protects a ceding company against an excessive amount of aggregate health insurance claim losses during a certain period of time or over a percentage of earned premium income.

STOP ORDER: A securities order from a customer to a broker that becomes a market order only if a transaction takes place at or through the price stated in the order. The sale that activates the order is called the trigger.

STOP PAYMENT: A request to a bank not to honor or allow the payment of a check after it has been delivered but before it has been presented.

STOPPING STOCK: A market specialist's guarantee of price to a stockbroker (for a customer order only), thus enabling the broker to try to improve upon that price without fear of missing the market.

STRADDLE: A securities trading position involving puts and calls on a one-to-one basis in which the puts and calls have the same strike price, expiration, and underlying entity. A long straddle is when both options are owned, and a short straddle is when both options are written.

STRAIGHT DEDUCTIBLE CLAUSE: Health or other insurance policy clause that specifies either the dollar amount or percentage of loss that the insurance does not cover.

STRAIGHT LINE DEPRECIATION: The depreciation method in which an equal amount of depreciation (noncash expense) is assigned to each year or period in a uniform fashion.

STREET: The slang term for Wall Street.

STREET NAME: When securities have been bought on margin (credit) or when the customer wishes the security to be held by the broker/dealer, the securities are registered and held in the broker's/dealer's firm name.

STRETCHING: Increase of the held duration for assets or liabilities.

STRIKE PRICE: The exercise price for securities sales.

STRIPS: Stripped Treasury Obligations. The principal and interest payments are separated from the underlying security. The stripped principal may be called the *corpus*. The stripped offerings are essentially Zero Coupon Bonds.

STRONG DOLLAR: U.S. dollar that can be exchanged for a large volume of foreign currency.

STRUCTURE: To rearrange cash flow components, both interest and principal, into new streams or structures. The breaking down of currency payments below Treasury Department reporting limits. The usual motivation is avoidance of income taxes or cloaking ownership. The quality and appropriateness of health care inputs.

STUDER, QUINT: Independent health care consultant in Pensacola, Florida. He is also former president and CEO of Baptist Hospital in Pensacola, Florida.

STYLE: Investment style is attributed to sophisticated institutional investors. Major styles include value, growth, and contrarian (going the opposite way of most investors at the time). Bottom-up and top-down, respectively, refer to picking stocks based exclusively on their individual characteristics or as a part of a broader economic view that predicts certain sectors will do better than others.

SUBCAPITATION: Any capitation or fixed-payment health care reimbursement method that is subordinate or secondary to global or full capitation.

SUBCHAPTER M: The section of the Internal Revenue Code that provides special tax treatment for regulated investment (mutual fund) companies.

SUBJECT: Slang term for negotiated offer/bid securities prices.

SUBJECT PREMIUM: A base or standard insurance premium.

SUBMITTED CHARGE: The charge submitted by a medical provider to the patient, insurance, or managed care plan, or a private payer.

SUBORDINATED DEBENTURES: Unsecured debts that are junior (more risky) or subordinate to debenture bonds.

SUBSCRIBERS: Those who buy usually new stock issues.

SUBSCRIPTION PRICE: The price at which a right or warrant is offered.

SUBSCRIPTION PRIVILEGE (PRE-EMPTIVE RIGHT): A shareholder's right to purchase newly issued shares (before the public offering). It must be exercised within a fixed period of time, usually 30 to 60 days, before the privilege expires and becomes worthless. Rights are exercisable at a value below the current market price. Rights have a market value and are actively traded. They differ from warrants in that they must be exercised within a relatively short period of time. They are proportionate to ownership, and a warrant's exercise price is always above the current market price.

SUBSEQUENT EVENT: Event that occurs after the end of the accounting period and before the publication of an entity's financial statements. Such events are disclosed in the notes to the financial statements. *See also* materiality.

SUBSIDIARY: A company owned by more than half of the voting shares of another company.

SUBSIDIARY LEDGER: A book of accounts for individual balances, the total of which appears in the general ledger.

SUBSIDY: Government payment based on health care output.

SUBSTANDARD BONDS: High yield and risky junk bonds.

SUBSTANTIAL RISK OF FORFEITURE: A facts and circumstances test that, if met, defers securities taxation under the economic benefit theory or under IRC §83.

SUBSTITUTE: Goods, products, and health care services that serve a purpose similar to other items.

SUBSTITUTE EFFECT: Ratio of a change in price of health care quantities consumed by patients when the consumer remains indifferent between the original and a new combination of health care goods or services.

SUICIDE PILL: Slang term for any anticorporate takeover strategy that puts itself (company) in jeopardy.

SUITABILITY: The decision made by a stockbroker if an investment in a particular security matches objectives and financial capital of the customer.

SUMMARY COMPLAINT PROCEEDINGS: In the event of a minor infraction of NASD Rules of Fair Practice, the District Business Conduct Committee may offer the accused member a penalty of censure and/or fine up to $2,500, if he wishes to plead guilty, waive formal hearings, and all rights of appeal.

SUM OF THE YEAR'S DIGITS (SOYD): An accelerated method of depreciation based on an inverted scale of total digits for the years of depreciate life. For 5 years of life, for example, the digits 1, 2, 3, 4, and 5 are added to produce 15. The first year's rate becomes 5/15 of the depreciable cost (33.3%), the second year's rate is 4/15 of depreciable cost (26.7%), the third year's rate 3/15, and so on.

SUNK COSTS: Expenses already incurred that are unchangeable.

SUNRISE INDUSTRIES: Slang term for small growth companies, such as emerging biotechnology companies or emerging health care organizations (EHOs).

SUPERBILL: A form that specifically lists all of the services provided by the physician. It cannot be used in place of the standard American Medical Association form.

SUPPLEMENTAL EXECUTIVE RETIREMENT PLAN (SERP): A nonqualified plan, primarily but not exclusively for executives, that provides for lost qualified pensions due to Internal Revenue Service restrictions.

SUPPLIER INDUCED DEMAND (SID): Discretionary influence of medical providers or the industry to induce changes in health care demand over patients or customers, such as in cosmetic and plastic surgery and direct-to-consumer pharmaceutical marketing.

SUPPLY: Relationship between the price of a health care good, product, or service and the quantity provided by medical sellers.

SUPPLY BUDGET: A projection of fixed and variable costs.

SUPPLY CURVE: Graphical representation of health care service quantity offered over time and at various price points.

SUPPLY SCHEDULE: Tabular illustration of how the quantity supplied of a health care good or service is related to the price.

SUPPLY SHOCK: A dramatic and unexpected increase in health care outputs. It is an abrupt change in aggregate medical supply.

SUPPLY SIDE ECONOMICS: Financial incentives used to influence the aggregate supply curve.

SUPPORT AND RESISTANCE: A technical market theory that attempts to predetermine price levels where eager investor purchases will develop (support) or aggressive selling may appear (resistance), based upon previous fluctuations for a particular security.

SUPPORT LEVEL: Security price level bottom caused by investor demand.

SUPPORTING: Form of securities market manipulation in which a broker/dealer with a short position in puts buys large blocks of the underlying security in an attempt to raise the price and reduce the loss potential on the naked puts.

SUPPORTING ORGANIZATIONS: A tax-exempt entity that is established by an individual or small group of donors for the purpose of supporting a public charity, such as a hospital or health care system.

SURCHARGE: An additional expense, cost, or tax.

SURPLUS: Occurs when the quantity of health care goods or services supplied exceeds the quantity demanded.

SURPLUS ACCOUNT: The difference between a company's assets and liabilities. Net surplus includes contingency reserves and unassigned funds, whereas gross surplus also includes surplus assigned for distribution as dividends.

SUSPENDED LOSS: Refers to a passive activity loss that may be held, without any time limitation, to offset passive income of future years or to offset a gain when the entire activity is relinquished through sale or other disposition.

SUSPENDED TRADING: Temporary halt in the trading of a security, or a financial market, usually ahead of material information.

SUSPICION FRAUD AND ABUSE: Fraud is illegal activity where someone obtains something of value without providing service for that value. In health care, this occurs when someone bills for services not provided by the physician. Abuse is the activity where someone overuses or misuses services. According to CMS, "Although some of the practices may be initially considered to be abusive, rather than fraudulent, activities, they may evolve into fraud." In the case of health care abuse, this occurs when a physician sees the patient for treatment more times than deemed medically appropriate. If there are reported issues or actions from other sources such as NPDB or a medical board, a health insurance program can take that opportunity to review health care providers' activities. Most participation agreements allow for this type of scrutiny. The preliminary review will usually request a sampling of specific medical records, which may progress to an on-site review of any and all medical records of patients that participate in a CMS program. These activities can be generated by the plan's quality assurance or quality improvement program and often are tied to the credentialing process for a provider's participation.

SUSTAINING CAPITAL REINVESTMENT: The recurring capital investment required of a health care or other business entity, sans the tax shield.

SWAP: A sale of a security and the simultaneous purchase of another security, for purposes of enhancing the investor's holdings. The swap may be used to achieve desired tax results, to gain income or principal, or to alter various features of a bond portfolio, including call protection, diversification or consolidation, and marketability of holdings.

SWAP OPTION: An interest rate exchange option.

SWEAT EQUITY: Equity produced by conscientious industry, such as employment and hard work.

SWEEP ACOUNT: Automatic investment of idle deposit balances.

SWEETENER: Any feature added in addition to a securities offering to make it more attractive to investors, for purchase.

SWITCH ORDER: A contingent market securities order awaiting some predetermined event.

SYNDICATE: A group of investment bankers usually organized along historical or social lines, with one member acting as manager who collectively insures the successful offering of a corporation's securities. It is a selling group that markets securities.

SYNERGY: Combination that produces more economic output than individual component inputs.

SYNTHETIC ASSETS: Something of value artificially created from other combined assets.

SYNTHETIC EQUIVALENT POSITIONS: Trades in options that have the same profit and loss potential as a stock and option strategy. Example: long stock + long put = long call.

SYNTHETIC POSITION: A strategy involving two or more instruments that has the same risk/reward profile as a strategy involving only one instrument. The following list summarizes the six primary synthetic positions:

- Synthetic long call—A long stock position combined with a long put.
- Synthetic long put—A short stock position combined with a long call.
- Synthetic long stock—A long call position combined with a short put.
- Synthetic short call—A short stock position combined with a short put.
- Synthetic short put—A long stock position combined with a short call.
- Synthetic short stock—A short call position combined with a long put.

SYSTEMATIC WITHDRAWAL PLAN: A program in which an investor receives regular payments from his or her portfolio or account.

SYSTEMIC (SYSTEMATIC) RISK: The market risk of all securities prices that cannot be reduced through business diversification or asset allocation It is a securities market risk.

T

T: time.

T + 1: Required securities settlement date, or the trade date plus one day.

T + N OR T PLUS N: Broader description of the stipulated settlement process. The T refers to the trade date, and the N is the number of days from the trade date to the settlement date.

T: Tax Rate.

T-ACCOUNT: A diagram used to illustrate changes in the assets and liabilities of a bank's balance sheet. A T-account is named because its perpendicular lines look like the letter T, and represent changes in assets on the left side, and changes in liabilities and net worth on the right side.

TABLE OF ALLOWANCES: A list of covered and payable health care products or services.

TACTICAL ASSET ALLOCATION: Active portfolio rebalancing based on relative market attractiveness.

TAILGATE: Unethical stockbroker practice of following a client's order for a personal brokerage account.

TAKE: Slang term for profit.

TAKE A POSITION: Purchase securities, usually as a long-term investment.

TAKEDOWN: Normally, the largest component of the spread on a municipal bond issue, similar to a commission, which represents the income derived from the sale of the securities. If bonds are sold by a member of the syndicate, the seller is entitled to the full takedown (also called the total takedown). If bonds are sold by a dealer who is not a member of the syndicate, such seller receives only that portion of the takedown known as the concession or dealer's allowance, with the balance (often termed the additional takedown) retained by the syndicate.

TAKEOVER: Usually a hostile change in the controlling interest of a corporation with a new management team. It is typically financed by debt, as in a leveraged buyout (LBO).

TANGIBLE ASSETS: Assets that exist in physical space.

TAPE: Older reporting services for securities prices using stock or ticker tape. It is now in electronic format.

TARGET COMPANY: A firm about to be acquired, usually in a hostile manner with debt financing.

TARGET COSTING: Services or products designed and produced with costs below predetermined levels.

TARGET FUNDS: Mutual funds that invest in specified categories, such as average timed maturities or durations, need for college tuition payments, retirement, and so forth.

TARGET INCOME HYPOTHESIS: Suggestion that medical providers seek to set target income levels and adjust utilization rates to achieve those targets, as in management-by-numbers.

TARGET PRICE: A price level for health care services that suggests a minimum price per unit of output.

TARIFF: Tax imposed on imported goods.

TAX AVOIDANCE: Legal steps to reduce taxation.

TAX BASIS: The accounting cost of an asset, adjusted for depreciation and/or improvements used for gain or loss determinations upon liquidation.

TAX COURT: A legislative court functioning to adjudicate controversies between taxpayers and the IRS, arising out of deficiencies assessed by the IRS for income, gift, estate, and windfall profit and certain excise taxes. It has no jurisdiction over other taxes such as employment taxes.

TAX CREDIT: A direct reduction in tax liability, one for one.

TAX DEDUCTION: A deductible tax expense at some pro-rated amount.

TAX DEFERRED: The absence of taxation until maturity, receipt, or disposition for profit.

TAX DEFERRED ANNUITY (TDA) OR 403(b): This typically is a defined contribution plan available to teachers, doctors, nurses, hospitals, clinics, and not-for-profit health care organizations. An organization must sponsor the plan. Once sponsored, insurance companies offer annuities through the company. Employees then select which insurance company will receive their contributions. The contributions are almost always on a pretax basis.

TAX EFFICIENT PORTFOLIOS: A securities portfolio with trading profits and tax minimization as goals. These portfolios recognize that the subsequent payment of taxes reduces the investor's after-tax returns. When holdings are held by pension plans or tax-deferred accounts, there is no immediate tax liability on realized gains. However, an investor holding mutual funds that have high rates of security turnover and significant realized gains are subject to immediate tax year liabilities.

TAX EQUITY AND FISCAL RESPONSIBILITY ACT OF 1982 (TEFRA): Legislation that established target rates of increase limits on reimbursements for inpatient operating costs per Medicare discharge. A facility's target amount is derived from costs in a base year updated to the current year by the annual allowable rate of increase. Medicare payments for operating costs generally may not exceed the facility's target amount. These provisions may still apply to hospitals and units excluded from PPS.

TAX EQUIVALENT YIELD: Municipal bond rate / (100% − tax bracket). It is a pretax yield of an equivalent tax-free investment.

TAX EVASION: Illegal steps used to reduce or eliminate taxation.

TAX EXEMPT: Free from any taxation liability. Without tax.

TAX EXEMPT BOND: Bond issued by a state or municipality whose interest payments (but not profits from purchase and sale) are exempted from federal taxation. Many hospital bonds are municipal bonds.

TAX EXEMPTED SECURITIES: Obligations issued by a state or municipality whose interest payments (but not profits from purchase and sale) are exempted from federal taxation. The interest payment may be exempted from local taxation, too, if purchased by a state resident, as is usual with public hospitals and clinics.

TAX FREE EQUIVALENT YIELD: Corporate bond rate $\times$ (100% − tax bracket) / Municipal bond rate.

TAX IDENTIFICATION NUMBER (TIN): The number used to identify an individual or business for federal income tax purposes. This would be an individual's Social Security number (SSN).

TAX LIEN: Claim placed on property as security for unpaid taxes.

TAX PREFERENCE ITEMS: Income or deductions, such as a portion of long-term capital gains that are not taxed, accelerated depreciation, depletion, intangible drilling costs, and tax-free interest received on certain municipal bonds. *See also* Alternative Minimum Tax (AMT).

TAX SHELTER: Allows tax deductions or exclusions in the deferral of income tax that would otherwise be currently due.

TAX YEAR: The period used to compute taxable income. It is an annual period that is a calendar year, fiscal year, or fractional part of a year for which the return is made.

TAXABLE BOND INTEREST: Fiscal year-to-date interest from government securities, mortgage-backed securities, and taxable short-term securities.

TAXABLE DIVIDEND: A taxable payment declared by a health care or other company's board of directors and given to its shareholders out of the company's current or retained earnings.

TAXABLE EQUIVALENT YIELD: The interest rate that must be received on a taxable security to provide the holder the same after-tax return as that earned on a tax-exempt security. Because interest earned on municipal securities is not subject to federal income taxation, a tax-exempt security does not have to yield to a holder as much as a taxable security to produce an equivalent after-tax yield. This differential is attributable to the effect of the tax liability incurred by the holder if it held a taxable security. The taxable equivalent yield varies according to the holder's marginal federal income tax bracket, and, where applicable, any state or local tax liability as well.

TAXABLE INCOME: Gross income minus certain deductions and exemptions, from which the income tax due is determined. All income after adjustments and allowances is subject to taxation, whether corporate or personal.

TAXABLE YEAR: A period of time for which a report is to be made by a person or business of income received allowable deductions, and so forth, for income tax purposes. This is generally a calendar year for individuals, but may be another acceptable 12-month period (fiscal year) for businesses. A taxpayer on the cash basis is required to include items in gross income in the taxable year received. A taxpayer on the accrual basis is required to include items in gross income in the taxable year they accrue.

TAXPAYER IDENTIFICATION NUMBER (TIN): A numerical code required to file a tax return or any other document with the IRS. Usually a social security number is used for an individual. A federal or employer ID number is assigned to other types of entities.

TEASER RATE: Slang term for a temporary and/or artificially low or high interest rate to induce a sale.

TECHNICAL ANALYSIS: An approach to market theory stating that previous price movements, properly interpreted, can indicate future price patterns, too. A technical analyst watches the market, not the company, and is sometimes called a chartist, for obvious reasons.

TED SPREAD: Commodity money price difference that occurs with interest rates between European denominated dollars (Euros) and U.S. Treasury bills, It is slang for *Treasury over Euro Dollars.*

TEENYO: Slang tem for 1/16th of a point. Also called Steenth.

TEMPORARY ACCOUNT: Expense and revenue accounts that are related to a specific accounting period and closed at the end of the period.

TEN BAGGER: An equity that grows in price by a factor of 10.

TENDER: To surrender shares.

TENDER OFFER: The offer to buy stock directly from its shareholders and usually over the opposition of management.

TERM: A specific period of time.

TERM BOND: A bond with maturity such that substantially all the issue is due at the same date. This is as opposed to a serial bond, although some bonds have serial and term maturities.

TERM ISSUE: An issue of municipal securities that has a single stated maturity.

TERM LOAN: A type of long-term financing usually paid off within a decade.

TERMINAL VALUE (TV): Residual value at the end of fixed or variable maturity, the sale of an asset, or the salvage price of a piece of equipment.

TERMINATION: To mature, end, or complete.

TESTAMENTARY TRUST: A trust created under an individual's will.

THALER, RICHARD H., PhD: Robert P. Gwinn Professor of Behavioral Science and Economics at the University of Chicago Graduate School of Business and Professor of Behavioral Science and Economics at the UCLA Anderson School of Management, who demonstrated that many investors hold naive notions about diversification and a pronounced lack of sophistication about portfolio asset selection.

THETA: Time value decay.

THETA PRICING MODEL: A mathematical pricing model for derivatives.

THIN ISSUE: Slang term for a small number or volume of securities transactions.

THIN MARKET: Slang term for a securities marketplace exchange with few offers to sell and few bids to buy.

THIRD MARKET: OTC for listed exchange securities.

THIRD-PARTY PAYER: An intermediary such as an insurance or managed care company, Medicare, or Medicaid that agrees to pay for medical services on behalf of a patient.

THIRTY-DAY WASH RULE: IRS rule that precludes securities loss sales to offset tax losses if made within 30 days of equivalent securities purchase.

THOMAS, WILLIAM: U.S. Representative (R-Calif.) and chairman of the Ways and Means Committee in Washington, D.C.

THOMPSON, TOMMY: Secretary of the Department of Health and Human Services (DHHS) in Washington, D.C.

THREE-DIGIT DIAGNOSTIC CODE: CPT code used, and usually not accepted, when no fourth or fifth digit is available or higher levels of specificity exist.

TICK: A transaction (up or down) on the stock exchange. It may be equal to 1, 5, or more basis points in terms of price. It may refer to a 1/8, 1/16, 1/32, 1/64, or other fraction of minimally acceptable change. The term is dependent on the rules of each market and exchange. Among other ticks are:

- Up-Tick,
- Down-Tick,
- Zero-Plus-Tick, and
- Zero-Minus-Tick.

TICK TEST: A stock market trading curb that allows only zero-plus and up-tick transactions in the face of a falling market.

TICKER SYMBOL: Stock symbol used on the ticker tape, in newspapers, or electronically, and so forth.

TIERED INTEREST RATE: An interest rate structure that allows for increased interest based on a higher tiered rate and increased account balance for that rate.

TIGHT MARKET: Narrow bid offer prices in a market, security, financial product, or other commodity.

TIGHT MONEY: A dearth of credit in an economic milieu. It is a restricted money supply.

TIME COSTS: Time value of money, especially through inactivity or sloth.

TIME DEPOSITS: Saving account at a bank.

TIME LIMIT: Number of days in which a health care claim may be filed.

TIME PERIOD CONCEPT: Suggests that accounting statements be reported at regular intervals.

TIME PREMIUM: The amount of money the price of an option exceeds its intrinsic value.

TIME VALUE: The part of an option premium that reflects the remaining life of the option. The more time that remains before the expiration date, the higher the premium, because there is more time available for the value of the underlying security to move up or down.

TIME VALUE OF MONEY: Money received in the present can earn money over a period of time (making the amount ultimately larger than if the same initial sum were received later). Therefore, both the amount of investment return and the length of time it takes to receive that return affect the rate of return (i.e., the value of the return).

TIME WEIGHTED RETURN: Performance measurement of capital at work void of additions, withdrawals, or other timing differences. The compounded periodic return with each period's return is calculated as follows:

$$R_t = \frac{EV - BV - CF}{BV = WCF} \qquad \text{for period } t$$

Where EV = Ending Market Value
   BV = Beginning Market Value
   CF = Cash Flow = Contributions − Withdrawals

$$WCF = \frac{[(\text{Day of CF}) - (\text{Total Days in Period})] \times CF}{\text{Total Days in Period}}$$

The time weighted return, R, over T periods is calculated as:

$$R = (1 + R_1) * (1 + R_2) * \ldots * (1 + R_T) - 1 \text{ for } t = 1, 2, \ldots, T$$

TIMES DIVIDEND EARNED RATIO: Stock earnings divided by preferred dividend requirements.

TIMES INTEREST EARNED RATIO (TIER): A financial ratio that suggests how much there is in profit before interest, for every dollar in interest expense [(excessive revenue over expenses + interest expense) / (interest expense)].

TIP: A voluntary payment that exceeds formal cost and usually for extraordinary service. Also called gratuity. It may also refer to information, usually financial, that is exchanged between parties and is not usually available to the public.

TITLE: Written evidence that proves the right of ownership of a specific asset. It declares the legal owner.

TITLE INSURANCE: Protection against financial loss resulting from legal defects in the title of an asset.

TITLE SEARCH: An investigation into the history of ownership of an asset to check for liens, unpaid claims, restrictions, or problems to prove that the seller can transfer free and clear ownership.

TOBIN TAX: Surcharge on foreign currency exchanges. Named for James Tobin, PhD, a Nobel-laureate economist at Yale University.

TOKEN PAYMENT: A form of co-payment, usually a nominal payment, made by the patient for a service or supply item.

TOMBSTONE AD: Slang term for an ad announcing a securities offering which merely gives the size of the offering, the name of the firm or underwriting group from which a prospectus is available, and a disclaimer that the ad is not an offer to sell nor a solicitation of an offer to buy.

TON: Slang for $100 million dollars.

TOOKER, JOHN: CEO of the American College of Physicians in Philadelphia, Pennsylvania.

TOP DOWN INVESTING: Investing method that first identifies general economic trends, then industries, then specific companies, and finally ingestible securities. It is the opposite of bottom-up investing.

TOP OUT: Maximum securities price plateau.

TORNQVIST INDEX: A discrete-time approximation in which averages over time fill in the quantities of health care capital and medical labor. The concept was developed by the Bank of Finland in the 1930s.

TOTAL ASSETS TURNOVER RATIO (TATR): Total revenues / total assets.

TOTAL BUDGET: Otherwise known as a global budget, it's a cap on overall health spending.

TOTAL COST: Sum value of all inputs used to produce health care goods or services over a given time period, or the sum of all fixed and variable costs. Holding costs plus transaction costs.

TOTAL DEMAND: All health care output buyers or purchasers, including all patients, third parties, or corporations.

TOTAL DIRECT AND OVERLAPPING DEBT: Total direct debt plus the issuer's applicable share of the total debt of all overlapping jurisdictions.

TOTAL EXPENDITURE: The number of purchased units of health care product over a given time period, multiplied by the price of the product, equals the total revenue to sellers.

TOTAL FIXED COST: The cost of all health care entity fixed inputs. Total fixed costs are not usually affected by changes in activity (i.e., clinic rent, taxes, insurance, depreciation, salaries of employees, and key personnel). Rent is still due even if no patients are seen. A fixed cost remains constant, over the relevant range, even if the activity changes (i.e., busy summer or winter slow down). However, fixed costs decrease per unit as the activity level rises and increase per unit as the activity level falls.

TOTAL MARGIN: A measure that compares total hospital revenue and expenses for inpatient, outpatient, and nonpatient care activities. Total margin may be calculated by subtracting total expenses from total revenue, and dividing by total revenue.

TOTAL MARKET VALUE: Total number of shares outstanding, multiplied by price per share.

TOTAL PRODUCT: All the aggregate output of a health care product, good, or service.

TOTAL RETURN: Measure of performance that includes capital appreciation (or depreciation) and reinvestment of dividends.

TOTAL RETURN CONCEPT: Income determining philosophy that includes interests, dividends, and capital appreciation.

TOTAL REVENUE: Medical service price multiplied by medical service or product quantity.

TOTAL SUPPLY: All the aggregate sellers, medical providers, or producers of a health care product, good, or service.

TOTAL SURPLUS: The sum of medical provider and patient health care service/product surplus.

TOTAL TREATMENT COSTS: (Patient Quantity in FFS plan) $\times$ (FFS costs/FFS enrollees) + (Patient Quantity in MCO or HMO, etc.) $\times$ (MCO or HMO Costs/MCO or HMO quantity enrollees). Health care system aggregate.

TOTAL UTILITY: Total satisfaction received by a patient from the use of health care products and services. It's enjoyment from health care consumption.

TOTAL VARIABLE COST: The price of variable health care inputs. Total variable cost increases and decreases in proportion to activity, while per-unit variable costs remain constant per unit.

TOUT: To promote a specific security or company.

TRACE: The accounting ability to assign a cost or expense to a particular cost object (heart surgery for patient X).

TRADE: To purchase or sell goods, products, securities, and/or services, and so forth. It's the process of a transaction exchange.

TRADE CREDIT: Credit gained from the purchase of products or services.

TRADE CURB: Temporary suspension of trading activities. A halt.

TRADE DATE: The actual date on which securities are purchased or sold.

TRADE DISCOUNT: Price reduction for the purchase of products or services.

TRADER: One who frequently sells and buys securities.

TRANCH: A multiclass security (French term). A slice.

TRANSACTION: Recordable event that affects the financial position of a company.

TRANSACTION COSTS: All fees such as brokerage commissions or mutual fund fees, that are charged when acquiring or selling financial or other assets. There are three types:

- research costs (locating information about opportunities for exchange)
- negotiation costs (negotiating the terms of the exchange)
- enforcement costs (enforcing contracts)

TRANSACTIONS DEMAND: Money need is positively related to income and negatively related to the interest rate.

TRANSACTIONS NOTE: A short-term and unsecured loan, for a specific transaction or event.

TRANSFER AGENT: An agent responsible for the registration of security share-owner names on the company records and the proper re-registration of new owners, when a transfer of stock occurs.

TRANSFER PAYMENT: A payment (transfer of money) from one group to another without use of any physical resource.

TRANSIT FLOAT: Elapsed time between check deposit and funds availability.

TRANSPARENCY: Presentation or announcement of positions. In portfolio and risk management it focuses on positions and the associated risk profiles.

TREASURER: Corporate official responsible for receipt, custody, release, and reporting of funds and securities market maintenance.

TREASURY BOND OPTION: An option representing the right to buy (call) or sell (put) $100,000 principal amount of each specific bond listed.

TREASURY SECURITIES: Treasury securities are issued by the federal government and are available in several types:

- Treasury Bills: Purchased at a discount from face value, treasury bills are sold in a minimum increment of $10,000, with multiples of $5,000 available above the minimum. Treasury bills are auctioned to the highest bidder, so the interest is not a set amount. Rather, it varies, depending on how high the bid. Treasury bills can be purchased through a commercial bank, a brokerage firm, or any Federal Reserve Bank.
- Treasury Bonds: Issued in denominations of $1,000 to $1,000,000 or more, treasury bonds mature in 11 to 30 years. Both notes and bonds may be purchased through commercial banks and brokerage firms or directly from the Federal Reserve Bank. Bills, notes, and bonds are very liquid and

can be readily sold. Bond funds have minimum investment requirements, which vary according to the fund's parameters. In 2001, 30-year Treasury bonds were discontinued, but they were reinstituted on February 9, 2006.

- Treasury Notes: Treasury notes mature in 2 to 10 years and interest is paid semiannually. Longer-maturing notes are sold in lots of $1,000 to $100,000 or more (see Figure 7).

TREASURY STOCK: Shares of stock reacquired by the corporation through purchase or donation, that are not used for dividend, voting, or earnings calculation purposes.

TREND: Financial pattern or direction. It may be an up or down movement, bullish or bearish.

TREYNOR INDEX: A risk-adjusted measure of financial performance that correlates with the return-in-excess of the risk-free rate of return, by a portfolio's systemic risk of the market.

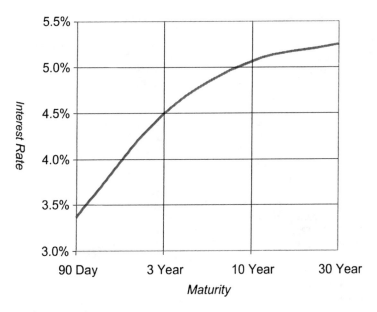

Figure 7: U.S. Treasury Yield.

TREYNOR, JACK, RATIO: Securities returns above or below the securities market line (SML), calculated as:

$$T = \frac{R_p - R_f}{\beta_p}$$

The ratio measures the excess return achieved over the risk free return per unit of systematic risk as identified by beta to the market portfolio. In practice, the Treynor ratio is often calculated using the T-Bill return for the risk-free return and the S&P 500 for a market basket portfolio.

TRIAL BALANCE: A low output point in the business cycle.

TRIN: A measurement of stock market strength using advance/decline ratios and volumes.

TRIPLE WITCH: Simultaneous expiration date for options, index options, and futures contracts. It is usually the third Friday in March, June, September, and December.

TROUGH: To bottom out, as in securities price level or business cycle.

TRUE INTEREST COST (TIC): Also known as Canadian Interest Cost. Under this method of computing borrowing costs, the interest cost is defined as the rate, compounded semiannually, necessary to discount the amount payable on the respective principal and interest payment dates to the purchase price received for the new issue of securities. TIC computations produce a figure slightly different from the net interest cost (NIC) method because TIC considers the time value of money (TVM), while NIC does not.

TRUST: A legal arrangement whereby control over property or funds is transferred to a trustee (a person or an organization) for the benefit of a designated person (the beneficiary). Trusts are created for a variety of reasons, including tax savings and improved asset management.

TRUST RECEIPT: A certification that the borrower holds goods in trust for a lender.

TRUSTEE: An appointed person or organization that manages the contents of a trust. It is the commercial banking institution charged with upholding the terms and conditions of a bond's indenture.

TRUSTOR: The creator of a trust, the person who transfers assets to a trust, or a person who encumbers his or her interest in real property by a transfer to a trustee under a deed of trust.

TRUTH IN LENDING ACT: A federal law requiring a disclosure of credit terms using a standard format (also known as Regulation Z). This is intended to facilitate comparisons between the lending terms of different financial institutions.

TURKEY: Slang term for a poor investment.

TURNAROUND: Positive reversal in the performance of a company.

TURNOVER: Quantity in a given time period that an item is represented by another exact or similar item.

TVERSKY, AMOS, PhD (d. 1996): Together with Daniel Kahnman, PhD, Tversky formulated the economic concept of *prospect theory* as an alternative that better accounts for observed behavior. He also discovered how human judgment may take heuristic shortcuts that systematically depart from basic principles of probability and finance.

TWENTY-BOND INDEX: General tracking index of 20 municipal bonds, 20-year maturities, with equivalent credit ratings.

TWENTY-DAY COOLING OFF PERIOD: A period of 20 calendar days following the filing of a registration statement with the SEC, during which the SEC examines the statement for deficiencies, the issuing corporation negotiates with an underwriting syndicate for a final agreement, and the syndicate prepares for the successful distribution of the impending issue. The final day of the period is normally considered the effective date, unless otherwise stated by the SEC.

TWISTING: Inducing the termination of a health or life insurance policy in order to purchase a new one, and/or the rapid turnover of securities to generate sales commissions for the agent or broker.

TWO-SIDED MARKET: A market with firm *bid* and *ask* prices, and often requiring a specialist to maintain a fair and orderly market.

TWO-TAIL TEST: A statistical test that evaluates both extreme sides, or tails, of a probability distribution. It considers both high rates of return and high rates of loss.

TYPE OF OPTION: Designation to distinguish between a put and a call option.

U

U: The commodity futures symbol for a September delivery month.

U4: Uniform Application for Securities Industry Registration or Transfer.

U5: Uniform Termination Notice for Securities Industry Registration.

UB-92 UNIFORM BILL 1992: Bill form used to submit hospital insurance claims for payment by third parties. Similar to HCFA (CMS) 1450 and 1500, but reserved for the inpatient component of health services.

UCR (USUAL, CUSTOMARY, AND REASONABLE) REDUCTION SAVINGS: The dollar amount or economic differential saved between the actual medical charges submitted for patient care and the allowed charges according to some proscribed payment schedule.

ULTIMATE NET LOSS: The total sum that a health care company becomes legally obligated to pay, such as legal, labor, and fringe benefits, operational costs, and so forth.

ULTRA-VIRES: Latin phrase meaning corporate actions unauthorized by its charter.

UNACCRUED: Most often describes income resulting from health care or other business payments received but not yet due.

UNALLOCATED BENEFIT: A reimbursement provision in health insurance policies, usually for miscellaneous hospital and medical expenses, that does not specify how much will be paid for each type of treatment, examination, or the like, but only sets a maximum that will be paid for all such treatments.

UNALLOCATED CLAIM EXPENSE: Expenses of loss adjustment that a health insurance company or other company incurs but cannot charge specifically to any single claim, such as claim department salaries and office overhead.

UNAUDITED FINANCIAL STATEMENTS: Financials that have not undergone a detailed examination by an independent CPA.

UNBUNDLED: Itemizing or fragmenting each component of a medical or health care service or procedure separately. This can often result in higher overall costs.

UNCERTAINTY: Financial or economic risk or volatility. A situation of unknown outcomes and their associated probabilities.

UNCOLLECTIBLE ACCOUNTS: Accounts and accounts receivable that will not be paid or satisfied in full.

UNCOLLECTIBLE ACCOUNTS EXPENSE: The cost to a seller of extending credit in ARs terms.

UNCOLLECTED FUNDS: Funds that have been deposited in an account or cashed against an account by a check that has not yet been cleared through the check collection process and paid by the drawee bank. Temporary holds are sometimes placed on their customer's uncollected funds. Funds are unavailable for withdrawal until the time period the hold expires.

UNCOMPENSATED CARE: Care rendered by hospitals or other medical providers without payment from the patient or a government-sponsored or private insurance program. It includes both charity care, which is provided without the expectation of payment, and bad debts, for which the provider has made an unsuccessful effort to collect payment due from the patient.

UNCOVERED CALL WRITER: A call writer is uncovered (naked) when that writer does not hold a long call of the same security class, with an equal or lower exercise price, or does not own an equivalent number of securities shares to the short position.

UNCOVERED EXPENSE: A cost incurred by the patient that his or her insurance policy or HMO contract does not cover, and was unknown previously.

UNCOVERED OPTION: A short securities option position that is not fully collateralized if notification of assignment should be received. A short call position is uncovered if the writer does not have a long stock position to deliver. A short put position is uncovered if the writer does not have the financial resources available in his or her account to buy the stock.

UNCOVERED PUT WRITER: A put writer is uncovered (naked) when that writer does not hold a long put of the same securities class, with an equal or higher exercise price.

UNDERCAPITALIZED: A health care or other firm with inadequate equity or debt financing for operations.

UNDERLYING MARKET PRICE: Price of a benchmark or index. For example, if a security had a call strike price of $110 and was trading at $107, the underlying market price would be $107 and that call would be $3 out-of-the-money.

UNDERLYING SECURITY: The security underlying an option contract against which a call or put is traded.

UNDERMARGINED ACCOUNT: A credit (margined) securities brokerage account that has fallen below minimum equity reserve requirements.

UNDERVALUED: Securities selling at a low fair market value price, usually below liquidation value levels.

UNDERWATER: Slang term for an investment that is losing money.

UNDERWRITER: A middleman between a securities company issuer and the public. There is usually an underwriting syndicate to limit risk and commitment of capital. There may also be contracts with selling groups to help distribute the issue for a concession. In the case of mutual funds, underwriters may also be known as a sponsor or distributor. Investment bankers also offer other services, such as advice and counsel on the raising and investment of capital. *See also* investment banker.

UNDERWRITER'S RETENTION: The percentage of a total securities issue to which each member of a securities syndicate is entitled and which is distributed to customers.

UNDERWRITER'S SYNDICATE: A group of investment bankers and firms that tout and/or sell various securities.

UNDERWRITING AGREEMENT: The contract between an investment banker and a corporate health care or other issuer, containing the final terms and prices of the issue. It is normally signed either on the evening before or early in the morning of the initial public offering date (effective date).

UNDERWRITING COMPENSATION (SPREAD): The profit realized by a securities underwriter that is equal to the difference between the price he paid to the issuer and the retail price of the public offering.

UNDERWRITING PERIOD: The period of time the underwriting process is considered to be continuing, and during which certain requirements of Municipal Securities Rule Board regulation are applicable. MSRB rules define the underwriting period as commencing at the time of the first submission to the underwriter(s) of an order for the new issue securities or the purchase of the new issue from the issuer, whichever occurs first, and ending at the time of the delivery of the securities to the underwriter(s) by the issuer or the sale of the last of the security by the underwriter(s), whichever occurs last.

UNDERWRITING PROFIT (OR LOSS): The profit (or loss) received from insurance or reinsurance premiums, as contrasted to that realized from investments. Also, the excess of premiums over claims paid and expenses (profit), or the excesses of claims paid and expenses over premiums (loss).

UNDIGESTED SECURITIES: Newly issued securities that remain unsold because of poor demand.

UNDIVIDED ACCOUNT (EASTERN ACCOUNT): A method for determining liability stated in a securities underwriting agreement in which each member of the underwriting syndicate is liable for any unsold portion of a securities issue according to each member's percentage participation in the syndicate.

UNEARNED INCOME/REVENUE: An individual's income derived from investments, as opposed to salary or wages.

UNENCUMBERED: Assets free of legal claims or liens.

UNFAVORABLE VARIANCE: When actual revenues and expenses are lower and higher than expected.

UNFUNDED PENSION PLAN: A traditional legacy defined benefit plan (DBP) for retirement that is not fully funded by its sponsoring corporation. It may be partially reinsured by the Pension Benefit Guarantee Corporation (PBGC).

UNI (INDIVIDUAL-K, SOLO- SINGLE-K™) 401(K) PLAN: An effective way for a single owner business to maximize retirement savings with tax-deductible, tax-deferred savings of up to $40,000+ a year as a result of tax law changes effective January 1, 2002. The plan combines the employee contribution of a 401(k) and the employer contribution of a profit sharing plan. The employee was able to contribute up to $14,000 in 2005 through salary deferral, although it may not exceed 100% of pay. The employer profit sharing contribution limit was up to 25% of pay, or 20% for self-employed. There is a total contribution limit, from both sources, of $42,000 in 2005, but only income up to $210,000 can be considered. However, under a catch up provision, individual's age 50+ may contribute an additional $4,000 in salary deferrals beyond the $14,000, allowing for a total contribution limit of $46,000 in 2005. A spouse is eligible to open an Individual(k) account provided a separate income is covered in the plan.

UNIFIED ESTATE AND GIFT TAX: A tax levied on an heir's inherited portion of an estate if the value of the estate exceeds an exclusion limit set by law. This estate tax is mostly imposed on assets left to heirs, but it does not apply to the transfer of assets to a surviving spouse. The right of spouses to leave any amount to one another is known as the unlimited marital deduction. States may also have similar taxes.

UNIFIED ESTATE AND GIFT TAX CREDIT: For Gift Tax Purposes in 2006, 2007, and 2008 the Unified Credit is $345,800, and the Applicable Exclusion Amount is $1,000,000. For Estate Tax Purposes in 2006, 2007, and 2008 the Unified Credit is $780,800, and the Applicable Exclusion Amount is $2,000,000. For Gift Tax Purposes in year 2009 the Unified Credit is $345,800, and the Applicable Exclusion Amount is $1,000,000. For Estate Tax Purposes in year 2009 the Unified Credit is $1,455,800, and the Applicable Exclusion Amount is $3,500,000. It is indexed through 2010–2011.

UNIFORM ACCOUNTANCY ACT (UAA): Framework for public accounting that was developed by the American Institute of Certified Public Accountants (AICPA) and the National Association of State Boards of Accountancy (NASBA) and is intended to enhance interstate reciprocity and practice across state lines by CPAs, meet the future needs of the profession, respond to the marketplace, and protect the public that the profession serves.

UNIFORM BILLING CODE OF 1982: See health care claim form; UB-82.

UNIFORM BILLING CODE OF 1992: See health care claim form; UB-92.

UNIFORM CAPITALIZATION RULES: Comprehensive set of rules to govern the capitalization, or inclusion in inventory and DME of direct and indirect cost of producing, acquiring, and holding property. Taxpayers are required to capitalize the direct costs and an allocable portion of the indirect costs attributable to real and tangible personal property produced or acquired for resale. Entities may not take current deductions for these costs but must be recovered through amortization or depreciation.

UNIFORM CLAIM FORM: All insurers and self-insurers would be required to use a single claim form and standardized format for electronic claims.

UNIFORM CLAIM TASK FORCE: An organization that developed the initial HCFA-1500 Professional Claim Form. The National Uniform Claim Committee later assumed the maintenance responsibilities.

UNIFORM GIFT/TRANSFER TO MINORS ACT (UGMA/UTMA): Securities or gift/transfers to a minor held in a custodial account and managed by an adult for the benefit of the minor.

UNIFORM COMMERCIAL CODE (UCC): A mostly state-wide, not federal, legal codification of commerce involving tangible and intangible business transactions.

UNIFORM PRACTICE CODE (UPC): A code established and maintained by the National Association of Securities Dealers (NASD) Board of Governors that regulates the mechanics of executing and completing securities transactions in the OTC market between members.

UNIFORM PRACTICE COMMITTEE: A National Association of Securities Dealers district subcommittee that disseminates information and interpretations landed down by the Board of Governors regarding the Uniform Practice Code (UPC).

UNISSUED STOCK: That portion of authorized stock not distributed (sold) to investors by a newly chartered corporation.

UNIT: A bundled securities or other position.

UNIT COST RISK POOL: A health care provider or medical facility bonus plan based on care utilization and efficiency, among other parameters, in isolation and the aggregate.

UNIT ELASTIC DEMAND: An elasticity of health care demand of one. It is the quantity of health care demanded and its price change in equal proportions. Price when the elasticity of health care demand equals one unit.

UNIT ELASTIC SUPPLY: Price when the elasticity of health care supply equals one unit.

UNIT ELASTICITY: Occurs when the health care elasticity co-efficient equals one, or the percentage change in health care quantity equals the percentage change in price.

UNIT INVESTMENT TRUST (UIT): Redeemable shares of a professionally selected and fixed portfolio of securities.

UNIT LABOR COSTS: Human resource costs per unit of health care output.

UNIT OF BENEFICIAL INTEREST (UBI): Shares of a Unit Investment Trust (UIT).

UNIT OF TRADING: The usual number of shares for a given securities financial transaction.

UNIT SHARE INVESTMENT TRUST (USIT): One *prime* and one *score* portion of a Unit Investment Trust (UIT).

UNITED STATES PER CAPITA COSTS: Per person (*capitus*-head) national Medicare average expense, per enrollee.

UNLIMITED PERSONAL LIABILITY: The use of personal, noncorporate assets, to satisfy a debt or other liability.

UNLISTED PROCEDURE: Medical description used when a procedure is not adequately described by an existing CPT code for reimbursement.

UNLISTED SECURITIES: Securities not formally listed on a securities exchange.

UNPAID DIVIDEND: A dividend of a corporation that has been declared but not distributed to shareholders.

UNQUALIFIED OPINION: Accounting and/or audit opinion not qualified for any material scope restrictions or departures from GAAP. The reviewer may issue an unqualified opinion only when there are no identified material weaknesses and when there have been no restrictions on the scope of the auditor's work. Clean option.

UNREALIZED APPRECIATION/DEPRECIATION: The amount by which the market value of portfolio securities or other holdings on a given date exceeds or falls short of their cost basis.

UNREALIZED GAIN OR LOSS: A gain or loss on paper that is not realized until an asset, security, or investment is sold.

UNRELATED BUSINESS INCOME: Income not related to the primary mission of a firm, entity, or corporation.

UNRESTRICTED FUNDS: Monetary resources of a not-for-profit entity, such as a medical center, clinic or public hospital, that has no fund restrictions as to use or purpose.

UNSECURED: A credit instrument or low priority of claim against a borrower.

UNSECURED CLAIM: A short-term loan that is not secured or only partially-backed by assets or collateral, such as credit card debt.

UNSECURED LOAN/BOND: A short-term or long-term loan that is not backed by assets or collateral.

UNSPECIFIED: ICD-9-CM term requesting additional medical payment information. The fourth digit is always 9. Fourth numbers 0–7 identify main trunk of specific medical condition. Fourth digit number 8 claimed for identifying other information.

UNSYSTEMATIC RISK: The business risk associated with individual securities rather than the whole marketplace (systematic or systemic risk).

UNWIND: To reverse a securities position.

UPCODING: Billing and code manipulation for increased reimbursement.

UPGRADE: An increase in the quality rating of a security, especially bonds. The raising, increase, or positive change in a health care or other company's credit rating.

UPSET PRICE: A seller's rock bottom and minimum auction price bid for securities.

UPSTAIRS MARKET: A securities transaction completed without the intermediation of a formalized stock exchange.

UPTICK: A positive change in price after a sequence of flat or down changes.

USEFUL LIFE: Physical assets that break down, deteriorate, or can be used up according to some predictable time period.

USUAL, CUSTOMARY, AND REASONABLE (UCR): Health insurance plans pay a physician's full charge if it is reasonable and does not exceed his or her usual charges and the amount customarily charged for the service by other physicians in the area.

USURY: Excess rate of interest over the legal rate charged to a borrower for use of money. Each state has its own definition of the exact rate and conditions that result in usury.

UTILITARIANISM: Moral philosophy holding the principle that the utility can be measured and summed over people and that utility comparisons between people are meaningful. Promotes universal health care.

UTILITY: Satisfaction patient-consumers receive from the health care or other products, goods, or services they acquire.

UTILITY THEORY: The relationship between money, risks, and happiness.

UTILIZATION: Amount of a health care resource divided by the amount available for use by patients.

UTILIZATION REVIEW (UR): Medical case evaluation for appropriateness of care, venue, timeliness, and other factors. Impacting clinical care and reimbursement.

V

V: The commodity futures symbol that represents an October delivery month.

V-CODE: Descriptors of patient health status and justification for medical encounters other than disease or injury already classified in the ICD-9-CM codes, for reimbursement.

VALUATION: Appraisal, as of a medical practice or clinic, as indicated by a *Statement of Fair Market Value*. Worth. It is the formal process of determining the worth of a health care or other business entity at a specific point in time, and the act or process of determining fair market value, often used as synonymous with appraisal. It is also a procedure whereby a securities certificate or coupon that has been torn or otherwise damaged (mutilated) is endorsed as being a valid or binding obligation of the issuer. Validation of damaged certificates is normally done by the issuer or its agent (e.g., the paying agent, trustee, registrar, or transfer agent). Validation of damaged coupons can also be done by a commercial bank.

VALUATION ALLOWANCE: Lowering or raising fair market current value by adjusting its acquisition cost to reflect its market value by use of a contra-account.

VALUATION APPROACH: A general method of business value determination using one or more conventional economic methods.

VALUATION DATE: The specific point in time when an *Opinion of Value* is given.

VALUATION METHOD: A specific method to determine health care or other business entity value.

VALUATION PERIOD: A period of years that is considered as a unit for purposes of calculating the status of a medical trust fund.

VALUATION SALES TERMS (MEDICAL PRACTICE):

- The *asking sale price* is often arbitrary, difficult to substantiate, and typically cut by as much as half during negotiations.
- The *realistic sale price* is one that both buyer and seller believe is fair.

- The *friendly sale price* is usually used for associates, partners, or other colleagues.
- The *creative sale price* is derived from creative financing, such as when a medical practice provides the down payment.
- The *emotional sale price* is either an inflated price paid by a motivated buyer or a depressed price accepted by a motivated physician seller.
- The *fair market sales value* is the standard used by most appraisers to derive a reasonable value for a medical practice.
- The *business enterprise sale* of a practice equals a combination of all assets (tangible and intangible) and the working capital of a continuing medical practice business.
- The value of *owner's sale equity* is the combined values of all practice assets (tangible and intangible), minus all practice liabilities (booked and contingent).

VALUE: The worth of anything, often expressed in terms of money, but not necessarily so. It indicates the present worth of all the rights to future benefits arising from ownership of the thing valued.

VALUE ADDED: The extra worth that a health care or other entity adds to intermediate products, goods, or services and is measured by the difference between the initial and later market value. It is a measure of incremental health care production or output.

VALUE ADDED TAX: A use or consumption surcharge. A levy.

VALUE CHAIN: The sequence of activities that add value to a health care firm's products, goods, or services.

VALUE CREATION: Net Present Value (NPV).

VALUE FUNDS: Mutual or hedge funds that invest in undervalued health care or other companies. These companies may temporarily exhibit lower-than-average ratios, such as price/earnings, price/sales, or book value.

VALUE HEALTH CARE PURCHASING: The bulk purchases of medical supplies, equipment, goods, or services in order to harvest economy of scale (bulk) cost savings.

VALUE INVESTING: A style of investing that searches for undervalued companies and buys their stock in hopes of sharing in the future gain when other analysts discover the company. It is the act of focusing on stocks selling at low prices relative to their assets, sales, and earnings. It is the opposite of growth investing.

VALUE STOCKS: Stocks that are considered to be inexpensive based on measures relative to their market value, such as current earnings or total assets. Often, these stocks are considered out of favor or undervalued by the market for some reason. It is the opposite of overvalued. It is trading below historic value.

VARIABLE: A dollar amount or quantity that can have more than a single value.

VARIABLE ANNUITY: A tax-deferred contract issued by an insurance company that offers a choice of investment options, allowing purchasers to choose from a number of subaccounts with various investment objectives. Variable annuities can offer diversification, flexibility, and estate benefits, and they are often used as a supplement to 401(k) and IRA plans, because contribution limits are much less restrictive.

VARIABLE BUDGET: A flexible budget.

VARIABLE CAPITATION: Incentive payment mechanism for health care providers and facilities using a corridor, such as 80–135% of estimated PM/PM fixed-fees, based on utilization costs with adjustments and other clinical quality measurements.

VARIABLE COST: Medical or health care services expense that remains the same per unit, but changes with variations in activity over the relevant range. Total variable costs increase and/or decrease in proportion to activity, while per-unit variable costs remain constant per unit. A variable cost changes in total in direct proportion to changes in the level of activity, but is constant on a per-unit basis. Clinic costs that are normally variable with respect to volume include: durable medical equipment (DME), indirect labor, and indirect materials such as utilities, air conditioning, clerical costs, and other medical supplies. Generally, variable costs change as a direct result of making a decision or altering a course of action.

VARIABLE INPUT: Those health care inputs whose quantity used may be varied in the short run.

VARIABLE INTEREST RATE BOND: Usually a long-term bond whose interest rate changes with shorter term interest rate fluctuations.

VARIABLE LABOR BUDGET: Labor expense projection that changes over time with overtime and work outages.

VARIABLE RATE: An interest rate that changes periodically in relation to an index. Payments may increase or decrease accordingly.

VARIABLE RATE LOAN: Debt whose interest rate changes over its life in relation to the level of an index.

VARIABLE RESOURCE: Any health care resource quantity that can be decreased or increased.

VARIANCE: The differences obtained from subtracting actual results from expected or budgeted results. It is a precursor to the standard deviation, or the square of the standard deviation, and is calculated by:

- computing the mean of the series,
- then taking the deviation or subtracting the mean from each observation,
- square the differences or deviations for each observation, and

- divide the sum of the squared deviations by the number of observations.

Note: The standard deviation is calculated by taking the square root of the variance.

VARIANCE ANALYSIS: Research into, and the study of, the differences between planned health care input quantities and actual output quantities.

VARIATION CALL: Issued when a margin account maintenance level is violated in order to obtain cash or securities equal to an amount to restore an account to the initial margin level.

VEGA: Change in an option given a change in volatility that measures the instantaneous change in premium to the instantaneous change in volatility. In reality, it is viewed as the change in premium given a 1% change in volatility. It is a letter of the Greek alphabet.

VEGA MODEL: A type of pricing model for derivatives.

VEGA RISK: Monetary exposure for a change in volatility for an option. For example, it might refer to a change from 6% to 7% or 6% to 5% depending on whether a party is short or long the option.

VELOCITY OF MONEY: The rate at which the money supply is used to make transactions for final goods and services.

VENTURE CAPITAL: Private capital supplied for a risky start-up business, usually in return for an equity share of the corporation.

VERIFIABILITY: To confirm, certify, or endorse.

VERMEER, THOMAS E., PhD, CPA: Treasurer for the International Society for Research in Healthcare Financial Management, Towson, Maryland.

VERTICAL ANALYSIS: A method of financial statement analysis that compares line item percentages rather than absolute amounts.

VERTICAL INTEGRATION: A health care entity that owns hospitals, clinics, medical practices, and/or the DME vendors used in various stages of patient care. It is down-line integration.

VERTICAL MERGER: The union of a health care entity with an input supplier.

VESTING: A timing schedule for when pension benefits come irrevocably due. It is the time at which certain benefits available to an employee are no longer contingent on the employee continuing to work for the employer.

VIRTUAL CORPORATION: Firms that conserve cash and limit financial risk by owning few assets and hiring few employees, such as internet-based or electronic health care firms.

VISIBLE SUPPLY: The total dollar volume of bond or debt-based securities offered over the next 30 days. The visible supply, which is compiled and published by *The Bond Buyer*, indicates the near-term activity in the municipal market.

VOLATILITY: A measure of the variability of security returns. Conventionally, volatility is defined as the annualized standard deviation of the logarithms of the asset's returns. An important aspect of volatility is that it measures the variability of returns and not the deviation.

VOLUME: The quantity or number of securities traded over a given timeperiod, or the number of medical goods or services. It is the quantity provided.

VOLUME OFFSET: Change in health care utilization service-mix based on a change in volume.

VOLUNTARY ACCUMULATION PLAN: An informal mutual fund investment program allowing a customer to arrange purchases in frequency and numbers of dollars at his own choosing, yet providing benefits normally available only to larger investors. Sales charge percentage requirements are constant throughout the life of the plan and, therefore, the plan is sometimes called a Level Charge Plan.

VON NEUMANN-MORGENSTERN: A utility function that has the expected utility property (i.e., patients become indifferent between receiving the same given bundle of health care services or gambling with the same future expected value of services).

VOTING CONTROL: The de facto control of a business, corporation, or health care enterprise.

VOTING RIGHT: Privilege attributed to most common stocks that allows a pro-rate input into corporate decision making.

VOUCHER: A document or receipt that authorizes a cash or asset disbursement. It is part of a managed care incentive program for patients to use cost efficient medical providers and health care facilities.

VOUCHER REGISTER: A list or record of payment vouchers.

VOUCHER SYSTEM: Use of vouchers for payment of goods, products, and services.

VULTURE CAPITALIST: Slang term for one who provides private capital for a risky start-up business, usually in return for a very large equity slice (ownership) of the corporation.

VULTURE FUND: A fund of depressed or below market rate securities or other assets.

W

WACHTER, ROBERT M., MD: Physician and health care economist from the University of California at San Francisco, who coined the term *hospitalist*.

WADE, RICHARD: Senior Vice President of Strategic Communications at the American Hospital Association in Chicago, Illinois.

WAGE: The price paid for human resources and labor.

WAGE BASE: The amount of gross earnings (employee) and or net earnings from self-employment (self-employed) to which FICA (Federal Insurance Contributions Act) and/or SECA (Self-Employment Contributions Act) is applied. The wage base is inflation indexed and based on average total wages and generally announced in November of the preceding year. For example, highly-paid earners saw a moderate increase on which Social Security taxes were due in 2006. The 2006 wage base of $94,200 was $4,200 higher than the 2005 amount, and the maximum additional Social Security tax collected above the 2005 wage base was $260.40. It was the largest increase since 2002 and reflects the largest increase in national average wages since 2000. The 2006 wage base reflected national average wages for 2004, the variable upon which the 2006 wage base formula is based. The 2004 national average wage index of $35,648.55 was 4.65% higher than the 2003 national average wage index, also the highest increase since 2000.

WAGE BRACKET: The usual, customary, and reasonable competitive market salary of a health care worker, of a specific type.

WAGE CURVE: The relation between the local rate of health care labor unemployment on the horizontal axis, and the local wage rate on the vertical axis. It is downward sloping because locally high wages and locally low unemployment are correlated.

WAGE DIFFERENTIAL: Salary difference among various health care workers.

WAGE PUSH INFLATION: The inflation induced by higher human resource employment costs (wages).

WALKER, JONATHAN, PhD: Economist originally from the Massachusetts Institute of Technology, and now President of Economists Incorporated in California.

WALLPAPER: Worthless, or near worthless securities.

WALL STREET: Slang term for the financial district in Manhattan, New York.

WALRASIAN AUCTIONEER: Hypothetical market maker who matches medical suppliers and patient demanders to get a single price for a health care good or service. A broker.

WANTS: The unlimited desire for health care products or services.

WARDEN, GAIL: President and CEO of Henry Ford Health System in Detroit, Michigan. Warden is also a former chairman of the American Hospital Association in Chicago, Illinois.

WARRANT: Certificates that allow the holder to buy a security at a set price, either within a certain time period or in perpetuity. Warrants are usually issued for common stock, at a higher price than current market price, in conjunction with bonds or preferred stock as an added inducement to buy. It is an inducement attached to new securities, giving the purchaser a long-term (usually 5 to 10 years) privilege of subscribing to one or more shares of stock reserved for him by the corporation from its unmissed or treasure stock reserve.

WASH SALE: When an investor sells a security at a loss, he can use that realized loss to offset a realized gain in order to reduce his tax liability on that gain. If the seller reacquires that or a substantially identical security within a 30-day period prior to or after the sale, he will lose the tax benefit of that realized loss.

WASTING ASSETS: Physical assets that can break down, deteriorate, or be used up.

WATERED STOCK: Equities in overvalued corporations.

WEAK DOLLAR: USD (U.S. Dollar) that has fallen in value against a foreign currency.

WEAK MARKET: Any market with declining prices and more sellers than buyers.

WEGMILLER, DONALD: President and CEO of Clark/Bardes Consulting Health Care Group in Minneapolis, Minnesota. He is also a former chairman of the American Hospital Association in Chicago, Illinois.

WEIGHTED AVERAGE COST OF CAPITAL (WACC): Mean cost of money determined by the percentage interest rate of cost of each class, in proportion to the total market value of an organization that each class represents. Proportional interest rate cost share.

WEIGHTED AVERAGE MATURITY: Average cost, interest rate, or data points based on the pro rata share of the data.

WEIGHTING: Assignment of more worth on a medical or health care fee based on the number of times it is charged (i.e., weighting the RBRVS fee for a procedure).

WELFARE LOSS: Slang term for net debit due to the misallocation of societal health care resources, or dead weight loss.

WENNBERG, JOHN, MD: Physician and health care economist who shocked the medical community in the 1970s when he compared disparate surgical rates among different counties, and in the 1980s when he proposed the need for physician incentives and cost reduction techniques. Currently, he is Director of the Center for Evaluative Clinical Sciences and the Peggy Y. Thomson Professor for the Evaluative Clinical Sciences at Dartmouth Medical School in Hanover, New Hampshire.

WESTERN ACCOUNT: A divided underwriting account.

WHEN, AS, AND IF ISSUED: A phrase used to describe the time period in the life of an issue of securities from the original date of the sale by the issuer to the delivery of the securities to, and payment by, the underwriter. Sales made during the *when, as, and if issued* period (also called the 'when-issued' period) are subject to receipt of the securities from the issuer by the underwriter in good form.

WHEN-ISSUED CONTRACT: A delivery contract involving securities (stocks or bonds) that have been proposed for distribution but not yet issued. The date of delivery is set for some time in the future by the National Association of Securities Dealers (NASD) Uniform Practice Committee (UPC) or the appropriate stock exchange, as the case may be.

WHIPSAWED: Slang term for the volatile up and down price movements of securities, markets, businesses, or assets.

WHISPER NUMBERS: Unofficial projected corporate earning estimates by Wall Street analysts. Wall Street financial performance gossip.

WHISPER STOCK: A company rumored to be an impending corporate take-over target.

WHITE KNIGHT: Slang term for a friendly investor sought to save a company from a hostile takeover.

WHITE MAIL: Below market stock sale to a friendly party. It is a corporate antitakeover method.

WHITE SHOE FIRM: A traditional, blue-blooded, and elite broker-dealer, legal, accounting, advisory, or investment banking firm. Upper crust.

WHITE SQUIRE: Slang term for a friendly (white knight) who acquires less than a majority interest in a company to thwart a hostile take-over attempt.

WIDE OPENING: A very large security spread.

WIDENING: An increased spread or price differential between an underlying cash market and the futures market.

WIDOW AND ORPHAN STOCK: A traditionally safe and secure stock that usually pays dividends.

WIENER PROCESS: A type of Markov Stochastic process that refers to changes in value over small time periods, as in Brownian motion. It is a slang term for a random walk.

WILDCARD: Unilateral choice of one party to a transaction.

WILENSKY, GAIL: Senior fellow of Project Hope in Millwood, Virginia. Wilensky is also a former HCFA administrator.

WILLIAMS, ALAN, PhD: Health care economist who suggested that all patients should be entitled to their "fair-innings" of life expectancy and good health.

WILLINGNESS TO PAY: The maximum amount of money that an individual is prepared to give up to ensure that a proposed health care measure is undertaken.

WILSHIRE INDEX: An equity stock index composed as a surrogate for 5,000 firms.

WINDFALL: A sudden and large profit.

WINDOW DRESSING: Portfolio manager year-end buying or selling for shareholder presentations.

WIRE HOUSE: A stockbrokerage firm, usually retail or boutique and/or national or regional in nature.

WIRE TRANSFER: An electronic transfer of funds from one financial institution to another. Wire transfers require the routing transit number, dollar amount, account number, and name of the account owner(s).

WITH RECOURSE: The legal ability to place a claim or a creditor.

WITHDRAWAL PLAN: Arrangement provided by many open-end mutual fund companies by which investors can receive monthly or quarterly payments in a designated amount, which may be more or less than actual investment income.

WITHHOLD: The portion of the monthly capitation payment to physicians withheld by the MCO or insurance plan until the end of the year or other time period to create an incentive for efficient care. The withhold is at risk, that is, if the physician exceeds utilization norms, he does not receive it. It serves as a financial incentive for lower utilization.

WITHHOLDING: Securities regulations require all hot issues be distributed to the public in insubstantial amounts. If the issue is not a hot issue, members of the industry can buy shares of the new issue and will be filled in the last priority. However, if the issue is hot, meaning the supply is insufficient to meet the public's demand, they cannot. If a member firm or representative tries to participate by reserving part of the new issue for themselves or other members they are guilty of withholding.

WITHHOLDING ALLOWANCE: A budgeted or estimated withholding amount. It is a taxpayer claim that exempts a certain amount of wages from being subject to withholding, and it is designed to prevent too much tax being withheld from a taxpayers wages. It may be obtained by completing form W-4 and submitting it to an employer.

WOLFE, SIDNEY, MD: Director of the Public Citizen's Health Research Group in Washington, D.C.

WORK: Conscientious industry and/or human physical or cognitive labor.

WORK IN PROGRESS: DME and inventory accounting consisting of partially completed goods awaiting completion and transfer to finished inventory.

WORK OUT: To cover a short or liquidate a long position. It is a return from bankruptcy. A troubled company taking measures to resurrect or restructure its financial and/or business operations.

WORK OUT MARKET: In the over-the-counter (OTC) market, a range of prices quoted by a market maker when he is not certain that there is an existing market available, but he feels he can "work one out" within a reasonable period of time.

WORK SHEET: Columnar document that assists in the movement of trial balances to financial statements.

WORKABLE: A bid price at which a dealer states its willingness to purchase securities from another dealer. A dealer soliciting a workable often is working to satisfy a customer's order to sell securities.

WORKING CAPITAL, NET: Current assets minus current liabilities.

WORKING CAPITAL CYCLE: The activities of a health care or other business entity that include:

- Securing cash;
- Turning cash into medical and other resources;
- Using resources for providing health care services; and
- Billing patients again to repeat the cycle.

WORKING CAPITAL RATIO: Ratio of short term assets to short term debt. Cash equivalent assets minus cash equivalent debts.

WORKING PAPERS: (1) Records kept by an auditor or accountant of the procedures applied, the tests performed, the information obtained, and the pertinent conclusions reached in the course of an audit or tax review. (2) Any records developed by a CPA, CVA, CMA, CFP©, CMA, or CMP© during an audit.

WORLD BANK: Many international organizations that aid countries in economic development with loans, advice, and research.

WRAP ACCOUNT: A discretionary brokerage securities account where all sales, administrative fees, and commissions are included in an annual percentage-based management fee. It is a separately managed account (SMA).

WRAP AROUND MORTGAGE: A second mortgage that expands the total amount of borrowing by a mortgagor without disturbing the original mortgage.

WRITE: To sell an option. An investor who sells an option is called the writer, regardless of whether the option is covered or uncovered.

WRITE DOWN: Net book value of corporate or business assets after depreciation and amortization expenses.

WRITE OFF: A bad debt expense. It consists of uncollected ARs.

WRITER OF AN OPTION: An investor who grants option privileges to a buyer in exchange for the premium.

X

X: The commodity futures symbol for a November delivery month.

X: A stock that is trading ex-dividend, ex-coupon, or ex-interest, or without its dividend, coupon, and/or interest payments.

X-INEFFICIENCY: Inability to produce a given health care output at the lowest average total cost possible.

X-TRADE (CROSS TRADE): A securities trade done in accordance with the rules and regulations of a particular exchange and other regulatory organizations. The letter X can indicate this type of transaction on a ticker tape, or be used on a stock ticket or blotter.

XR: A stock that is trading ex-rights, or without its terms and conditions (i.e., voting) or other rights.

XW: A stock that is trading ex-warrants, or without warrants as an enticement to buy a sweetener.

XX: Trading without warrants or securities.

XENOCURRENCY: Currency of foreign nations.

Y

Y: X-dividend and sale in full. Newspaper listing.

YANKEE BOND: American debt securities on the London Stock Exchange.

YARD: One billion units of a currency.

YARDSTICK COMPETITION: Pricing policy and benchmark based on average marginal health care costs in order to induce managed care cost cutting machinations.

YELLOW BOOK: Slang term for the Government Accounting Organization manual of standards for auditing the financial statements of entities receiving federal financial assistance. Yellow Book is the name given to *Government Auditing Standards* issued by the Comptroller General of the United States which contains standards for audits of government organizations, programs, activities and functions, and of government assistance received by contractors, nonprofit organizations such as medical clinics and hospitals, and other nongovernment organizations. It includes British stock exchange listing requirements.

YELLOW DOG CONTRACT: Agreement that health care workers not engage in collective labor union action.

YELLOW KNIGHT: Slang term for a corporate merger following a takeover attempt.

YELLOW SHEETS: Pink-sheet bid and ask OTC price listings for a market maker in corporate bonds.

YIELD (RATE OF RETURN): The dividends or interest paid by a company on its securities, expressed as percentage of the current price or of the price of original acquisition.

YIELD (7-DAY OR 30-DAY): The annualized current rate of mutual fund investment income calculated by a Securities and Exchange Commission formula that includes the fund's net income (based on the yield to maturity of each bond it holds), the average number of outstanding fund shares during the 7-day or 30-day period shown, and the maximum offering price per share on the last day of the period.

YIELD CURVE: Curvilinear relationship between time to maturity and yield, for a specific asset class. It is a graph that plots market yields on securities of equivalent quality but different maturities, at a given point in time. The vertical axis represents the yields, while the horizontal axis depicts time to maturity. The term structure of interest rates, as reflected by the yield curve, will vary according to market conditions, resulting in a variety of yield curve configurations:

- Normal or Positive Yield Curve—Indicates that short-term securities have a lower interest rate than long-term securities.
- Inverted or Negative Yield Curve—Reflects the situation of short-term rates exceeding long-term rates.
- Flat Yield Curve—Reflects the situation when short- and long-term rates are about the same.

YIELD SPREAD: Yield differential between different (bond) debt securities.

YIELD TO CALL: The rate of return to the investor earned from payments of bond (debt) principal and interest, with interest compounded semiannually at the stated yield, presuming that the security is redeemed prior to its stated maturity date. (If the security is redeemed at a premium call price, the amount of the premium is also reflected in the yield.)

YIELD TO CRASH: Debt yield to adjusted minimum maturity.

YIELD TO MATURITY: The yield earned on a bond from the time it is purchased until it is redeemed.

YIELD TO PUT: Bond return, if held, and sold to the issuing company on a specific date.

YOUNG, QUENTIN, MD: National Coordinator of the Physicians for a National Health Program in Chicago, Illinois.

YOUNIS, MUSTAFA Z., DrPH, MBA, MA: Executive committee member for the International Society for Research in Healthcare Financial Management, Towson, Maryland.

YO-YO STOCK: Slang term for an equity whose price fluctuates in an often wild manner.

Z

Z: Commodities future symbol for a December delivery month.

Z-ACCRUAL BOND: A security that has accretion characteristics and grows much like a zero coupon bond, however it is subject to prepayments or other events.

Z-CERTIFICATE: Bank of England short term certificate to facilitate transactions.

Z-R: Zero coupon security sold at a deep discount, without interest payments until maturity.

ZERHOUNI, ELIAS, MD: Director of the National Institute of Health in Bethesda, Maryland.

ZERIAL: Serial zero coupon bonds with optional maturity dates.

ZERO BASED BUDGETING: A budgeting method that requires accountability for the line item existence and funding needs of existing and new health or other services programs.

ZERO COST COLLAR: A transaction with little or zero cash outlay or cost. Often it is a security held as some protection is sought by a hedging transaction.

ZERO COUPON BOND: A bond that pays both principal and interest at maturity. These debt instruments pay interest only at maturity, as compared with semiannual interest payments on treasuries. Zero coupon bonds generate no coupon payments whatsoever throughout the life of the security. They are sold at a discount to the face value of the bond, and as the maturity date moves closer, the price of the bond will move toward par. Therefore, the investment return comes entirely from the price increase between the time of purchase and the maturity date (or redemption date, if it is sold prior to maturity). The coupon income is not reinvested and thus the potential income derived from reinvestment is not considered in valuing the zero's investment performance. Zero coupon bonds can be applied in a variety of ways:

- STRIPS are an acronym for Separate Trading of Registered Interest and Principal Securities. STRIPS consist of either the interest or principal on U.S. Treasury bonds. They are direct obligations of the U.S. government and are considered the safest and most liquid of all zero coupon bonds. They have maturities from 6 months to 30 years.
- CATS are an acronym for Certificates of Accrual on Treasury Securities. These are physical certificates representing cash flows of U.S. Treasury bonds that are held in a separate trust. Because CATS represent cash flows of treasury bonds, they are considered to be backed by the government. They have maturities from 1 to 22 years.

ZERO CURVE: A yield curve comprised of the yields of zero coupon bonds arranged over time. Frequently, this arrangement is graphically portrayed starting with the shortest maturities and progressing to the longest maturities.

ZERO MINUS TICK: A transaction on the Stock Exchange at a price equal to that of the preceding transaction but lower than the last different price.

ZERO PLUS TICK: A transaction on the Stock Exchange at a price equal to that of the preceding transaction but higher than the last different price.

ZERO PREMIUMS: Medicare managed care plans in which there is no extra premium payment for a member above the monthly Medicare Part B payment for all beneficiaries.

ZERO SUM GAME: A matching set of competitive winners and losers.

ZETA: A type of volatile derivative pricing model. Synonymous with vega, kappa, omega or sigma. It is a letter of the Greek alphabet.

ZOMBIES: Slang term for insolvent or bankrupt companies that are still in operation (i.e., dot com zombies).

Acronyms/Abbreviations

The limits of your language are the limits of your world.
—Ludwig Wittgenstein

A: Includes extras (in newspapers)
AA: Accumulation Account
AAA: American Academy of Actuaries
AAA: American Accounting Association
AAA: American Arbitration Association
AAAHC: Accreditation Association for Ambulatory Health Care
AACPD: Adjusted Average Charge Per Day
AACPD: Adjusted Average Charge Per Discharge
AACTQ: Abbreviated Account Query
AAD: At A Discount
AAE: Affirmative Action Employer
AAHAM: American Association of Health Care Administrative Management
AAHC: American Association of Health Care Consultants
AAHE: Association for the Advancement of Health Education
AAHP: American Association of Health Plans
AAI: Accredited Advisor in Insurance
AAI: Alliance of American Insurers
AAII: American Association of Individual Investors
AAIS: American Association of Insurance Services
AAL: Actuarial Accrued Liability
AAMA: American Academy of Medical Administration
AAMS: Accredit Asset Management Specialist
AAPC: American Academy of Professional Coders
AAPCC: Adjusted Annual Per Capita Cost
AAPCC: Adjusted Average Per Capita Cost
AAPP: American Association of Preferred Providers
AAR: After-hours Activity Report

AAR: Annual Average Rate
AARF: Additional Adjusted Reduction Factor
AB: Bachelor of Arts (latartium baccalaureus or artium baccalaureatus) degree
ABA: Accredited Business Accountant
ABA: Adjusted Blind Account
ABA: American Banker's Association
ABA: American Bar Association
ABA: American Business Accountant
ABC: Activity-Based Costing
ABCM: Activity-Based Cost Management
ABHES: Accrediting Bureau of Health Education Schools
ABLA: American Business Law Association
ABM: Activity-Based Management
ABN: Advanced Beneficiary Notice
ABO: Accumulation Benefit Obligation
ABS: Asset Backed Securities
ABS: Automated Bond System
ABT: American Board of Trade
ABV: Accredited in Business Valuation
ABVM: Adjusted Book Value Method
AC: Akaike's Criterion
AC: Appeals Council
AC: Account
AC: Average Cost
ACATS: Automated Customer Account Transfer Service
ACB: Account Cash Balance
ACC: Ambulatory Care Center
ACD: Alternate Care Determination
ACE: Aetna Claims Exchange
ACE: Adjusted Current Earnings
ACE: AMEX Commodities Exchange
ACE: Average Current Earnings
ACG: Adjusted Clinical Group
ACH: Automated Clearing House
ACHE: American College of Health Care Executives

387

ACI: Audit Controls Integrity
ACI: Average Cost of Illness
ACME: American College of Medical Executives
ACP: Accelerated Claims Process
ACP: Average Collection Period
ACPC: Average Cost Per Claim
ACPE: American College of Physician Executives
ACPPD: Average Charge Per Patient Day
ACPPD: Average Cost Per Patient Day
ACPS: Advanced Claims Processing System
ACR: Accelerated Cost Recovery
ACR: Adjusted Community Rating
ACRS: Accelerated Cost Recovery System
ACS: Ambulatory Care Services
ACS: Average Charge per Stay
ACT: Automated Confirmation Transaction
ACV: Actual Cash Value
AD: Admission and Discharge
AD: Admitting Diagnosis
AD: Advance-Decline Line
AD: Aggregate Demand
ADB: Adjusted Debt Balance
ADC: Average Daily Census
ADFS: Alternate Delivery and Financing System
ADP: Automatic Data Processing
ADPL: Average Daily Patient Load
ADPL-BAS: Average Daily Patient Load-Bassinet
ADPL-IP: Average Daily Patient Load-Inpatient
ADPL-T: Average Daily Patient Load-Total
ADR: Advance Decline Ratio
ADR: Asset Depreciation Range
ADR: Automatic Dividend Reinvestment
ADR/ADS: American Depository Receipt/Share
ADRG: Adjacent Diagnostic Related Group
ADRG: Adjusted Diagnostic Related Group
ADRG: Alternative Diagnostic Related Group

ADS: Advanced Detection System
ADS: Alternative Delivery System
ADSC: Average Daily Service Charge
ADT: Admission Discharge/Transfer
AE: Account Executive
AECHO: Aetna Electronic Claim Home Office
AEDC: American Economic Development Council
AEP: Accredited Estate Planner
AEP: Appropriates Evaluation Protocol
AES: Spanish Health Economics Association
AET: Annual Earnings Test
AEX: Amsterdam Exchange
AFC: Accredited Financial Counselor
AFC: Average Fixed Cost
AFDC: Aid to Families with Dependent Children
AFDS: Alternate Finance Delivery System
AFEHCT: Association for Electronic Health Care Transactions
AFS: Alternative Financing System
AFT: Automatic Funds Transfer
AG: Affiliated Group
AGI: Adjusted Gross Income
AGPA: American Group Practice Association
AGPAM: American Guild of Patient Account Managers
AH: Academy Health
AHA: American Hospital Association
AHCA: American Health Care Association
AHCPR: Agency for Health Care Policy and Research
AHES: Australian Health Economics Society
AHIA: Association of Health Insurance Agents
AHIMA: American Health Information Management Association
AHP: Accountable Health Plan
AHPA: American Health Planning Association
AHSR: Association for Health Services Research

AI: Accrued Interest

AIBD: Association of International Bond Dealers

AICPA: American Institute of Certified Public Accountants

AIM: Advanced Informatics in Medicine

AIM: American Institute of Management

AIME: Average Indexed Monthly Earnings

AIMR: Association for Investment Management and Research

AIP: Automatic Investment Program

AIR: Assumed Interest Rate

ALC: Alternate Level of Care

ALCO: Asset Liability Committee

ALM: Assets and Liability Management

ALOH: Average Length Of Hospitalization

ALOS: Average Length Of Stay

AM: Active Market

AM: After Market

AM: Allied Member

AMA: Asset Management Account

AMA: American Management Association

AMAA: Alliance of Merger & Acquisition Advisors

AMBAC: American Municipal Bond Assurance Corporation

AMCRA: American Managed Care Review Association

AMD: Aggregate Monetary Demand

AME: Average Monthly Earnings

AMEX: American Stock Exchange

AMGA: American Medical Group Association

AMI: Alternate Mortgage Instrument

AMIA: American Medical Informatics Association

AMLOS: Arithmetic Mean Length of Stay

AMOSS: Amex Options Switching System

AMP: Automated Medical Payment

AMP: Average Manufacturer's Price

AMPS: Auction Market Preferred Stock

AMT: Alternate Minimum Tax

AMW: Average Monthly Wage

AN: Account Number

ANSI: American National Standards Institute

AO: At Occupation

AOB: Assignment Of Benefits

AOC: Administrator On Call

AOC: Ambulatory Outpatient Center

AOD: Administrator On Duty

AOES: Automatic Order Entry System

AON: All Or None

AOS: Automated Order System

AOTP: Automated One Time Payment

AP: Accounts Payable

AP: Accumulation Period

AP: Accumulation Plan

AP: Additional Premium

AP: Administrative Proceedings

AP: Affiliated Person

AP: Associated Person

AP: Average Product

APB: Accounting Principles Board

APC: Ambulatory Patient Classification

APC: Ambulatory Payment Classification

APC: Amended Payroll Certification

APC: Average Propensity to Consume

APCC: Adjusted Per Capita Cost

APDRG: All Patient-Diagnostic Related Groups

APES: Portuguese Health Economics Association

APG: Ambulatory Patient Groups

APG: Ambulatory Payment Groups

APHA: American Public Health Association

APHP: Acute Partial Hospitalization Program

APPAM: Association for Public Policy Analysis and Management

APR: Adjusted Payment Rate

APR: Annual Percentage Rate

APR: Average Percent Rate

APR: Average Payment Rate

APR-DRG: All Patient Refined-Diagnostic Related Group

APS: Auction Preferred Stock

APS: Average Propensity to Save

APT: Admissions Per Thousand

APT: Arbitrage Pricing Theory

APT: Automated Pit Trading

APTC: Association of Publicly Traded Companies
APY: Annual Percentage Yield of Interest
AR: Accounts Receivable
AR: Acknowledged Receipt
AR: Annual Report
ARB: Arbitrager
ARI: Accounts Receivable Insurance
ARM: Adjustable Rate Mortgage
ARPS: Adjustable Rate Preferred Stock
ARR: Average Rate of Return
ART: Accredited Records Technician
ART: Accounts Receivable Turnover
AS: Accumulated Surplus
AS: Active Securities
AS: Administrative Simplification
AS: Admission Scheduling
AS: Aggregate Supply
AS: Assessable Stock
ASA: Accredited Senior Appraiser
ASA: American Society of Appraisers
ASA: Association of the Society of Actuaries
ASC: Administrative Services Contract
ASCS: Admission Scheduling and Control System
ASCII: American Standard Code for Information Interchange
ASCX12N: American Standard Committee standard for claims and reimbursement
ASE: American Stock Exchange
ASE: Amsterdam Stock Exchange
ASE: Athens Stock Exchange
ASHE: American Society of Health Economics
ASO: Administrative Services Only
ASR: Age, Sex, Rate
ASX: Australian Stock Exchange
ATA: Accredited Tax Advisor
ATB: Across the Board
ATC: Average Total Cost
ATCPC: Approximate Trade Credit Percentage Cost
ATM: Automated Teller Machine
ATP: Accredited Tax Planner
ATP: Arbitrage Trading Program

ATR: Acid Test Ratio
AUM: Assets Under Management
AUR: Ambulatory Utilization Review
AV: Actual Value
AVA: Accredited Valuation Analyst
AVC: Average Variable Cost
AVG: Ambulatory Visit Group
AVI: Average Cost of Illness
AWC: Acceptance, Waiver, and Consent
AWI: Area Wage Index
AWI: Average Wage Index
AWP: Any Willing Provider
AWP: Average Wholesale Price
AWPL: Any Willing Provider Law

B: Annual Rate plus Stock Dividends
B: Beta coefficient

- **Bl:** Beta of a levered firm
- **Bu:** Beta of an unlevered firm

B: Bid
B2B: Business to Business
B2C: Business to Consumer
B2P: Business to Patient
BA: Banker's Acceptance
BA: Budget Authority
BAA: Business Agency Announcement
BAC: Business Advisory Council
BAC: Business Associate Contract
BAN: Bond Anticipation Note
BAR: Billing, Accounts Receivable
BAS: Block Automation System
BB: Big Board
BB: Bond Baby
BB: Bond Bearer
BB: Buy Back
BBA: Balanced Budget Act, of 1997
BBB: Better Business Bureau
BBRA: Balanced Budget Refinement Act, of 1999
BC: Blue Chip
BC: Blue Cross
BCA: Blue Cross Association
BCD: Binary Code Decimal
BCEP: Board Certified in Estate Planning

BCHS: Bureau Community Health Services
BCI: Board Certified in Insurance
BCM: Billing and Collection Master
BCMF: Board Certified in Mutual Funds
BCS: Board Certified in Securities
BD: Bad Delivery
BD: Bank Draft
BD: Bill Discontinued
BD: Broker-Dealer
BDE: Bad Debt Expense
BDO: Bottom Dropped Out
BDOC: Bed Days of Care
BDR: Bearer Depository Receipt
BE: Bill of Exchange
BEA: Break Even Analysis
BEA: Bureau of Economic Affairs
BEA: Bureau of Economic Analysis
BEAD: Break Even Analysis in Dollars
BEAP: Break Even Analysis in Patients
BEAP: Break Even Analysis in Procedures
BEC: Benefit Entitlement Code
BEC: Benefits Executive Council
BEER: Benefits Estimate Earnings Record
BEP: Basic Earning Power
BEP: Break Even Point
BEPD: Break Even Point in Dollars
BEPP: Break Even Point in Patients
BEPP: Break Even Point in Procedures
BEPIPD: Break Even Point in Patient Dollars
BEPIPU: Break Even Point in Patient Units
BEPR: Basic Earning Power Ratio
BF: Brought Forword
BF: Backdoor Financing
BHCA: Bank Holding Company Act
BHU: Basic Health Unit
BIC: Bank Investment Contract
BIF: Bank Insurance Fund
BL: Bill of Lading
BLN: Billion
BLS: Bureau of Labor Statistics
BM: Bear Market
BM: Budget Month
BM: Buyer's Market
BMA: Bond Market Association

BMAD: Part B Medicare Annual Data file
BNI: Beneficiary Notice Initiative
BO: Buy Order
BO: Buyer's Option
BOM: Beginning of Month
BOM: Buy On Margin
BOML: Bill Of Medical Lading
BOP: Balance Of Payments
BOPUD: Benefit Overpayment/Underpayment Data
BOT: Balance Of Trade
BOT: Board Of Trustees
BOT: Bought
BR: Bills Receivable
BR: Bond Rating
BR: Business Risk
BRA: Bankruptcy Reform Act
BRI: Benefit Rate Increase
BS: Back Spread
BS: Balance Sheet
BS: Bellwether Stock
BS: Bill of Sale
BS: Block Sale
BS: Blue Shield
BS: Bureau of Standards
BS: Butterfly Spread
BSE: Boston Stock Exchange
BSE: Brussels Stock Exchange
BSR: Bill Summary Record
BTG: Beat the Gun
BTM: Benefit Termination Month
BTM: Bulling the Market
BUR: Billing Update Record
BV: Book Value
BVA: Book Value per Asset
BVS: Book Value per Share
BVPS: Book Value Per Share
BW: Bid Wanted
BY: Base Year

C: Liquidation Dividend
C2C: Consumer to Consumer
C2C: Customer to Customer
CA: Callable
CA: Capital Account
CA: Chartered Accountant
CA: Claims Authorizer

CA: Commercial Agent
CA: Credit Account
CA: Current Account
CA: Current Assets
CAA: Certified Annuity Advisor
CAA: Corporate Accountability Act
CACM: Central American Common Market
CAD: Cash Against Documents
CAES: Computer Assisted Executions System
CAF: Civil Assets Forfeiture
CAF: Cost Assurance and Freight
CAGR: Compound Annual Growth Rate
CAH: Critical Access Hospital
CAHSPR: Canadian Association of Health Services and Policy Research
CalPERS: California Public Employee Retirement System
CAM: Chartered Asset Manager
CAMPS: Cumulative Auction Market Preferred Stocks
CAN: Claimant Account Number
CAO: Chief Accounting Officer
CAO: Chief Administrative Officer
CAP: Capitation
CAP: Capitated Ambulatory Plan
CAP: Competitive Allowance Program
CAPM: Capital Asset Pricing Model
CAPS: Claims Adjusted Processing System
CAPS: Convertible Adjustable Preferred Stock
CAR: Certification of Automobile Receivables
CAR: Cumulative Average Return
CARA: Constant Absolute Risk Aversion
CARD: Certificates for Amortizing Revolving Debt
CASB: Cost Accounting Standards Board
CAT: Catastrophic Claim
CATS: Certificates of Accrual on Treasury Securities
CAWR: Combined Annual Wage Reporting
CBA: Capital Builder Account
CBA: Certified Business Appraiser

CBA: Cost Benefit Analysis
CBC: Certified Business Consultant
CBC: Certified Business Counselor
CBC: Cost Benefit Criteria
CBD: Cash Before Delivery
CBI: Certified Business Intermediary
CBO: Collateral Bond Obligation
CBO: Congressional Budget Office
CBO: Cost Budget Office
CBOE: Chicago Board Options Exchange
CBOT: Chicago Board of Trade
CBP: Cost-Based Payment
CBPPMI: Cain Brothers Physician Practice Management Index
CBR/P: Cost-Based Reimbursement/ Payment
CBT: Chicago Board of Trade
CC: Complications and Comorbidities
CAP: Comorbidity Affecting Payment
CAP: Complication Affecting Payment
CC: Controllable Cost
CCA: Certified Cost Accountant
CCA: Claims Adjustment and Analysis
CCA: Current Cost Accounting
CCC: Cash Conversion Cycle
CCD: Component Cost of Debt
CCG: Check Claim Group
CCH: Commercial Clearing House
CCI: Consumer Confidence Index
CCI: Correct Coding Initiative
CCN: Community Care Network
CCO: Chief Compliance Officer
CCPA: Consumer Credit Protection Act
CCPS: Component Cost of Preferred Stock
CCR: Cost to Charge Ratio
CCR: Cost of Carrying Receivables
CCRC: Continuing Care Retirement Community
CD: Certificate of Deposit
CDFA: Certified Divorce Financial Analyst
CDFI: Community Development Finance Institute
CDHP: Consumer Driven Health Plan
CDO: Collateralized Debt Obligation

CDP: Certified Divorce Planner

CDSC: Contingent and Deferred Sales Charge

CDT: Current Dental Terminology

CE: Cash Earnings

CE: Commodity Exchange

CE: Covered Entity

CEA: Council of Economic Advisors

CEA: Certified Estate Advisor

CEA: Cost Effectiveness Analysis

CEBS: Certified Employee Benefit Specialist

CED: Cross Elasticity of Demand

CEDR: Center for Economic Development and Research

CEF: Closed End Fund

CEIC: Closed End Investment Company

CEIR: Center for Economic and Industry Research

CEO: Chief Executive Officer

CEP: Certified Estate Planner

CER: Capital Expenditure Review

CERT: Center for Education and Research in Therapeutics

CES: French Health Economists Society

CF: Carried Forward

CF: Cash Flow

CF: Conversion Factor

CFA: Cash Flow Analysis

CFA: Chartered Financial Accountant

CFA©: Chartered Financial Analyst©

CFAA: Computer Fraud and Abuse Act

CFC: Certified Financial Consultant

CFC: Charted Financial Consultant

CFC: Consolidated Freight Classification

CFFA: Certified Forensic Financial Analyst

CFI: Cost, Freight, and Insurance

CFM: Certified Financial Manager

CFM: Cash Flow Management

CFO: Certified Financial Officer

CFO: Chief Financial Officer

CFP©: Certified Financial Planner©

CFR: Code of Federal Regulations

CFS: Cash Flow Statement

CFS: Certified Fund Specialist

CFS: Consolidated Financial Statements

CFSSP: Certified Financial Services Specialty Professional

CFTC: Commodities Futures Trading Commission

CG: Capital Goods

CGT: Capital Gains Tax

CHAMPUS: Civilian Health and Medical Program for Uniformed Services

CHAP: Community Health Accreditation Program

CHC: Certified Health Consultant

CHC: Community Health Center

CHE: Certified Health Care Executive

CHECCS: Clearing House Electronic Check Clearing System

CHFC: Chartered Financial Consultant

CHFP: Certified Health Care Financial Professional

CHHP: Coordinated Home Health Program

CHIM: Center for Health Information Management

CHMSA: Critical Health Manpower Shortage Area

CHIME: College of Health Information Management Executives

CHIN: Community Health Information Network

CHN: Community Health Network

CHP: Comprehensive Health Planning

CHRIS: Computerized Human Resource Information System

CHX: Chicago Stock Exchange

CI: Coding Institute

CI: Compound Interest

CIA: Certified Internal Auditor

CIAO: Critical Infrastructure Assurance Office

CIC: Certified Insurance Consultant

CIC: Chartered Investment Counselor

CIF: Cost, Insurance, and Freight

CIF: Corporate Income Fund

CIMA: Certified Investment Management Analyst

CIMC: Certified Investment Management Consultant

CIO: Chief Information Officer

CIO: Chief Investment Officer

CIPB: Critical Infrastructure Protection Board

CIS: Computer Information System

CISN: Community Integrated Service Network

CISP: Certified IRA Services Professional

CLEAR: Consolidated Licensure for Entities Assuming Risk

CLD: Called-in

CLN: Construction Loan Note

CLT: Capitation Liability Theory

CLTC: Certified in Long Term Care

CLU: Chartered Life Underwriter

CM: Call Money

CM: Case Management

CM: Case Mix

CMA: Certified Management Accountant

CMA: Chartered Market Analyst

CMA: Certified Merger Advisor

CMA: Cost Minimization Analysis

CMA: Current Month Accrual

CMAC: CHAMPUS Maximum Allowable Charge

CMAR: Current Money Amount of Reduction

CMBA: Currently Monthly Benefit Amount

CME: Chicago Mercantile Exchange

CMFC: Chartered Mutual Fund Counselor

CMHC: Community Mental Health Center

CMI: Case Mix Index

CML: Capital Market Line

CMM: Cumulative Member Month

CMN: Certificate of Medical Necessity

CMO: Collaterized Mortgage Obligation

CMP©: Certified Medical Planner©

CMP: Competitive Medical Plan

CMR: Contribution Margin Ratio

CMS: Care Management System

CMS: Centers for Medicare and Medicaid Services

CMS-1500: CMS standard claim form

CMT: Constant Maturity Treasury

CMV: Current Market Value

CN: Consignment Note

CN: Credit Note

CNH: Community Nursing Home

CNHI: Committee for National Health Insurance

CNS: Continuous Net Settlement

CO: Call Option

CO: Cash Order

CO: Certificate of Origin

CO: Coinsurance

CO: Covered Option

COA: Certificate Of Authority

COB: Close Of Business

COB: Coordination Of Benefits

COBRA: Consolidated Omnibus Budget Reconciliation Act

COC: Certificate Of Coverage

COD: Cash On Demand/Delivery

CODA: Cash Or Deferred Arrangement

COFI: Cost Of Funds Index

COI: Cost Of Illness

COL: Cost Of Living

COLA: Cost Of Living Adjustment

COLTS: Continuously Offered Long-Term Securities

COM: Current Operating Month

COMEX: Commodity Exchange

COMSP: Cost Of Medical Service Provided

CON: Certificate Of Need

COO: Chief Operating Officer

COPA: Certificate Of Public Advantage

COPN: Certificate Of Public Need

CORF: Comprehensive Outpatient Rehabilitation Facility

CORP: Corporation

COT: Chain Of Trust

CP: Closing Price

CP: Closing Purchase

CP: Collar Price

CP: Commercial Paper

CP: Conversion Price

CPA: Certified Public Accountant

CPC: Certified Pension Consultant

CPCU: Chartered Property Casualty Underwriter

CPD: Central Processing Department
CPEP: Carrier Performance Evaluation Program
CPF: Current Principal Factor
CPFF: Cost Plus Fixed Fee
CPhD: Certified in Philanthropic Development
CPI: Consumer Price Index
CPM: Chartered Portfolio Manager
CPM: Cost Per Thousand
CPMI: Consumer Price Medical Index
CPPC: Cost Plus Percentage Cost
CPR: Computerized Patient Record
CPR: Customary, Prevailing, and Reasonable
CPS: Convertible Preferred Stock
CPS: Cumulative Preferred Stock
CPS: Current Population Survey
CPT: *Current Procedural Terminology*
CPT-4: Current Procedural Terminology, Fourth Edition
CPU: Central Processing Unit
CPV: Current Principle Value
CPVA: Cost Profit Volume Analysis
CQS: Consolidated Quotation System
CR: Capitation Rate
CR: Carrier Replacement
CR: Carrier's Rate
CR: Class Rate
CR: Company Risk
CR: Conversion Ratio
CR: Credit
CR: Current Rate
CR: Current Ratio
CRA: Certified Retirement Administrator
CRA: Certified Review Appraiser
CRA: Corporate Responsibility Act of 2002
CRAT: Charitable Remainder Annuity Trust
CRB: Commodity Research Bureau
CRC: Community Rating by Class
CRC: Certified Retirement Counselor
CRCM: Certified Regulatory Compliance Manager
CRD: Central Registration Depository

CRFA: Certified Retirement Financial Advisor
CRORC: Common Return On Regulatory Capital
CRPC: Certified Retirement Planning Counselor
CRPS: Chartered Retirement Plan Specialist
CRRA: Constant Relative Risk Aversion
CRSP: Center for Research in Securities Prices
CRT: Charitable Remainder Trust
CRUT: Charitable Remainder Unit Trust
CRVS: California Relative Value Studies
CS: Capital Stock
CS: Closing Sale
CS: Common Stock
CS: Complexity-Severity
CS: Corporate Securities
CSA: Certified Senior Advisor
CSE: Chicago Stock Exchange
CSE: Copenhagen Stock Exchange
CSE: Cincinnati Stock Exchange
CSOP: Certified Securities Operations Professional
CSR: Cost Summary Review
CSTSA: Certified Specialist in Tax Sheltered Accounts
CT: Cash Trade
CTA: Commodity Trading Advisor
CTB: Collateralized Trust Bond
CTEP: Certified (Chartered) Trust and Estate Planner
CTFA: Certified Trust and Financial Advisor
CTO: Chief Technology Officer
CUA: Cost Utility Analysis
CUNA: Credit Union National Association
CUPR: Customary Usual Prevailing Rate
CUPR: Customary Usual Prevailing Reasonable
CUR: Current Unreduced Rate
CUREX: Current Unreduced Expenses
CUSIP: Committee on Uniform Security Identification Procedures
CUWI: Current Unvalidated Wage Items
CV: Co-efficient of Variation

CV: Cost Variance
CV: Convertible Security
CVA: Certified Valuation Analysts
CVPA: Cost Volume Profit Analysis
CWO: Cash With Order
CWM: Chartered Wealth Manager
CXL: Cancel
CY: Calendar Year
CY: Current Yield

D: Delivery
D: Delta or difference
D: Discount
D: Dividend
DA: Date of Admission
DA: Deposit Account
DA: Disability Assistance
DA: Discretionary Account
DA: Document against Acceptance
DAC: Delivery Against Cost
DAF: Defined Asset Fund
DAR: Days in Accounts Receivable
DAW: Dispense As Written
DB: Debit
DB: Direct Broker
DB: Dun & Bradstreet
DBA: Doing Business As
DBC: Defined Benefit Coverage
DBMS: Data Base Management System
DBP: Defined Benefit Plan
DC: Diagnostic Code
DC: Differential Cost
DC: Direct Cost
DC: Dual Choice
DCA: Deferred Compensation Administrator
DCA: Deferred Compensation Arrangement
DCA: Dependent Care Account
DCC: Defined Contribution Coverage
DCF: Discounted Cash Flows
DCFA/M: Discounted Cash Flow Analysis/Method
DCG: Diagnostic Cost Group
DCI: Duplicate Coverage Inquiry
DCOH: Days Cash On Hand
DCP: Defined Contribution Plan

DCP: Deferred Compensation Plan
DD: Data Dictionary
DD: Declaration Date
DD: Deferred Delivery
DD: Delayed Delivery
DDBDM: Double Declining Balance Depreciation Method
DDE: Direct Data Entry
DDI: Deep Discount Issue
DDM: Discount Dividend Model
DDR: Discharge During Referral
DDS: Disability Determination Services
DEA: Data Envelope Analysis
DEA: Designated Examination Authority
DEAR: Daily Earnings At Risk
DEERS: Defense Enrollment Eligibility Reporting System
DEFRA: Deficit Reduction Act
DFFC: Discounted From Full Charges
DFFS: Discounted Fee-For-Service
DHHS: Department of Health and Human Services
DI: Disability Insurance
DI: Disposable Income
DIA: Diamonds
DISA: Data Information Standards Association
DJ: Dow Jones
DJA: Dow Jones Averages
DJIA: Dow Jones Industrial Average
DJTA: Dow Jones Transportation Average
DJUA: Dow Jones Utility Average
DK: Don't Know
DLP: Date of Last Payment
DM: Direct Measurement
DME: Durable Medical Equipment
DMEPOS: Durable Medical Equipment, Prosthetics, Orthotics, and Supplies
DMERC: Durable Medical Equipment Regional Carrier
DMW: Deemed Military Wages
DN: Debit Note
DNI: Do Not Increase
DNR: Do Not Reduce
DOA: Date Of Admission
DO: Delivery Order
DOJ: Department of Justice

DOL: Department of Labor
DOS: Date of Service
DOT: Designated Order Turnaround
DP: Data Processing
DP: Document against Payment
DPH: Department of Public Health
DPI: Disposable Personal Income
DPMM: Designated Primary Market Makers
DPP: Direct Participation Program
DPR: Dividend Payout Ratio
DPR: Drug Price Review
DPT: Days Per Thousand
DR: Debit
DR: Debt Ratio
DRA: Deficit Reduction Act
DRC: Diagnostic Related Category
DRG: Diagnostic Related Group
DRIP: Dividend Reinvestment Plan
DRM: Direct Reduction Mortgage
DRS: Data Retrieval System
DS: Debenture Stock
DSH: Disproportionate Share Hospital
DSM-IV: *Diagnostic and Statistical Manual of Mental Disorders, Fourth Edition*
DSO: Days Sales Outstanding
DSO: Debt Service Obligation
DSR: Days Sales Receivable
DT: Dow Theory
DTC: Depository Transfer Check
DTC: Depository Trust Company
DTC: Direct to Consumer
DUR: Drug Utilization Review
DVP: Delivery Versus Payment
DXNNH: Diagnosis Not Normally Hospitalized

E: Declared or paid in preceding 12 months
EA: Enrolled Agent
EA: Evaluate and Advise
EAC: Estimated Acquisition Cost
EACH: Essential Access Community Hospital
EAFE: Europe and Australia, Far East equity index
EM: Evaluate and Manage

EAP: Employee Assistance Program
EAR: Effective Annual Rate
EBCDIC: Extended Binary Code Decimal Information Code
EBI: Effective Buying Income
EBIT: Earnings Before Interest and Taxes
EBITDA: Earnings Before Interest, Taxes, Depreciation, and Amortization
EBRI: Employee Benefit Research Institute
EBT: Earnings Before Taxes
EC: Electronic Claim
EC: Electronic Commerce
EC: Enterprise Community
EC: European Community
EC: Exchange Control
ECB: European Central Bank
ECD: Equity-linked Certificate of Deposit
ECF: Extended Care Facility
ECI: Employment Cost Index
ECM: European Common Market
ECM: Emerging Company Marketplace
ECN: Electronic Communication Network
ECOA: Equal Credit Opportunity Act
ECT: Estimated Completion Time
ECU: European Currency Unit
ED: Euro Dollar
EDD: Estimated Deliver Date
EDGAR: Electronic Data Gathering, Analysts, and Retrieval (SEC)
EDI: Electronic Data Interchange
EDIFACT: EDI For Admission, Commerce, and Trade
EDP: Electronic Data Processing
EDR: European Depository Receipts
EEC: European Economic Community
EFP: Exchange for Physical
EFT: Electronic Funds Transfer
EGARCH: Exponential Generalized Autoregressive Conditional Heteroskedasticity
EGHP: Employer Group Health Plan
EGTRRA: Economic Growth and Tax Relief and Reconciliation Act of 2001
EHIP: Employee Health Insurance Plan
EHO: Emerging Health Care Organization
EI: Exact Interest
EI: Economic Index

EIB: European Investment Bank
EIN: Employer Identification Number
EL: Even Lots
ELOC: Equity Line Of Credit
ELOS: Estimated Length Of Stay
ELS: Estate Law Specialist
EM: End of Month
EM: Evaluation and Management
EMC: Electronic Medical Claims
EMCC: Emerging Market Clearing Corporation
EMF Index: Emerging Market Free Index
EMP: End of Month Payment
EMR: Electronic Medical Records
EMS: European Monetary System
EMU: European Monetary Unit
EO: Executive Order
EO: Errors and Omissions
EOA: Effective On or About
EOB: Explanation Of Benefits
EOC: Episode Of Care
EOD: Every Other Day
EOE: Errors and Omissions Expected
EOE: European Options Exchange
EOI: Evidence of Insurability
EOMB: Explanation Of Medical Benefits
EOMB: Explanation Of Medicare Benefits
EOQ: Economic Order Quantity
EOQC: Economic Order Quantity Cost
EOS: Economy Of Scale
EOY: End Of Year
EP: Earned Premium
EP: Earnings Price
EPEA: Expense Per Equivalent Admission
EPFT: Electronic Payment Funds Transfer
EPMPM: Encounters Per Member Per Month
EPMPY: Encounters Per Member Per Year
EPO: Exclusive Provider Organization
EPPS: Earnings Per Preferred Share
EPR: Earnings Price Ratio
EPRA: Ethics in Patient Referral Act
EPS: Earnings Per Share
EPSDT: Early and Periodic Screening, Diagnosis, and Treatment
EPYTB: Equivalent Pretax Yield on Taxable Bond

ER: Exchange Rate
ERISA: Employee Retirement Income Security Act of 1974
ERM: Exchange Rate Mechanism
ERTA: Economic Recovery Tax Act of 1981
ES: Earned Surplus
ES: Emergency Service
ES: Exempt Securities
ESOP: Employee Stock Ownership Plan
ESOT: Employee Stock Ownership Trust
ESP: Exchange Stock Portfolio
ESPP: Employee Stock Purchase Plan
ET: Expenditure Target
ETA: Estimated Time of Arrival
ETD: Estimated Time of Departure
ETF: Electronically Traded Fund
ETF: Exchange Traded Fund
ETG: Episode Treatment Group
ETLT: Equal To or Less Than
ETM: Escrowed To Maturity
EU: European Union
EUR: Economic Utilization Review
EURCO: European Composite Unit
EUS: Earning Utilization Statement
EV: Expected Value
EVA: Economic Value Added
EMVA©: Economic Medical Value Added©
EVOIL: Economic Value Of Individual Life
EXIMBANK: Export/Import Bank

F: Commodity futures symbol for a January delivery month
F: Dealt in Flat (bond listing)
FA: Fiscal Agent
FA: Foreign Associate
FA: Fraud and Abuse
FA: Free Alongside
FAcct: Foundation for Accountability
FAC: Face Amount Certificate
FACC: Face Amount Certificate Company
FACT: Factor Analysis Chart
FANS: Funds Available Notification System
FAQ: Full Account Query
FAQ: Firm Access and Query

FAR: Federal Acquisitions Regulations

FAS: Free Alongside

FASAC: Financial Accounting Standards Advisory Council

FASB: Financial Accounting Standards Board

FAT: Fixed Asset Transfer

FATR: Fixed Assets Turnover Ratio

FB: Freight Bill

FB: Fringe Benefits

FBO: For the Benefit Of

FBP: Flexible Benefit Plan

FC: Factor Cost

FC: Fixed Capital

FC: Fixed Cost

FC: Futures Contract

FCA: False Claims Act

FCBA: Fair Credit Billing Act

FCBI: Fellow Certified Business Intermediary

FCC: Fixed Charge Coverage

FCCCDA: Fair Credit and Charge Card Disclosure Act

FCCR: Fixed Charge Coverage Ratio

FCER: Full Claims Earnings Record

FCFAC: Federal Credit Financial Assistance Corporation

FCM: Futures Commission Merchant

FCN: Financial Control Number

FCOP: Foreign Currency Options Principal

FCRA: Fair Credit Reporting Act

FCS: Full Capacity Sales

FDCPA: Fair Debt Collection Practices Act

FDI: Foreign Direct Investment

FDIC: Federal Deposit Insurance Corporation

FDO: Formula Driven Overpayment

FE: Futures Exchange

FECA: Federal Employee's Compensation Act

FED: Federal Reserve Bank

FEHB: Federal Employee Health Benefits

FEHBAR: Federal Employee Health Benefits Acquisition Regulations

FEHBG: Federal Employees Health Benefit Guide

FEHBP: Federal Employee Health Benefits Program

FEI: Financial Executives Institute

FEIN: Federal Employee Identification Number

FET: Federal Excise Tax

FFB: Federal Financing Bank

FFC: Federal Funding Criteria

FFIEC: Federal Financial Institutions Examination Council

FFO: Funds From Operations

FFP: Federal Financial Participation

FFS: Fee-For-Service

FFSS: Fee-For-Service System

FFY: Federal Fiscal Year

FGIC: Financial Guarantee Insurance Company

FHB: Federal Home Bank

FHFMA: Fellow Health Care Financial Management Association

FHLMC: Federal Home Loan Mortgage Corporation

FHMOA: Federal Health Maintenance Organization Act

FI: Financial Institution

FI: Fiscal Intermediary

FIA: Fellow of the Institute of Actuaries

FIBBA: Fellow International Business Brokers Association

FIBOR: Frankfort Interbank Offered Rate

FIC: Fraternal Insurance Counselor

FICA: Federal Insurance Contributions Ac

FICA: Fellow, Institute of Chartered Accountants

FICB: Federal Intermediate Credit Bank

FICO: Financing Corporation

FIFO: First-In, First-Out

FIG: Fiscal Intermediary Group

FIN: Federal Identification Number

FIPS: Fixed Income Pricing System

FIR: Futures Initial Requirement

FIRREA: Financial Institutions Reform, Recovery, and Enforcement Act of 1989

FIT: Federal Income Tax

FITW: Federal Income Tax Withholding
FLB: Federal Loan Bank
FLEX: Flexible Exchange Options
FLMI: Fellow Life Management Institute
FLUX: Flow Uncertainty Index
FM: Fee Maximum
FMAN: February, May, August, and November cycle
FMAP: Federal Medical Assistance Percentage
FMFIA: Federal Manager's Fiscal Integrity Act
FMFIA: Federal Manager's Financial Integrity Act
FMO: Financial Management Office
FMV: Fair Market Value
FNMA: Federal National Mortgage Association
FOB: Free-On-Board
FOC: Free-Of-Charge
FOIA: Freedom Of Information Act
FOK: Fill Or Kill
FOMC: Federal Open Market Committee
FOOTSIE: Financial Times SE 100 Index UK Stocks
FOR: Free-On-Rail
FOT: Free-On-Truck
FP: Floating Policy
FP: Fixed Price
FP: Fully Paid
FPA: Financial Planning Association
FPL: Federal Poverty Level
FPP: Faculty Practice Plan
FQAM: Financial Quality Assurance Manager
FQC: Firm Quote Composite
FQCHC: Federally Qualified Community Health Center
FQHMO: Federally Qualified Health Maintenance Organization
FR: *Federal Register*
FR: Financial Risk
FRA: Federal Reserve Act
FRA: Forward Rate Agreement
FRB: Federal Reserve Banks
FRB: Federal Reserve Board

FRCD: Floating Rate Certificate of Deposit
FREIT: Finite Life Real Estate Investment Trust
FRN: Floating Rate Note
FRS: Federal Reserve System
FS: Final Settlement
FS: Frankfurt Stock Exchange
FS: Futures Spread
FSA: Fellow of the Society of Actuaries
FSA: Flexible Spending Account
FSI: Financial Strength Index
FSMA: Financial Services Modernization Act of 1999
FSP: Flexible Spending Plan
FSR: Financial Status Report
FTA: Fair Trade Act
FTC/A: Federal Trade Commission/Act
FTE: Full Time Equivalent
FTEP: Full Time Equivalent Provider/Practitioner
FTI: Federal Tax Included
FUTA: Federal Unemployment Tax Act
FV: Face Value
FV: Future Value
FVF: Future Value Factor
FVO: For Valuation Only
FX: Foreign Exchange
FY: Fiscal Year
FYA: For Your Attention
FYI: For Your Information

g: Growth rate
G: Commodity futures symbol for a February delivery month
G-8: Group of Eight Finance Ministers
GA: General Account
GAAP: Generally Accepted Accounting Principles
GAAS: Generally Accepted Auditing Standards
GAB: General Adjustment Bureau
GAF: Geographic Adjustment Factor
GAI: Guaranteed Annual Income
GAO: General Accounting Office
GARCH: Generalized Autoregressive Conditional Heteroskedasticity
GARP: Generally Accepted Risk Principles

GASB: Government Accounting Standards Boards

GATT: General Agreement on Tariffs and Trade

GD: Good Delivery

GD: Gross Debt

GDP: Gross Domestic Product

GDR: Global Deposit Receipt

GERP: Geographic Expense Reimbursement Plan

GHAA: Group Health Association of America

GHI: Group Health Insurance

GIC: Guaranteed Income Contract

GIC: Guaranteed Investment Contract

GL: Go Long

GLBA: Gramm-Lech-Bliley Act

GMLOS: Geometric Mean Length Of Stay

GNMA: Government National Mortgage Association

GNP: Gross National Product

GO: General Obligation

GO: Government Obligation

GOCO: Government Owned Contract Operated

GOE: General Office Expense

GOX: Gold Index

GP: Going Public

GPA: General Public Assistance

GPAM: Graduated Payment Adjustable Mortgage

GPCI: Geographic Practice Cost Index

GPDI: Gross Private Domestic Investment

GPM: Gross Profit Margin

GPR: Gross Profit Ratio

GPWW: Group Practice Without Walls

GRAT: Grantor Retained Annuity Trust

GRIT: Grantor Retained Income Trust

GRUT: Grantor Retained Uni Trust

GS: Glamour Stock

GS: Government Securities

GS: Growth Stock

GSCC: Government Securities Clearing Corporation

GSE: Government Sponsored Enterprise

GTC: Good-Till-Canceled

GTM: Good This Month

GTW: Good This Week

H: Commodity futures symbol for a March delivery month

H: Declaration or Paid after stock dividend (in newspapers)

HAP: Hospital Accreditation Program

HAS: Hospital Administrative Services

HAT: Hospital Arrival Time

HB: Hospital Based

HBA: Health Benefits Advisor

HBA: Hill Burton Act

HBCS: Hospital Billing and Collection Service

HBO: Hospital Benefits Organization

HBP: Hospital Based Physician

HC: Health Care

HC: Holding Company

HCA: Health Care Account

HCA: Health Care Accountant

HCA: Hospital Cooperation Acts

HCC: Health Care Clearinghouse

HCC: Health Care Corporation

HCD: Health Care Delivery

HCF: Health Care Finder

HCFA: Health Care Financing Administration

HCFA 1500: Universal billing form

HCFAR: Health Care Financing Administration Ruling

HCIA: Health Care Investment Analysts

HCMA: Health Cost Minimization Analysis

HCPCS: Health Care Common Procedural Coding System

HCPCS: HCFA Common Procedure Coding System

HCPP: Health Care Prepayment Plan

HCQIA: Health Care Quality Improvement Act

HCRIS: Hospital Cost Reporting Information System

HCTA: Health Care Trust Account

HCUA: Health Cost Utility Analysis

HCUP: Hospital Cost and Utilization Project

HDHP: High Deductible Health Plan

HDS: Health Care Delivery System
HEAL: Health Education Assistance Loan
HEDIS: Health Employers and Data Information Set
HEF: Health Education Foundation
HEL: Home Equity Loan
HERC: Health Economic Research Center
HESG: Health Economists Study Group
HEX: Helsinki Stock Exchange
HEZ: Health Economic Zone
HF: Held For
HFMA: Health Care Financial Management Association
HFR: Hold for Release
HFSG: Health Care Finance Study Group
HH: Hold Harmless
HHA: Home Health Agency
HHI: Herfindahl-Hirschman Index
HHRG: Home Health Care Resources Group
HHS: Health and Human Services (Department)
HI: Hospital Insurance (Part A: Medicare)
HI: Hot Issue
HIAA: Health Insurance Association of America
HIBAC: Health Insurance Benefits Advisory Council
HIBCC: Health Care Industry Business Communications Council
HIBOR: Hong Kong Interbank Offered Rate
HIC: Health Information Center
HIC: Health Insurance Claim
HIMSS: Health Care Information and Management Systems Society
HINN: Hospital Issued Notice of Noncoverage
HIP: Health Insurance Plan
HIPAA: Health Insurance Portability and Accountability Act of 1996
HIPC: Health Insurance Purchasing Cooperative
HIPPS: Health Insurance Prospective Payment System
HISAC: Health Care Information Sharing and Analysis Center
HITF: Health Insurance Trust Fund

HL7: Health Level 7
HLT: Highly Leveraged Transaction
HMO: Health Maintenance Organization
HMPSA: Health Manpower Shortage Area
HOA: Health Oversight Agency
HP: Hospital Peer Review
HPAC: Health Policy Advisory Center
HPB: Historic Payment Basis
HPC: Health Policy Council
HPC: Health Purchasing Cooperative
HPFSA: Health Plan Flexible Spending Account
HPO: Hospital Physician Organization
HPPC: Health Plan Purchasing Cooperative
HPSA: Health Professional Shortage Area
HQ: Headquarters
HR: Hospital Record
HRA: Health Reimbursement Arrangement
HRA: Health Risk Assessment
HRET: Hospital Research and Education Trust
HRSA: Health Resources and Services Administration
HS: Health Status
HSA: Health Savings Account
HSA: Health Security Act
HSA: Health Services Administration
HSA: Health Services Agreement
HSA: Health Service Area
HSR: Health Services Research
HSRC: Health Services Research Center
HUD: Housing and Urban Department
HUR: Hospital Utilization Review
HURA: Health Underserved Rural Area
HURT: Hospital Utilization Review Team
HV: Hospital Visit

i: interest rate, also known as k
I: Imports
I: Paid this Year, Dividend Omitted, Deferred, or No Action Taken at Last Meeting
I: Interest
I-BONDS: Indexed Savings Bonds

IAA: Investment Advisors Act

IAFP: International Association for Financial Planning (now FPA)

IASC: International Accounting Standards Committee

IB: Introducing Broker

IBA: Institute of Business Appraisers

IBA: Investment Bankers Association

IBBA: International Business Brokers Association

IBES: Institutional Brokers Estimate System

IBF: International Banking Facility

IBFS: Interim Billing and Follow-up System

IBNR: Incurred But Not Reported

IBNRL: Incurred But Not Reported Losses

IC: Indifference Curve

IC: Indirect Cost

IC: Information Coefficient

IC: Internal Controls

ICA: International Claim Association

ICA: Investment Company Act

ICBA: Institute of Certified Business Appraisers

ICBC: Institute of Certified Business Counselors

ICD: *International Classification of Diseases*

ICD-9-CM: *International Classification of Diseases, Ninth Edition, Clinical Modification*

ICD-10-CM: *International Classification of Diseases, Tenth Edition, Clinical Modification*

ICE: International Commercial Exchange

ICF: Intermediate Care Facility

ICFP: Institute of Certified Financial Planners

ICI: Investable Commodity Index

ICI: Investment Company Institute

ICMA: Institute of Cost and Management Accountants

ICN: Internal Control Number

ICON: Index Currency Option Note

ICP: Inventory Conversion Period

ICS: Issued Capital Stock

ICSD: International Council of Securities Dealers

ID: Immediate Delivery

ID: Income Debenture

ID: Interim Dividend

IDB: Industrial Development Bond

IDC: Indirect Costs

IDN: Integrated Delivery Network

IDS: Integrated Delivery System

IE: Investment Executive

IED: Income Elasticity of Demand

IET: Interest Equalization Tax

IFA: Independent Financial Advisor

IFC: International Finance Corporation

IG: Inspector General

IGARCH: Integrated Generalized Autoregressive Conditional Heteroskedasticity

***i*HEA:** *International* Health Economics Association

IHDN: Integrated Health Delivery Network

IHO: Integrated Health Organization

IHS: Indian Health Services

II: Institutional Investor

IIA: Institute of Internal Auditors

IIC: Inflation Index Charge-Customary

IID: Investment In Default

IIHI: Individually Identifiable Health Information

IMA: Institute of Management Accountants

IMAB: International Markets Advisory Board

***i*MBA:** Institute of Medical Business Advisors, Inc.[©]

***i*MBA-VN[©]:** *Institute* of Medical Business Advisors Virtual Network[©]

***i*MBA-VU[©]:** *Institute* of Medical Business Advisors Virtual University[©]

IMF: International Monetary Fund

IMM: International Monetary Market

IMS: Information Management System

INC: Incorporation/Incorporated

INSTINET: International Networks Corporation (now Instinet Group, Inc.)

INT: Interest Payment in U.S. Dollars

IO: Implicit Option
I/O: Input/Output
IO: Interest Only
IO: Investor Owned
IOC: Immediate Or Cancel order
IOI: Indication Of Interest
IOM: Index Or Market option
IOS: Investment Opportunity Schedule
IOU: I Owe You
IO-ette: A small principal IOU
IOV: Initial Office Visit
IP: In Patient
IP: Issue Price
IPA: Independent Physician Association
IPA: Independent Practice Association
IPA: Independent Provider Association
IPA: Individual Practice Association
IPA: Individual Provider Association
IPL: Investment Product Line
IPO: Initial Public Offering
IPS: Internent Payment System
IPS: Investment Policy Statement
IR: Interest Rate
IR: Investor Relations
IRA: Individual Retirement Account
IRB: Industrial Revenue Bond
IRC: Internal Revenue Code
IRP: Interest Rate Parity
IRR: Internal Rate of Return
IRR: Internal Rate of Return, where:

- K = discount rate, rate of return, or cost of capital
- K_{nom} = nominal rate of return
- K_d = before tax cost of debt
- K_e = cost of new common stock
- K_m = required rate of market return
- K_{ps} = cost of preferred stock
- K_{rf} = rate of return for a risk-less asset
- K_{ks} = cost of retained earnings
- K_{sl} = cost of equity for a levered firm
- K_{su} = cost of equity for an unlevered firm

IRR: Implied Repo Rate

IRS: Internal Revenue Service
IRX: 13 week Treasury Bill Index
IS: Information Services
ISB: Independent Standards Board
ISB: Investors Service Bureau
ISBN: International Standard Book Number
ISCC: International Securities Clearing Corporation
ISDA: International Swaps Dealers Association
ISE: Irish Stock Exchange
ISE: Italian Stock Exchange
ISFDs: Indexed Sinking Fund Debentures
ISG: Intermarket Surveillance Group
ISID: International Securities Identification Directory
ISM: Institute for Supply Management
ISMA: International Securities Market Association
ISMP: Institute for Safe Medication Practices
ISO: Incentive Stock Option
ISRHFM: International Society for Research in Health Care Financial Management
ISRO: International Securities Regulatory Organization
IT: Income Tax
IT: Information Technology
ITC: Investment Tax Credit
ITR: Inventory Turnover Ratio
ITS: Intermarket Trading System
ITS/CAES: Intermarket Trading System/ Computer Assisted Execution System

J: Commodity futures symbol for an April delivery month
JA: Joint Account
JAJO: January, April, July, October cycle
JC: Joint Cost
JCAHO: Joint Commission on Accreditation of Health Care Organizations
JCWAA: Jobs Creation and Worker Assistance Act
JD: Juris Doctorate
JI: Jensen Index
JIT: Just In Time

JITI: Just In Time Inventory
JSE: Johannesburg Stock Exchange
JT: Joint Tenants
JTE: Joint Tenants by the Entirety
JTIC: Joint Tenants In Common
JTWROS: Joint Tenants With Rights Of Survivorship
JUA: Joint Underwriting Association
JV: Joint Venture

K: Commodity futures symbol for a May delivery month
K: Prefix meaning multiplied by one thousand
K: Declared or Paid this Year on a Cumulative Issue with Dividends in Arrears
K: Kilo, meaning × 1,000
KCBT: Kansas City Board of Trade
KD: Knock Down
KS: Kiting Stocks
KYC: Know Your Customer

L: Listed; securities
LA: Legal Assets
LA: Liquid Assets
LAC: Long Run Average Cost
LB: Legal Bond
LBO: Leveraged Buy Out
LC: Letter of Credit
LC: Leverage Contract
LC: Loan Crowd
LCE: London Commodity Exchange
LCM: Least Common Multiple
LCM: Lower of Cost or Market
LEAPS: Long-term Equity Anticipation Securities
LEI: Leading Economic Indicator
LESOP: Leveraged Employee Stock Ownership Plan
LFS: Laboratory Fee Schedule
LI: Letter of Intent
LIBID: London Interbank Bid
LIBOR: Lisbon Interbank Offered Rate
LIBOR: London Interbank Offered Rate
LIFFE: London International Financial Futures and Options Exchange
LIFO: Last In, First Out

LL: Limited Liability
LLC: Limited Liability Company
LLP: Limited Liability Partnership
LLM: Masters in Law
LMI: Labor Market Information
LMT: Limit
LMV: Long Market Value
LO: Limited Order
LO: Lowest Offer
LOB: Line Of Business
LOC: Letter Of Credit
LOI: Letter Of Intent
LOINC: Logical Observations Identifiers, Names, and Codes
LOIS: Limited Order Information System
LOS: Length Of Stay
LP: Limited Partnership
LP: Long Position
LR: Listing Requirement
LRA: Linear Regression Analysis
LRAC: Long Run Average Cost
LRAS: Long Run Average Supply
LS: Letter Security
LS: Listed Securities
LSE: London Stock Exchange
LTC: Long Term Care
LTCL: Long Term Capital Loss
LTCG: Long Term Capital Gain
LTCU: Long Term Care Unit
LTV: Loan to Value
LTVR: Loan to Value Ratio
LUPA: Low Utilization Payment Adjustment
LUTCF: Life Underwrite Training Council Fellow
LYON: Liquid Yield Options Note

M: Imports
M: Matured Bonds (in newspapers)
M: Mega
M: Money Supply
M: Prefix meaning divided by 1,000
M: Prefix meaning multiplied by 1,000,000
MA: Margin Account
MA: Market Averages
MA: Mergers Acquisitions

MAA: Medicare Approved Amount

MAAA: Member of the American Academy of Actuaries

MAAC: Maximum Allowable Actual Charge

MABC: Medical Activity Based Costing

MAC: Major Ambulatory Category

MAC: Maximum Allowable Charge

MAC: Maximum Allowable Cost

MAC: Municipal Assistance Corporation

MACD: Moving Average Convergence/ Divergence

MACL: Maximum Allowable Cost List

MACRS: Modified Accelerated Cost Recovery System

MADC: Mean Average Daily Census

MAX: Maximum

MB: Market Basket

MB: Market to Book ratio

MBA: Master in Business Administration

MBAᵉ: Medical Business Advisors, Inc.ᵉ

MBA: Mortgage Banker's Association

MBARS: Municipal Bonds Acceptance and Reconciliation Services

MBA-VNᵉ: Medical Business Advisors Virtual Networkᵉ

MBA-VUᵉ: Medical Business Advisors Virtual Universityᵉ

MBIA: Municipal Bond Insurance Association

MBO: Management Buy Out

MBP: Monthly Benefit Payment

MBS: Mortgage Backed Security

MBSCC: Mortgage Backed Securities Clearing Corporation

MC: Margin Call

MC: Marginal Change

MC: Marginal Cost

MC: Marginal Credit

MC: Medicare + Choice

MC: Mixed Cost

MCAMP: Municipal Check A Month Portfolio

MCATS: Municipal Certificates of Accrual on Tax-exempt Securities

MCBA: Masters Certified Business Appraiser

MCC: Marginal Cost of Capital

MCC: Medicare Cost Contract

MCC: Mutual Capital Certificate

MCI: Medicare Cost Index

MCO: Managed Care Organization

MCR: Medical Cost Ratio

MCR: Medicare Cost Report

MCR: Modified Community Rating

MD: Maturity Date

MD: Month after Date

MDA: Management Discussion and Analysis

MDC: Major Diagnostic Category

MDDRG: Physician Diagnostic Related Group

MDG: Major Diagnostic Group

MDH: Medicare Dependent Hospital

MDS: Minimum Data Set

MEB: Marginal External Benefit

MEB: Medical Economics Bureau

MEC: Marginal Efficiency of Capital

MECA: Medicare Expanded Choice Act

MEDISGPS: Medical Illness Severity Grouping System

MEDLARS: Medical Education Literature Analysis and Retrieval System

MedPAC: Medicare Payment Advisory Commission

MedPAR: Medicare Provider Analysis and Review file

MEI: Marginal Efficiency of Investment

MEI: Medicare Economic Index

MERC: Chicago Mercantile Exchange; slang term

MeSH: Medical Staff Hospital Organization

MESOP: Management Enrichment Stock Ownership Plan

MET: Multiple Employee Trusts

MEVAᵉ: Medical Economic Value Addedᵉ

MEWA: Multiple Employer Welfare Association

MF: Mutual Fund

MFA: Medical Fiscal Agent

MFAIC: Medicare Fraud and Abuse Information Coordinator
MFC: Monetary and Financial Code
MFP: Master Financial Professional
MFS: Medicare Fee Schedule
MGMA: Medical Group Management Association
MGP: Medical Group Practice
MHA: Master of Health Care Administration
MHB: Maximum Hospital Benefit
MHS: Manufactured Housing Securities
MIA: Medically Indigent Adult
MIBOR: Madrid Interbank Offered Rate
MICEX: Moscow Interbank Currency
MIDAS: Market Information Data Access System
MIE: Meals and Incidental Expenses
MIG: Medically Insured Group
MIG: Moody's Investment Grade
MIMC: Member of the Institute Management Consultants
MIN: Minimum
MIPS: Monthly Income Preferred Security
MIP: Mortgage Insurance Premium
MIRR: Modified Internal Rate of Return
MIS: Management Information System
MIS: Moody's Investment Service
MISER: Massachusetts Institute for Social and Economic Research
MIT: Market If Touched
MIT: Master of Information Technology
MIT: Municipal Investment Trust
MJSD: March, June, September, December cycle
ML: Matched and Lost
MLN: Million
MLP: Master Limited Partnership
MLP: Mid-Level Provider
MLR: Medical Loss Ratio
MM: Member Month
MMA: Money Market Account
MMDA: Money Market Deposit Account
MMF: Money Market Fund
MMM: Master of Medical Management
MMMF: Money Market Mutual Fund

MMSA: Medicare Medical Savings Account
MNC: Multinational Corporation
MO: Money Order
MOB: Municipals Over Bonds
MOC: Market On Close
MODD: Modified Duration
MOO: Market On Opening
MOS: Margin Of Safety
MOU: Memorandum Of Understanding
MP: Marginal Product
MP: Market Price
MPB: Marginal Private Benefit
MPC: Market Performance Committee
MPC: Marginal Private Cost
MPC: Marginal Propensity to Consume
MPCA: Medical Practice Cost Analysis
MPCA: Medical Project Cost Analysis
MPFS: Medicare Physician Fee Schedule
MPFSDB: Medicare Physician Fee Schedule Data Base
MPI: Master Patient Index
MPI: Master Person Index
MPI: Master Provider Index
MPRC: Medicare Payment Review Commission
MPS: Marginal Propensity to Save
MPT: Modern Portfolio Theory
MPV: Minimum Price Variance
MPY: Member Per Year
MR: Marginal Revenue
MRDF: Machine Readable Data File
MRP: Marginal Revenue Product
MRP: Maximum Reimbursement Point
MRP: Minimum Risk Portfolio
MRS: Marginal Rate of Substitution
MRT: Marginal Rate of Tax
MS: Majority Stockholder
MS: Master of Science
MS: Minority Stockholder
MSA: Medical Savings Account
MSA: Metropolitan Statistical Area
MSB: Marginal Social Benefit
MSD: Master of Science in Dentistry
MSE: Madrid Stock Exchange
MSE: Mexican Stock Exchange

MSE: Midwest Stock Exchange

MSFS: Master of Science in Financial Services

MSO: Medical Services Organization

MSP: Medicare Secondary Payer

MSRB: Municipal Securities Rulemaking Board

MTA: Monthly Treasury Average

MTDC: Modified Total Direct Costs

MTF: Military Treatment Facility

MTN: Medium Term Note

MUA: Medically Underserved Area

MU: Marginal Utility

MUD: Municipal Utility District

MUNI: Municipal Security

MV: Market Value

MVA: Medical Value Added

MVPS: Medicare Volume Performance Standard

MY: Member Year

N: New Issue

N: Number of time periods

NA: National Association

NA: No Approval

NABE: National Association for Business Economics

NACHA: National Automated Clearing House Association

NACVA: National Association of Certified Valuation Analysts

NAFE: National Association of Forensic Economists

NAFTA: North American Free Trade Agreement

NAHC: National Association of Health Care Consultants

NAHMOR: National Association of Health Maintenance Organization Regulators

NAIC: National Association of Investment Clubs

NAIC: National Association of Investors Corporation

NAIRU: Nonaccelerating Inflation Rate of Unemployment

NAPFA: National Association of Personal Financial Advisors

NAPH: National Association of Public Hospitals

NAPHS: National Association of Psychiatric Health Systems

NAR: Net Accounts Receivable

NAS: Nonavailability Statement

NASAA: North American Securities Administrators' Association

NASBA: National Association of State Boards of Accountancy

NASD: National Association of Securities Dealers, Inc.

NASDAQ: National Association of Securities Dealers Automated Quotation system

NASDIM: National Association of Securities Dealers and Investment Managers

NAV: Net Asset Value

NAVPS: Net Asset Value Per Share

NBIA: National Business Incubation Association

NBS: National Bureau of Standards

NBVG: National Business Valuation Group

NC: Net Capital

NC: No Charge

NC: Noncallable

NCAHC: National Council on Alternative Health Care

NCCBH: National Council for Community Behavioral Health Care

NCH: National Claims History

NCHS: National Center for Health Statistics

NCN: Net Cost per Nurse

NCPAHAA: National CPA Health Advisory Association

NCQA: National Committee for Quality Assurance

NCS: Noncallable Securities

NCV: No Commercial Value

ND: Next Day

NDC: National Drug Code

NDF: Nondeliverable Funds

NE: Net Earnings

NEC: Not Elsewhere Classified

NEMS: National Exchange Market System
NEO: Nonequity Options
NFA: National Futures Association
NFE: Net Fixed Expenses
NFP: Not-for-Profit
NFPC: Not-for-Profit Corporation
NH: New High
NH: Not Held
NHCAA: National Health Care Antifraud Association
NHCQA: National Health Care Cost and Quality Association
NHCT: National Health Care Trust
NHCTF: National Health Care Trust Fund
NHDS: National Hospital Discharge Survey
NHE: National Health Expenditures
NHF: National Health Fund
NHI: National Health Insurance
NHIP: National Health Insurance Plan
NHO: National Hospital Organization/ Operation
NHS: National Health Service
NI: Negotiable Instrument
NIBT: Net Income Before Tax
NIC: Net Interest Change
NIC: Net Interest Cost
NIEO: New International Economic Order
NIH: National Institute of Health
NIM: Net Interest Margin
NIP: Normal Investment Practice
NIPA: National Income and Product Accounts
NIRF: NASD Information Request Form
NIS: Net Income Statement
NISAC: National Infrastructure Simula- tion and Analysis Center
NIT: Negative Income Tax
NL: No Load
NLF: No Load Fund
NLO: No Limit Order
NM: Narrow Market
NMAB: National Marketing Advisory Board
NMES: National Medical Expenditure Survey
NMF: Nonmember Firm

NMS: National Market System
NMS: Normal Market Size
NOA: Notice Of Admission
NOB: Notes Over Bonds
NOBA: Notice Of Budget Authority
NOI: Net Operating Income
NOI: Notice Of Intent
NOL: Net Operating Loss
Non-PAR: Nonparticipating Physician (Provider)
NOR: Non-Operating Revenue
NORC: National Opinion Research Center
NOS: Not Otherwise Specified
NOW: Negotiable Order of Withdrawal
NP: Net Position
NP: No Protest
NP: Nonprofit
NP: Notary Public
NP: Note Payable
NPDA: National Practitioner Data Bank
NPI: National Physician (Provider) Identification
NPO: Nonprofit Organization
NPP: Nonparticipating Physician/ Provider
NPP: Nonparticipating Practitioner
NPP: Nonprofessional Provider
NPR: Notice of Program Reimbursement
NPR: Notice of Proposed Rulemaking
NPSR: Net Patient Services Revenue
NPV: Net Present Value
NPV: No Par Value
NPVS: Nonpar Value Stock
NQB: National Quotation Bureau
NQB: No Qualified Bidders
NQDC: Nonqualified Deferred Compensation
NQDS: NASD Quotation Dissemination Service
NR: Not rated
NR: Note Receivable
NRHA: National Rural Health Association
NRO: Nonresident Owned
NRPMP: Net Revenue Per Medical Provider
NRPP: Net Revenue Per Physician
NSBA: National Small Business Association

NSCC: National Securities Clearing Corporation
NSE: National Stock Exchange
NSF: National Standard Format
NSF: Nonsufficient Funds
NSTA: National Securities Trade Association
NSTS: National Securities Trading Systems
NTU: Normal Trading Units
NUBC: National Uniform Billing Committee
NUCC: National Uniform Claim Committee
NUCO: New Company
NV: Nominal Value
NVS: Nonvoting Stock
NW: Net Worth
NWC: Net Working Capital
NWCRP: National Workers Compensation Reinsurance Pool
NY: Net Yield
NYACH: New York Automated Clearing House
NYBOT: New York Board Of Trade
NYCE: New York Curb Exchange (ASE)
NYCHA: New York Clearing House Association
NYFE: New York Futures Exchange
NYM: New York Mercantile Exchange
NYME: New York Mercantile Exchange
NYMEX: New York Mercantile Exchange
NYSE: New York Stock Exchange

O: Old options listing
OA: Open Access
OARS: Opening Automated Report Service
OASM: Option Adjusted Spread Model
OASDHI: Old Age Survivors and Disability Health Insurance
OATS: Orders Audit Trail Systems
OB: Or Better
OBO: Order Book Official
OBRA: Omnibus Budget Reconciliation Act

OBV: On Balance Value
OC: Opportunity Cost
OC: Overhead Cost
OCA: Outstanding Claims Account
OCBOA: Other Comprehensive Basis Of Accounting
OCC: Options Clearing Corporation
OCO: One Cancels the Other
OD: Other Diagnosis
OD: Overdraft, overdrawn
ODR: Office of Direct Reimbursement
ODS: Organized Delivery System
OECD: Organization of Economic Cooperation and Development
OEF: Open End Fund
OEIC: Open End Investment Company
OEIT: Open End Investment Trust
OEX: Standard & Poor's 100 Stock Index
OF: Offshore Funds
OHI: Other Health Insurance
OI: Ordinary Interest
OID: Original Issue Discount
OIG: Office of the Inspector General
OL: Odd Lot
OL: Operating Leverage
OM: On Margin
OM: Open Market
OM: Outcomes Management
OMB: Office of Management and Budget
ONAS: Out-Patient Nonavailability Statement
ONS: Out-Patient Nonavailability Statement
OO: Open Order
OOA: Out Of Area
OOAB: Out Of Area Benefit
OON: Out Of Network
OOP: Out Of Pocket
OOPC: Out-Of-Pocket Charges
OOPC: Out-Of-Pocket Costs
OP: Offering Price
OP: Opening Price
OP: Opening Purchase
OP: Out Patient
OP: Over Payment
OPD: Out Patient Department

OPL: Operational Policy Letter
OPL: Other Party Liability
OPHC: Office of Prepaid Health Care
OPHCOO: Office of Prepaid Health Care Operations and Oversight
OPM: Office of Personnel Management
OPM: Options Pricing Model
OPM: Other People's Money
OPPS: Outpatient Prospective Payment System
OPRA: Options Pricing Reporting Authority
OPREB: Other Post-Retirement Employment Benefit
OR: Occupancy Rate
OR: Operating Room
OSC: Outpatient Surgery Center
OSG: Office of the Surgeon General
OSHA: Occupational Safety and Health Administration
OSJ: Office of Supervisory Jurisdiction
OSS: Order Support System
OT: Outlier Threshold
OT: Over Time
OTB: Off The Board
OTC: Over The Counter
OTCBB: Over The Counter Bulletin Board
OTS: Office of Thrift Supervision
OW: Offer Wanted
OWC: Owner Will Carry
OWCP: Office of Worker's Compensation Program

P: Paid this year
P: Put, in options newspaper listing
P: Price, or probability of occurrence
P = MC: Price equals marginal cost
P2P: Patient to Patient
P2P: Patient to Physician
P2P: Peer to Peer
PA: Paying Agent
PA: Patriot Act
PA: Per Anum
PA: Physician Assistant
PA: Power of Attorney

PA: Privacy Act
PA: Purchasing Agent
PA: Purchasing Alliance
PAAF: Pre-Admission Assessment Form
PAB: Private Activity Bond
PAC: Planned Amortization Class
PAC: Pre-Admission Certification
PAC: Pre-Authorized Check
PAC: Put and Call Options market
PACE: Performance And Cost Efficiency
PAL: Passive Activity Loss
PAM: Patient Accounts Manager
PAR: PARticipating Physician (Provider) or Supplier
PAR: Price Adjusted Rate
PATH: Physician At Teaching Hospital
PAYE: Pay As You Earn
PAYERID: Medicare Pre-HIPAA National Payer ID Initiative
PAYSOP: Payroll-based Stock Ownership Plan
PdeB: Paris Bourse
PB: Patient Broker
PBC: Pro Bono Care
PBGC: Pension Benefit Guarantee Corporation
PBL: Point Balance
PBM: Pharmacy Benefits Manager
PBM: Prescription Benefits Manager
PBO: Pension Benefit Obligation
PBP: Prescription Benefits Pharmacy
PBVR: Price to Book Valuation Ratio
PC: Paid Claim
PC: Participation Certificates
PC: Per Case
PC: Perfect Competition
PC: Plus Commission
PC: Pre-existing Condition
PC: Prepaid Care
PC: Price to Cash flow ratio
PC: Professional Corporation
PC: Per Capita
PC: Purchasing Coalition
PC: Purchasing Cooperative
PCAOB: Public Company Accounting Oversight Board

PCCM: Primary Care Case Management
PCLR: Paid Claim Loss Ratio
PCCO: Physician-sponsored Coordinated Care Organization
PHO: Physician (Provider) Hospital Organization
PCM: Primary Care Manager
PCP: Primary Care Physician
PCP: Primary Care Provider
PC/PM: Per Contract/Per Month
PC/PM: Pharmacy Contract/Per Month
PCR: Per Case Review
PCR: Physician Contingency Reserve
PCR: Policy Contingency Reserve
PCX: Pacific Exchange
PDP: Payables Deferral Period
PDV: Present Discounted Value
PE: Physician Expenses
PE: Practice Expense
PE: Price Earnings Ratio
PE: Provider Expenses
PEBES: Personal Earnings and Benefit Statement
PEC: Pharmaco-Economics Center
PEC: Pre-Existing Condition
PED: Price Elasticity of Demand
PEG: Prospective Earnings Growth
PEL: Permanent Employer Leasing
PEL: Physician Employer Leasing
PEO: Permanent Employer Outsourcing
PEO: Physician Employer Outsourcing
PEPM: Per Employee Per Month
PEPP: Payment Error Prevention Program
PER: Price Earnings Ratio
PERLS: Principal Exchange Rate-Linked Securities
PFCRA: Program Fraud Civil Remedies Act
PFD: Preferred Stock
PFP: Personal Financial Planner
PFS: Personal Financial Specialist
PHCO: Physician Hospital Community Organization
PHLX: Philadelphia Stock Exchange
PHO: Physician Hospital Organization
PHP: Prepaid Health Plan

PhRMA: Pharmaceutical Research and Manufacturers of America
PHS: Public Health Service
PI: Principle and Interest
PI: Profitability Index
PIA: Patient Income Account
PIA: Personal Incidental Allowance
PIBOR: Paris Interbank Offered Rate
PIK: Payment-in-Kind
PIKS: Payment-in-Kind Securities
PIN: Personal Identification Number
PIP: Periodic Interim Payment
PITI: Principal, Interest, Taxes, and Insurance
PL: Price List
PL: Public Law
P&L: Profit and Loss
PLAM: Price Level Adjusted Mortgage
PLC: Public Liability Company
PLI: Professional/Physician Liability Insurance
PM: Primary Market
PM: Program Memorandum
PMC: Physician Management Corporation
PME: Point of Maximum Efficiency
PMM: Purchase Money Mortgage
PMOS: Profit Margin On Sales
PMPM: Per Member Per Month
PMPY: Per Member Per Year
PMS: Profit Margin on Sales
PMT: Payment
PMV: Private Market Value
PN: Project Note
PN: Promissory Note
PNA: Personal Needs Allowance
PNI: Participate, Not Initiate
PO: Physician (Provider) Organization
PO: Principal Only
PO: Purchase Order
POA: Power of Attorney
POB: Point of Business
POB: Public Oversight Board
POP: Public Offering Price
POR: Pay On Return
POS: Point Of Sale

POS: Point Of Service
POTGR: Point Of Total Government Responsibility
PP: Paper Profit
PP: Percent of Premium
PP: Purchase Price
PPA: Patient Protection Act
PPA: Preferred Provider Arrangement
PPA: Partnership for Prescription Assistance
PPD: Per Patient Day
PPF: Production Possibilities Frontier
PPGP: Pre-Paid Group Practice
PPI: Producer Price Index
PPM: Physician Practice Management
PPMC: Physician Practice Management Corporation
PPN: Preferred Provider Network
PPO: Preferred Provider Organization
PPP: Purchasing Power Parity
PPR: Physician (Provider) Patient Relationship
PPRC: Physician Payment Review Commission/Comparison
PPS: Prospective Payment System
PR: Peer Review
PR: Periodic Rate
PR: Pro Rata
PRA: Paperwork Reduction Act
PRC: Physician Review Committee
PRE-RE: Pre-Refunded Municipal Note
PRG: Procedure Related Group
PRIME: Prescribed Right to Income and Maximum Equity
PRO: Peer Review Organization
ProPAC: Prospective Payment Assessment Commission
PRRB: Physician (Provider) Reimbursement Review Board
PRV: Practice (Expense) Relative Value
PS: Penny Stock
PS: Pink Sheets
PS: Preferred Stocks
PS: Price Spread
PS: Price to Sell ratio

PS: Purchase/Sale
PSA: Public Securities Association
PSE: Pacific Stock Exchange
PSID: Panel Study of Income Dynamics
PSLRA: Private Securities Litigation Reform Act
PSO: Physician (Provider) Sponsored Organization
PT: Paper Title
PT: Passing Title
PT: Perfect Title
PT: Profit Taking
PTA: Prior To Admission
PTMPY: Per Thousand Members Per Year
PUFF: Proposed Use of Federal Funds
PUHCA: Public Utility Holding Company Act
PV: Present Value
PVF: Present Value Factor
PVH: Private Voluntary Hospital
PVR: Profit/Volume Ratio
PVSG: Practice Valuation Study Group
PX: Price

Q: Quarterly
Q: Unit sales
QA: Quick Assets
QAPI: Quality Insurance and Performance Improvement
QARI: Quality Assurance Reform Initiative
QB: Qualified Buyer
QC: Quality Control
QDCP: Qualified Deferred Compensation Plan
QDRO: Qualified Domestic Relations Order
QDS: Quote Dissemination System
QFP: Qualified Financial Planner
QI: Quarterly Index
QIRI: Quality Insurance Reform Initiative
QLY: Quality of Life Year
QMB: Qualified Medicare Beneficiary
QP: Quoted Price
QPA: Qualified Pension Administrator
QPP: Qualified Pension Plan

QQQQ: Qubes (ETFs)
QR: Quick Ratio
QS: Quality Stock
QT: Quotation Ticker
QT: Questionable Trade

r: Correlation coefficient
R: Declared or paid in preceding 12 months plus stock dividend
R: Option not traded in newspapers
R: Range
R: Register
R: Right
RA: Remittance Advice
RA: Restricted Account
RADAR: Research And Data Analysis Reporting system
RADT: Registration, Admission, Discharge, and Transfer
RAM: Receipts of Accrual on Municipal Securities
RAM: Reverse Annuity Mortgage
RAN: Revenue Anticipation Note
RAPS: Resource Analysis and Planning System
RAROC: Rate Adjusted Return On Capital
RAROE: Rate Adjusted Return On Equity
RATS: Regression Analysis of Time Series
RB: Rating Board
RBC: Real Business Cycle
RBE: Risk Bearing Entity
RBNI: Reported But Not Incurred
RBRVS: Resource Based Relative Value Scale
RC: Reasonable Charges
RC: Reasonable & Customary
RC: Risk Capital
RCC: Reasonable & Customary Charge
RCC: Ratio of Charges to Costs
RCC: Ratio of Costs to Charges
RCCAC: Ratio of Charges to Charges (or Costs to Charges) Applied to Costs (Charges)
RCMM: Registered Competitive Market Maker
RCP: Receivables Collection Period
RD: Research and Development

RDRG: Revised Diagnostic Related Group
REB: Reportable Economic Benefit
REBC: Registered Employee Benefits Consultant
RED: Refund Escrow Deposit
REIT: Real Estate Investment Trust
REMIC: Real Estate Mortgage Investment Conduit
REMM: Registered Equity Market Maker
REPO: Repurchase agreement
RETRO: Retrospective rate derivation
RFA: Registered Financial Analyst designate
RFA: Registered Financial Associate
RFA: Regulatory Flexibility Act
RFC: Registered Financial Consultant
RFG: Registered Financial Gerontologist
RFP: Registered Financial Planner
RFP: Request for Proposal
RFQ: Request for Quotation
RH: Red Herring
RHA: Regional Health Administrator
RHFM: Research in Health Care Financial Management
RHIA: Registered Health Information Administrator
RHIE: Rand Health Insurance Experiment
RHIT: Registered Health Information Technologist
RHPC: Responsible Health Policy Coalition
RHU: Registered Health Underwriter
RI: Residual Income
RIA: Registered Investment Advisor
RIC: Regulated Investment Company
RICO: Racketeer Influenced and Corrupt Organization Act
RIF: Reduction In Force
RL: Round Lot
RM: Risk Management
ROA: Return On Assets
ROC: Return On Capital
ROCE: Return On Capital Employed
ROD: Return On Debt
ROE: Return On Equity
ROI: Return On Investment
RONA: Return On Net Assets

RONW: Return On Net Worth
ROP: Registered Options Principal
ROR: Rate Of Return
ROS: Return On Sales
ROTA: Return On Total Assets
RP: Risk Premium
RPA: Retirement Protection Act
RPI: Residual Practice Income
RPI: Retail Price Index
RPm: Risk Premium of the Market
RPQ: Request for Price Quotation
RR: Rate Regulations
RR: Rate Review
RR: Registered Representative
RRA: Registered Record Administrator
RRP: Reverse Repurchase Agreement
RS: Redeemable Stock
RSA: Risk Sensitive Analysis
RSA: Risk Sensitive Assets
RSL: Risk Sensitive Liabilities
RTC: Resolution Trust Corporation
RTS: Russian Trading System
RTU: Relative Time Unit
RTW: Right To Work
RUG: Resource Utilization Group
RVS: Relative Value Scale
RVS: Relative Value Study/Scale/
    Schedule
RVU: Relative Value Unit
RVW: Relative Value Weight
RWP: Relative Weighted Product

S&P: Standard & Poor's
S: No option offered
S: Sales in U.S. dollars
S: Signed
SA: Seasonally Adjusted
SA: Society of Actuaries
SAA: Single Audit Act
SAA: Special Arbitrage Account
SAAR: Seasonally Adjusted Annual Rate
SAB: Special Assessment Bond
SAI: Statement of Additional Information
SAIF: Savings Association Insurance
    Fund
SAR: Stock Appreciation Rights

SARBOX: Sarbanes-Oxley Act
SARSEP: Salary Reduction Simplified
    Employee Pension Plan
SAS: Statement of Auditing Standards
SAV: Small Area Variation
SAYE: Save as You Earn
SB: Savings Bond
SBA: Small Business Administration
SBA: Small Business Association
SBI: Share of Beneficial Interest
SBIC: Small Business Investment
    Corporation (Company)
SBU: Strategic Business Unit
SCC: Stock Clearing Corporation
SCH: Sole Community Hospital
SCOR: Small Corporate Offering
    Registration
SCORE: Special Claims On Residual
    Equity
SCP: Sole Community Provider
SD: Settlement Date
SD: Standard Deduction
SD: Stock Dividend
SDC: Secondary Diagnostic Category
SDFS: Same Day Funds Settlement
SDP: Single Drug Pricer
SE: Self Employed
SE: Shareholder's Equity
SE: Standard Error
SE: Stock Exchange
SEAQ: Stock Exchange Automated
    Quotations
SEC: Securities Exchange Commission
SECO: Securities Exchange Commission
    Organization
SECPS: Securities Exchange Commission
    Practice Section
SEP: Simplified Employee Plan
SERIES 3: Commodities license
SERIES 4: Registered options principle
    license
SERIES 5: Interest rate options license
SERIES 7: General securities license
SERIES 8: General securities sales super-
    vision license
SERIES 15: Foreign currency options
    license

SERIES 16: Supervisory analyst license

SERIES 24: General securities principal license

SERIES 26: Investment company and variable contracts principal license

SERIES 27: Financial and options principal license

SERIES 28: Introducing broker/dealer financial operations principal license

SERIES 52: Municipal securities representative license

SERIES 53: Municipal securities principal license

SERIES 62: Corporate securities representative

SERIES 63: Mutual fund license

SERIES 65: Uniform securities agent state license

SERP: Supplemental Executive Retirement Plan

SF: Sinking Fund

SFA: Stochastic Frontier Analysis

SFAS: Statement of Financial Accounting Standards

SFE: Sydney Futures Exchange

SFR: Substantial Financial Risk

SFSP: Society of Financial Service Professionals

SG: Surgeon General

SGA: Sales, General, and Administrative

SGA: Sustainable Growth Adjustments

SGE: Substantial Gainful Employment

SGR: Sustainable Growth Rate

SH: Shareholder

SH: Stockholder

SHPM: Society for Health Care Planning and Marketing

SI: Severity Index

SI: Simple Interest

SIA: Securities Industry Association

SIAC: Securities Industry Automation Corporation

SIBOR: Singapore Interbank Offered Rate

SIC: Split Investment Company

SIC: Standard Industrial Classification

SICA: Securities Industry Committee on Arbitrage

SID: Supplier Induced Demand

SIMPLE: Savings Incentive Match Plan for Employees

SIMPLE-IRA: Savings Incentive Match Plan for Employees-IRA

SIP: Sharebuilder Investment Plan

SIPC: Securities Investment Protection Corporation

SIT: State Income Tax

SL: Sales and Leaseback

SL: Savings and Loan

SL: Sold

SLA: Savings and Loan Association

SLD: Sold

SLMA: Student Loan Marketing Association; Sallie Mae

SLO: Stop-Loss Order

SLS: Sold Last Sale

SMA: Society of Management Accountants

SMA: Special Miscellaneous Account

SMART: Securities Market Automated Regulated Trading architecture

SMI: Supplemental Medical Insurance

SML: Security Market Line

SMS: Socioeconomic Monitoring System

SMV: Short Market Value

SN: Stock Number

SNOM: Systematized Nomenclature of Medicine

SO: Stock Option

SOB: Statement Of Benefit

SOC: Standard Of Care

SOES: Small Order Entry System

SOP: Standard Operating Procedure

SOP: Statement Of Policy

SOR: Stockholder Of Record

SORP: Senior Options Registered Principal

SOW: Statement Of Work

SOYD: Summary Of the Years' Digits method

SP: Salary Payable

SP: Short Position

SP: Standard of Performance
SP: Standards & Poor's
SP: Stock Price
SPD: Summary Plan Description
SPDA: Single Premium Deferred Annuity
SPDR: Standard & Poor's Depository Receipt
SPP: Select Provider (Physician) Program
SPP: Stock Purchase Price
SPX: Standard & Poor's 500 Stock Index
SRAC: Short Run Aggregate Cost
SRAS: Short Run Aggregate Supply
SRO: Self-Regulatory Organization
SRP: Salary Reduction Plan
SRT: Spousal Remainder Trust
SS: Selling Short
SS: Senior Securities
SS: Short Sale
SS: Shrinking Stocks
SS: Social Security
SSA: Social Security Administration
SSAE: Statements on Standards for Attestation Engagements
SSARS: Special Standards for Accounting and Review Services
SSE: Stockholm Stock Exchange
SSI: Supplemental Security Income
SSN: Social Security Number
SSOP: Second Surgical Opinion Program
ST: Standard Treatment
ST: Stock Transfer
STD: Short Term Disability
STP: Stop
STP LMT: Stop-Limit Order
STRIPS: Separate Trading of Registered Interest and Principle of Securities
SU: Set up
SUBC: State Uniform Billing Committee
SUR: Seemingly Unrelated Regressions
SUTA: State Unemployment Tax Act
SWARCH: Switching Autoregressive Regime Conditional Handle
SWAT: Stock Watch Automatic Tracking
SWG: Sub Work Group

t: Time
T: Number of transactions
T: Tax rate
T: Treasury
TA: Tax Abatement
TA: Technical Analyst
TA: Trade Acceptance
TA: Transfer Agent
TAB: Tax Anticipation Bill
TAC: Targeted Amortization Class
TAI: Tax Advantaged Investment
TAN: Tax Anticipation Note
TANF: Temporary Assistance to Needy Families
TASE: Tel Aviv Stock Exchange
TAT: Turn Around Time
TATR: Total Assets Turnover Ratio
TBE: Tenancy By the Entirety
TC: Total Cost
TCM: Treasury Constant Maturity
TD: Time Deposit
TD: Trade Date
TDA: Tax Deferred Annuity
TDA: Two (Three) Day Average
TDC: Total Direct Costs
TE: Travel and Expenses
TE: Trial and Error
TED: Treasury to Euro Dollar
TEFRA: Tax Equity and Fiscal Responsibility Acts of 1982–1983
TFC: Total Fixed Cost
TIC: Tenancy In Common
TIC: True Interest Cost
TIE: Time Interest Earned
TIER: Times Interest Earned Ratio
TIF: Tax Increment Funding
TIGR: Treasury Investors Growth Receipt
TIL: Truth In Lending
TIN: Tax Identification Number
TIP: Tax-based Income Policy
TIPS: Treasury Inflation Protected Securities
TL: Trade Last
TL: Trade Limit
TM: Third Market
TM: Trade Mark

TMTR: Third Market Trade Reporting
TO: Treasury Obligation
TPA: Third Party Administrator
TPO: Treatment, Payment, or Health Care Operations
TPR: Third Party Reimbursement
TRA: Taxpayer Relief Act of 1997
TR: Total Return
TR: Total Risk
TR: Treasury Receipt
TRACES: Trust Automatic Common Exchange Securities
TRS: Total Return Swaps
TSA: Tax Sheltered Annuity
TSE: Tokyo Stock Exchange
TSS: Trade Support System
TSX: Toronto Stock Exchange
TT: Transfer To
TT: Turnover Time
TU: Total Utility
TV: Terminal Value
TVA: Tennessee Valley Authority
TYX: Thirty Year Treasury Bonds

U&C: Usual and Customary
UAA: Uniform Accountancy Act
UAAL: Underfunded Actuarial Accrued Liability
UAL: Underfunded Actuarial Liability
UB: Uniform Bill, or Billing
UB-82: Uniform Billing Code, 1982
UB-92: Uniform Billing Code, 1992
UBI: Unit of Beneficial Interest
UBIT: Unrelated Business Income Tax
UCAS: Uniform Cost Accounting Standard
UCC: Uniform Commercial Code
UCF: Uniform Claim Form
UCR: Usual, Customary, and Reasonable
UCR/PACE: Usual, Customary, and Reasonable/Performance And Cost Efficiency
UCRS: Utilization Control Reporting System
UFCTF: Uniform Claim Task Force
UGMA: Uniform Gift to Minors Act

UHCIA: Uniform Health Care Information Act
UI: Unearned Income
UI: Unemployment Insurance
UIT: Unit Investment Trust
UL: Unauthorized Leave
UM: Utilization Management
UMA: Unified Management Account
UME: Un-reimbursed Medical Expense
UOM: Uniform Options Market
UOT: Unit Of Trading
UP: Unrealized Profit
UPC: Uniform Practice Code
UPC: Uniform Price (Product) Code
UPIN: Unique Patient Identification Number
UPIN: Unique Physician Identification Number
UPL: Upper Payment Limit
UR: Under Review
UR: Utilization Review
URO: Utilization Review Organization
US: Underlying Security
US: Unregistered Stock
USD: United States Dollar
USFMG: United States Foreign Medical Graduate
USIT: Unit Share Investment Trust
USPCC: United States Per Capita Cost
USSG: United States Surgeon General
USTF: Uniformed Service Treatment Facility
USU: Unbundled Stock Unit
UTMA: Uniform Transfer to Minors Act
UTP: Unlisted Trading Privileges
UW: Underwriter

V: Value

- **VI:** Value of a levered firm
- **Vu:** Value of an un-levered firm

V: Velocity of Money
V-CODE: Supplementary classification of factors influencing health status and contact with health services (VO1–V82)

VA: Veterans Administration
VA: Veteran Affairs
VADM: Very Accurately Defined Maturity
VAH: Veterans Affair Hospital
VAR: Value at Risk
VAT: Value Added Tax
VC: Variable Cost
VC: Venture Capitalist
VC: Voluntary Closing
VC: Voluntary Cost
VCF: Venture Capital Fund
VD: Volume Deleted
VD: Volume Discount
VI: Vested Interest
VI: Voluntary Insolvency
VIP: Voluntary Insurance Program
VLIS: Value Line Investment Survey
VOL: Volume
VPS: Volume Performance Standard
VRM: Variable Rate Mortgage
VSE: Vancouver Stock Exchange
VSP: Versus Purchase
VT: Voting Trust
VTC: Voting Trust Certificate

W: Proportion, or Weight

- **Wd** = Weight of debt
- **Wps** = Weight of preferred stock
- **Wce** = Weight of common equity

W: Wage Earner
WAC: Weighted Average Cost
WAC: Weighted Average Coupon
WACC: Weighted Average Cost of Capital
WCE: Winnipeg Commodity Exchange
WACM: Weak Axiom of Cost
   Minimization
WAL: Weighted Average Life
WAM: Weighted Average Maturity
WC: Worker's Compensation
WCA: Working Capital Account
WCA: Workmen's Compensation Act
WCB: Worker's Compensation Board
WD: When Distributed (in stock listing in
   newspapers)

WEBS: Worldwide Equity Benchmark
   Shares
WHO: World Health Organization
WI: When Issued
WIB: When Issued Basis
WL: Waiting List
WOTC: Work Opportunity Tax Credit
WOW: Written Order of Withdrawal
WPI: Wholesale Price Index
WPO: Weakly Pareto Optimal
WR: Warehouse Receipt
WS: Wall Street
WS: Watered Stock
WSE: Warsaw Stock Exchange
WSJ: Wall Street Journal
WT: Warrant
WTO: World Trade Organization
WV: Work Relative Value
WW: With Warrants

X: Exports
X: Ex-Interest (in newspapers)
XAM: AMEX Market Value Index
XC: Ex-Coupon
XCH: Ex-Clearing House
XD: Ex-Dividend (in newspapers)
X-DIS: Ex-Distribution (in newspapers)
XDIV: Ex-Dividend
XI: Ex-Interest
XMI: AMEX Major Market Index
XR: Ex-Rights
XR: X-Ray
XW: Ex-Warrants
XX: Without Securities, or Without Warrants

Y: Ex-Dividend and Sales in Full
Y: Yield
YLD: Yield
YR: Year
YS: Yield Spread
YTB: Yield To Broker
YTC: Yield To Call
YTD: Year To Date
YTD: Yield To Date
YTM: Yield To Maturity

YTM: Year To Month
YYS: Yo-Yo Stock

Z: Zero
ZBA: Zero Bracket Account

ZBB: Zero Based Budgeting
ZPG: Zero Population Growth
ZPHMO: Zero Premium Health Maintenance Organization
ZR: Zero Coupon Issue

Bibliography

PRINT MEDIA TEXTBOOKS

American Medical Association. (2001). *Benchmark capitation rates: The physician's how-to guide for calculating Fee-for-service equivalents.* Chicago, IL: Author.

American Organization of Nurse Executives (AONE). (2000). *Nurse recruitment and retention study.* Chicago, IL: Author.

Austin, C. J., & Boxerman, S. B. (1995). *Quantitative analysis for health services administration.* Arlington, VA: AUPHA Press; Ann Arbor, MI: Health Administration Press.

Austrin, M. S. (1999). *Managed healthcare simplified.* Albany, NY: Delmar Thomson Learning.

Baker, J. (2006). *Management accounting for health care organizations: Tools and techniques for decision support.* Sudbury, MA: Jones and Bartlett Publishers.

Baker, J. (2006). *Health care finance: Basic tools for nonfinancial managers* (2nd ed.). Sudbury, MA: Jones and Bartlett Publishers.

Baker, J. J. (1998). *Activity-based costing and activity-based management for health care.* Gaithersburg, MD: Aspen.

Berkowitz, E. N. (2006). *Essentials of health care marketing* (2nd ed.). Sudbury, MA: JB Publishers.

Bode, G. L. (2000). Medical practice economic report card. In D. E. Marcinko (Ed.), *The business of medical practice.* New York: Springer Publishing.

Bode, G. L. (2003). Employee benefits and stock options. In D. E. Marcinko (Ed.), *Financial planner's library on CD-ROM.* New York: Aspen Publishing.

Bode, G. L. (2003). Using deductions and credits to reduce taxable income. In D. E. Marcinko (Ed.), *Financial planner's library on CD-ROM.* New York: Aspen Publishing.

Bode, G. L. (2004). Medical practice financial benchmarking. In D. E. Marcinko (Ed.), *The advanced business of medical practice.* New York: Springer Publishing.

Brigham, E., & Gapenski, L. G. (1999). *Financial management.* New York: Dryden Press.

Britt, T., Schraeder, C., & Shelton, P. (1998). *Managed care and capitation: Issues in nursing practice.* Washington, D.C.: American Nurses Publishing.

Broyles, R. (2006). *Fundamentals of statistics in health administration.* Sudbury, MA: Jones and Bartlett Publishers.

Cimasi, R. J. (in press). Lessons in market competition for healthcare organizations. In D. E. Marcinko (Ed.), *Financial management of healthcare organizations.* Blaine, WA: Specialty Technical Publications.

Cimasi, R. J. (in press). Valuation of healthcare entities. In D. E. Marcinko (Ed.), *Financial management of healthcare organizations*. Blaine, WA: Specialty Technical Publications.

Cleverley, W. (2003). *Essentials of health care finance*. Sudbury, MA: Jones and Bartlett Publishers.

Committee on Quality of Health Care in America. (2001). *Crossing the quality chasm: A new health system for the 21st century*. Washington, DC: National Academy Press.

Council on Graduate Medical Education. (1995). *Managed health care: Implications for the physician workforce and medical education. Sixth report*. Rockville, MD: U.S. Department of Health and Human Services, Public Health Service, Health Resources and Services Administration.

Council on Graduate Medical Education. (1999). *Physician education for a changing health care environment. Thirteenth report*. Rockville, MD: U.S. Department of Health and Human Services, Public Health Service, Health Resources and Services Administration.

The Commonwealth Fund Task Force on Academic Health Centers. (2002). *Training tomorrow's doctors: The medical education mission of academic health centers*. New York: The Commonwealth Fund.

Culyer, A. J. (2005). *The dictionary of health economics*. Cheltenham, Glos.: Edward Elgar Publishing.

Dacso, S. T., & Dacso, C. C. (1999). *Risk contracting and capitation answer book: Strategies for managed care*. Gaithersburg, MD: Aspen.

Drummond, M., Sculpher, M. J., Torrance, G. W., O'Brien, B. J., & Stoddart, G. L. (2005). *Methods for the economic evaluation of health care programs* (3rd ed.). Oxford: Oxford University Press.

Eastaugh, S. (2004). *Health care finance and economics*. Sudbury, MA: Jones and Bartlett Publishers.

Eastaugh, S. R. (1998). *Health care finance: Cost, productivity, and strategic design*. Gaithersburg, MD: Aspen.

Feldstein, P. J. (1999). *Health care economics* (5th ed.). Albany: Delmar Publishers.

Feldstein, P. J. (2002). *Health policy issues: An economic perspective* (3rd ed.). Chicago, IL: Health Administration Press.

Filippone, S. R. (1996). *Elementary mathematics*. Boston, MA: Houghton Mifflin.

Fine, A. (in press). *Health care technology assessment handbook*. Sudbury, MA: JB Publishers.

Finkler, S. (2004). *Essentials of cost accounting for health care organizations*. Sudbury, MA: Jones and Bartlett Publishers.

Finkler, S. (2006). *Accounting fundamentals for health care management*. Sudbury, MA: Jones and Bartlett Publishers.

Finkler, S. A., & Ward, D. M. (1999). *Cost accounting for health care organizations: Concepts and applications* (2nd ed.). Gaithersburg, MD: Aspen.

Finkler, S. A., & Ward, D. M. (1999) *Issues in cost accounting for health care organizations* (2nd ed.). Gaithersburg, MD: Aspen.

Firebaugh, W., & Marcinko, D. E. (in press). Hospital endowment fund management. In D. E. Marcinko (Ed.), *Financial management of healthcare organizations*. Blaine, WA: Specialty Technical Publications.

Foland, S., Goodman, A., & Stano, M. (2001). *The economics of health and healthcare*. New York: Prentice-Hall.

Francis, B. (2003). Valuing the closely held business. In D. E. Marcinko (Ed.), *Financial planner's library on CD-ROM*. New York: Aspen Publishing.

Frank, C. (2000). *Physician empowerment through capitation*. Sudbury, MA: Jones and Bartlett Publishers.

Gapenski, L. C. (1999). *Healthcare finance: An introduction to accounting and financial management*. Chicago, IL: Health Administration Press.

Getzen, T. (1990). Macro forecasting of national health expenditures. In L. Rossiter & R. Scheffler (Eds.), *Advances in health economics*, (vol. 11, pp. 27–48).

Getzen, T. (1997). *Health economics: Fundamentals and flow of funds*. New York: John Wiley & Sons.

Getzen, T. E. (2004). *Health economics: Fundamentals and flow of funds* (2nd ed.). New York: John Wiley & Sons.

Ginn, G. (2006). Sarbox and patriot acts for hospitals. In D. E. Marcinko (Ed.), *Financial management of healthcare organizations*. Blaine, WA: Specialty Technical Publications.

Gold, M. R., Siegel, J. E., Russell, L. B., & Weinstein, M. C. (1996). *Cost-effectiveness in health and medicine*. New York: Oxford University Press.

Goldfield, N. (1999). *Ambulatory care services and the prospective payment*. Sudbury, MA: Jones and Bartlett Publishers.

Goldfield, N. (1999). *Physician profiling and risk adjustment* (2nd ed.). Gaithersburg, MD: Aspen.

Grodzki, L. (2000). *Building your ideal private practice—How to love what you do and be highly profitable too*. New York: WW Norton and Company.

Guillem Lapez-Casasnovas, B. R., & Currais, L. (2005). *Health and economic growth: Findings and policy implications*. Boston, MA: The MIT Press.

Hermanson, R. H., & Edwards, J. D. (2001). *Financial accounting*. Homewood, IL: Irwin.

Herzlinger, R. (1994). *Financial accounting and managerial control for non-profit organizations*. Gaithersburg, MD: Aspen.

Hetico, H. R. (2004). Choosing medical management consultants wisely. In D. E. Marcinko (Ed.), *The advanced business of medical practice*. New York: Springer Publishing.

Hetico, H. R. (2003). Selecting your financial advisory team. In D. E. Marcinko (Ed.), *Financial planning for physicians and healthcare professionals.* New York: Aspen Publishing.

Hetico, H. R. (2004). Selecting financial planners and business consultants wisely. In D. E. Marcinko (Ed.), *Financial planning for physicians and advisors.* Sudbury, MA: Jones and Bartlett Publishers.

Hetico, H. R. (2005). Selecting insurance advisors wisely. In D. E. Marcinko (Ed.), *Insurance and risk management strategies for physicians and advisors.* Sudbury, MA: Jones and Bartlett Publishers.

Horngren, C. T. (1999). *Accounting.* Upper Saddle River, NJ: Prentice-Hall.

Hyman, D. N. (1998). *Economics.* Boston, MA: Irwin Press.

Institute of Certified Public Accountants (1998). *AICPAs Audit and Accounting Guides for Healthcare Organizations.* Chicago, IL: Author.

Isenberg, S. F., & Gliklich, R. E. (1999). *Profiting from quality: Outcomes strategies for medical practice.* San Francisco, CA: Jossey-Bass.

Jacobs, P. (2004). *The economics of health and medical care.* Sudbury, MA: Jones and Bartlett Publishers.

Javier, J., Marcinko, D. E., & Hetico, H. R. (2003). Post mortem estate planning. In H. S. Margolis (Ed.), *The elder law portfolio series.* New York: Aspen Publishing.

Kongstvedt, P. (2003). *Best practices in medical management: The managed health care handbook series.* Sudbury, MA: Jones and Bartlett Publishers.

Kongstvedt, P. (2004). *The managed health care handbook* (3rd ed.). [CD-ROM]. Sudbury, MA: Jones and Bartlett Publishers.

Krider, B. (1997). *Valuation of physician practices and clinics.* Sudbury, MA: Jones and Bartlett Publishers.

Lee, D. W. (1995). *Capitation: The physicians' guide.* Chicago, IL: American Medical Association.

Lexicon: Dictionary of heath care terms, organizations, and acronyms. (2nd ed.). (1998). Oakbrook Terrace, IL: Joint Commission on Accreditation of Healthcare Organizations.

Mansfield, E. (1998). *Principles of macroeconomics.* New York: WW Norton and Company.

Marcinko, D. E. (2000). *The business of medical practice.* New York: Springer Publishing.

Marcinko, D. E. (Ed.). (2003). *Financial planner's library on CD-ROM.* New York: Aspen Publishing.

Marcinko, D. E. (2003). *Financial planning for physicians and healthcare professionals.* New York: Aspen Publishing.

Marcinko, D. E. (2004). *The advanced business of medical practice.* New York: Springer Publishing.

Marcinko, D. E. (Ed.). (2004). *Financial planning for physicians and advisors.* Sudbury, MA: Jones and Bartlett Publishers.

Marcinko, D. E. (2005, March). Do not make these investment mistakes. *Physicians Practice.* p. 61.

Marcinko, D. E. (Ed.). (2005). *Insurance and risk management strategies for physicians and advisors.* Sudbury, MA: Jones and Bartlett Publishers.

Marcinko, D. E. (2005, February 15). How much is your medical practice worth? *Physician's Money Digest,* p. 26.

Marcinko, D. E. (2005, March). Recognizing new medical practice risks. *OB-GYN Physician's Money Digest.* p. 26.

Marcinko, D. E. (2005, June). Hedge your fund bets. *Physician Practice,* p. 67.

Marcinko, D. E. (2005, July–August). Appraising a medical practice. *Physician Practice,* p. 61.

Marcinko, D. E. (2005, October). Add more value to your medical practice. *Physician's Money Digest,* p. 18.

Marcinko, D. E. (Ed.). (2006). *Dictionary of health insurance and managed care.* New York: Springer Publishing.

Marcinko, D. E. (Ed.). (in press). *Financial management of healthcare organizations.* Blaine, WA: Specialty Technical Publications.

Marcinko, D. E., & Hetico, H. R. (2003). Financial planning for the elderly. In H. S. Margolis (Ed.), *The elder law portfolio series.* New York: Aspen Publishing.

Marcinko, D. E., & Hetico, H. R. (in press). Cash flow, budgeting and working capital management for hospitals. In D. E. Marcinko (Ed.), *Financial management of healthcare organizations.* Blaine, WA: Specialty Technical Publications.

Marcinko, D. E., & Piasecki, D. (in press) EOQC in healthcare inventory management. In D. E. Marcinko (Ed.), *Financial management of healthcare organizations.* Blaine, WA: Specialty Technical Publications.

Mayo, H. (2000). *Investments—An introduction.* New York: Dryden Press.

Med Stat Group. (1998). *The 1998 MedStat Quality Catalyst Physician Study.* Ann Arbor, MI: MedStat Group.

Medicare. (2006). *Medicare drug coverage 101: Everything you need to know about the new medicare prescription drug benefits,* and the *2006 guide to health insurance for people with medicare.* Available at: 1–800–MEDICARE (1–800–633–4227) and, for hearing and speech impaired, at TTY/TDD: 1–877–486–2048.

McConnell, C. R. (2000). *Economics.* New York: McGraw-Hill.

Osborn, C. (2006). *Statistical applications for health information management.* Sudbury, MA: Jones and Bartlett Publishers.

Parker, M. (1993). *Microeconomics.* Menlo Park, CA: Addison-Wesley Publishing.

Passtrak Series 6 Investment Company/Variable Contract Limited Representative. (2000). Chicago, IL: Dearborn Financial, Inc.

Puig-Junoy, J. (2005). *The public financing of pharmaceuticals: An economic approach.* Edward Elgar Publishing Limited.

Rattiner, J. (2003). Personal and business cash flow planning. In D. E. Marcinko (Ed.), *Financial planner's library on CD-ROM.* New York: Aspen Publishing.

Rettig, R. A. (1996). *Health care in transition: Technology assessment in the private sector.* Santa Monica, CA: RAND.

Rice, T. H. (1998). *The Economics of Health Reconsidered.* Chicago, IL: Health Administration Press.

Rognehaugh, R. (1998). *The managed health care dictionary* (2nd ed.). Sudbury, MA: Jones and Bartlett Publishers.

Rosenberg, J. M. (2004). *The essential dictionary of investing and finance.* New York: Barnes & Noble Books.

Schmuckler, E. (2007). Workplace violence costs. In D. E. Marcinko (Ed.), *Financial management of healthcare organizations.* Blaine, WA: Specialty Technical Publications.

Scott, C. (2001). *Public and private roles in health care systems: Reform experience in seven OECD countries.* Buckingham, UK: Open University Press.

Shortell, S. M., & Kaluzny, A. D. (2006). *Essentials of health care management.* Albany, NY: Delmar Publishing.

Sloan, F. A. (1995). *Valuing health care: Costs, benefits, and effectiveness of pharmaceuticals and other medical technologies.* Cambridge, NY: Cambridge University Press.

Sparrow, M. K. (2000). *License to steal: How fraud bleeds America's health care system: Vol. 2.* Boulder, CO: Westview Press.

Stahl, M. J. (1999). *The physician's essential MBA: What every physician leader needs to know.* Gaithersburg, MD: Aspen.

Sturm, Arthur C., Jr. (1998). *The new rules of healthcare marketing: 23 strategies for success.* Chicago, IL: Health Administration Press.

Sultz, H. (2006). *Health care USA: Understanding its organization and delivery* (5th Ed.). Sudbury, MA: JB Publishers.

Surpin, J., & Weideman, G. (1999). *Outsourcing in health care: The administrator's guide.* Chicago, IL: AHA Press.

Tinsley, R. (2004). *Medical practice management handbook.* New York: Harcourt-Brace.

Trites, P., Chinn, S., & Hetico, H. R. (in press). Hospital compliance. In D. E. Marcinko (Ed.), *Financial management of healthcare organizations.* Blaine, WA: Specialty Technical Publications.

Walker, D. L., & Gans, D. N. (2003). *Rightsizing: Appropriate staffing for your medical practice.* Dubuque, IA: Kendall/Hunt Publishing.

Weinberg, D. A. (2001). *Code green—Money driven hospitals and the dismantling of nursing.* Ithaca, NY: Cornell University Press.

Weston, J. F. (1991). *Essentials of managerial finance.* New York: Hold, Rinehart and Winston, Inc.

White, K. (in press). Managing and enhancing hospital revenue cycles. In D. E. Marcinko (Ed.), *Financial management of healthcare organizations.* Blaine, WA: Specialty Technical Publications.

Wiese, C. W. (in press). Capital formation for hospitals. In D. E. Marcinko (Ed.), *Financial management of healthcare organizations.* Blaine, WA: Specialty Technical Publications.

Zimer, D. (1999). *Physician compensation arrangements: Management and legal trends.* Sudbury, MA: Jones and Bartlett Publishers.

PRINT MEDIA PUBLICATIONS

Bodenheimer, T. (1999). The American health care system: The movement for improved quality in health care. *New England Journal of Medicine, 340,* 488–492.

Blumenthal, D. (1996). Their SO. Managed care and medical education. The new fundamentals. *Journal of the American Medical Association, 276,* 725–727.

Blumenthal, D. (1999). Health care reform at the close of the 20th century. *New England Journal of Medicine, 340,* 1916–1920.

Campbell, E. G., Weisman, J. S., & Blumenthal, D. (1997). Relationship between market competition and the activities and attitudes of medical school faculty. *Journal of the American Medical Association, 278,* 222–226.

Canby, J. B., IV. (1995). Applying activity-based costing to healthcare settings. *Healthcare Financial Management, 49*(2), 50–52, 54–56.

Cherry, J., & Sridhar, S. (2000). Six sigma: Using statistics to reduce variability and costs in radiology. *Radiology Management, 6,* 1–5.

Fiscella, K., Franks, P., Gold, M. R., & Clancy, C. M. (2000). Inequality in quality: Addressing socioeconomic, racial, and ethnic disparities in health care. *Journal of the American Medical Association, 283,* 2579–2584.

Friedman, E. (1997). Managed care and medical education: Hard cases and hard choices. *Academic Medicine, 72,* 325–331.

Getzen, T., & Poullier, J.-P. (1992). International health spending forecasts: Concepts and evaluation. *Social Science and Medicine, 34*(9), 1057–1068.

Greenlick, M. R. (1992). Educating physicians for population-based clinical practice. *Journal of the American Medical Association, 267,* 1645–1648.

Halpern, R., Lee, M. Y., Boulter, P. R., & Phillips, R. R. (2001). A synthesis of nine major reports on physicians' competencies for the emerging practice environment. *Academic Medicine, 76,* 606–615.

Heffler, S., Smith, S., Won, G., Clemens, M. K., Keehan, S., & Zezza, M. et al. (2002). Health spending projections for 2001–2011: The latest outlook. *Health Affairs, 21*(2), 207–218.

Iglehart, J. K. (1999). The American health care system—Expenditures. *New England Journal of Medicine, 340*, 70–76.

Kohn, L. T., Corrigan, J. M., & Donaldson, M. S. (Eds.). (1999). *To err is human. Building a safer health system.* Washington, D.C.: National Academy Press.

Kuttner, R. (1999). The American health care system—Health insurance coverage. *New England Journal of Medicine, 340*, 163–168.

Kuttner, R. (1999). Managed care and medical education. *New England Journal of Medicine, 341*, 1092–1096.

Ludmerer, K. M. (1999). *Time to heal: American medical education from the turn of the century to the era of managed care.* New York: Oxford Press.

Lurie, N. (1996). Preparing physicians for practice in managed care environments. *Academic Medicine, 71*, 1044–1049.

Meyer, G. S., Potter, A., & Gary, N. (1997). A national survey to define a new core curriculum to prepare physicians for managed care practice. *Academic Medicine, 72*, 669–676.

Moore, G. T. (1986). HMOs and medical education: Fashioning a marriage. *Health Affairs, 5*, 147–153.

Phillips, J., Rivo, M. L., & Talamonti, W. J. (2004, January). Partnerships between health care organization and medical school in a rapidly changing environment: A view from the delivery system. *Archives of Family Medicine, 36*(suppl 1), 138–145.

Rabinowitz, H. K., Babbott, D., Bastacky, S., Pascoe, J. M., Patel, K. K., Pye, K. L., & Rodak, J. (2001). Innovative approaches to educating medical students for practice in a changing healthcare environment: The national UME-21 project. *Academic Medicine, 76*, 587–597.

Rivo, M. L., Keller, D. R., Teherani, A., O'Connell, M. T., Weiss, B. A., & Rubenstein, S. A. (2004, January). Practicing effectively in today's health system: Teaching systems-based care. *Archives of Family Medicine, 36* (suppl), S63–S67.

Schroeder, S. A. (2001). Prospects for expanding health insurance coverage. *New England Journal of Medicine, 344*, 847–852.

Shea, J. A., Bridge, P. D., Gould, B. E., & Harris, I. B. (2004, January). UME-21 local evaluation initiatives: Contributions and challenges. *Archives of Family Medicine, 36*(suppl), S133–S137.

Smedley, B. D., Stith, A. Y., & Nelson, A. R. (Eds.). (2002). *Unequal treatment: Confronting racial and ethnic disparities in health care.* Washington, D.C.: National Academy Press.

Simon, S. R., Pan, R., Sullivan, A. M., Clark–Chiarelli, N., Connelly, M. T., Peters, A. S., et al. (1999). Views of managed care: A survey of students, residents, faculty, and deans at medical schools in the United States. *New England Journal of Medicine, 340*, 928–936.

Veloski, J. J., & Barzansky, B. (2004, January). Evaluation of the UME-21 initiative at 18 medical schools between 1999 and 2001. *Archives of Family Medicine, 36*(suppl), S138–S145.

Wood, D. L. (1998). Educating physicians for the 21st century. *Academic Medicine, 73*, 1280–1281.

Yedidia, M. J., Gillespie, C. S., & Moore, G. T. (2000). Specific clinical competencies for managing care: Views of residency directors and managed care medical directors. *Journal of the American Medical Association, 284*, 1093–1098.

PRINT MEDIA JOURNALS

- *Health Economics:* Wiley.
- *Journal of Healthcare Economics:* Elsevier.
- *European Journal of Health Economics:* Springer.
- *Economics and Human Biology:* Elsevier.
- *Applied Health Economics and Health Policy:* ADIS.
- *International Journal of Healthcare Finance and Economics:* Kluwer.
- *Journal of Mental Health Policy and Economics:* Kluwer.

ELECTRONIC INTERNET MEDIA

www.amosweb.com
www.ashrm.org
www.aima.org
www.bloomberg.com
www.businessweek.com
www.careworks.com
www.cms.hhs.gov
www.economist.com
www.efficientfrontier.com
www.ei.com
www.finance.yahoo.com
www.findce.com
www.glossarist.com
www.healtheconomics.org
www.hoovers.com
www.investopedia.com
www.irahelp.com
www.KFF.org

www.marketguide.com
www.mcareol.com
www.mcres.com
www.Medicare.gov
www.MedicareRights.org
www.ModernHealthcare.com
www.morningstar.com
www.nim.nih.gov
www.ostinato.stanford.edu
www.pharma-lexicon.com
www.rhfm.org
www.safetyandquality.org
www.sec.gov
www.stanford.edu/~wfsharpe
www.thestreet.com
www.wsj.com
www.yardeni.com

RELATED ASSOCIATIONS

- **FPA—Financial Planning Association.** This group, officially formed January 1, 2000, is the result of the merger between the Institute of Certified Financial Planners (ICFP) and the International Association of Financial Planning (IAFP). This creates a central organization for the financial planning profession. Tel: 800-322-4237. www.fpanet.org.
- **AIMR**—The Association for Investment Management Research confers the title Charted Financial Analyst to those who have passed the three-pronged Certified Financial Analyst© examination or the self-administered standards of professional practice examination. Tel: 800-247-8132. www.aimr.org.
- **SFSP—Society of Financial Service Professionals.** This is the new name for what was the American Society for CLU and ChFC, both popular designations in the insurance community. Accordingly, its membership is dominated by insurance agents and is tied to The American College in Bryn Mawr, Pennsylvania, that grants those designations. Holding a designation is not a requirement for membership. Tel: 610-526-2500. www.financialpro.org.
- *i*MBA—*Institute* of Medical Business Advisors, Inc. Offers an asynchronous live online professional designation program integrating personal financial planning and medical practice management for financial advisors: Certified Medical Planner© (CMP©). Tel: 770-448-0769; Fax: 775-361-8831. www.MedicalBusinessAdvisors.com.
- **IMCA—The Investment Management Consultants Association.** Members must pass the Certified Investment Management Analyst (CIMA) course. Tel: 800-599-9462. www.imca.org.
- **AICPA—American Institute of Certified Public Accountants.** The primary membership organization for CPAs. Tel: 212-596-6200. www.aicpa.org.
- **NAPFA—National Association of Personal Financial Advisors.** A membership organization comprised entirely of fee-only financial advisors. Tel: 888-333-6659. www.napfa.org.

Alliance for Healthcare
  Strategy
Tel: 312-704-9700
www.alliancehlth.org

American Academy of Medical
  Administrators
Tel: 248-540-4310
www.aameda.org

American Association of Healthcare Administrative Management
Tel: 202-857-1179
www.aaham.org

American College of Healthcare Administrators
Tel: 703-549-5822
www.achca.org

American College of Healthcare Executives
Tel: 312-424-2800
www.ache.org

American College of Physician Executives
Tel: 813-287-2000
www.acpe.org

American Medical Group Association
Tel: 703-838-0033
www.amga.org

American Society of Health Economics (ASHE)
Tel: 902-461-4432
www.healtheconomics.org

Association for Financial Planning and Counseling
Tel: 614-485-9650
www.afcpe.org

Center for Fiduciary Studies
Tel: 866-390-5080
www.cfstudies.com

Center for Healthcare Information
Tel: 734-973-6166
www.chim.org

Certified Financial Planner Board of Standards
Tel: 800-487-1497
www.cfp.net

Certified Medical Planner© Online Education for Healthcare Financial Advisors and Consultants (CMP©)
Tel: 770-448-0769
www.CertifiedMedicalPlanner.com

Chartered Financial Analysts Institute
Tel: 800-247-8132
www.cfainstitute.org

Healthcare Financial Management Association
Tel: 708-531-9600
www.hfma.org

Institute of Medical Business Advisors, Inc.© (*i*MBA)
Tel: 770-448-0769
www.MedicalBusinessAdvisors.com

International Health Economics Association (*i*HEA)
Tel: 902-461-4432
www.healtheconomics.org

Investment Management
    Consultants Association
Tel: 303-770-3377
www.imca.org

National Institute for Financial
    Counseling Education
Tel: 321-727-2233
www.nifce.org

Medical Group Management
    Association
Tel: 303-799-1111
www.mgma.com

Research in Healthcare Financial
    Management
Tel: 305-348-2861
www.rhfm.org

National Association of Healthcare
    Access Management
Tel: 202-857-1125
www.naham.org

SECURITIES EXCHANGE COMMISSION

SEC Headquarters
450 Fifth Street, NW
Washington, D.C. 20549
Office of Investor Education and Assistance:
Tel: 202-942-7040
E-mail: help@sec.gov

NASD DISTRICT OFFICES

District 1
525 Market Street, Suite 300
San Francisco, CA 94105-2711
Tel: 415-882-1200
Fax: 415-546-6991

Elisabeth P. Owens, Director
Northern California (the counties of Monterey, San Benito, Fresno, and Inyo, and the remainder of the state north or west of such counties), northern Nevada (the counties of Esmeralda and Nye, and the remainder of the state north or west of such counties), and Hawaii

District 2
300 South Grand Avenue, Suite 1600
Los Angeles, CA 90071
Tel: 213-627-2122
Fax: 213-617-3299

Lani M. Sen Woltmann, Director
Southern California (that part of the state south or east of the counties of
Monterey, San Benito, Fresno, and Inyo), southern Nevada (that part of the
state south or east of the counties of Esmeralda and Nye), and the former U.S.
Trust Territories

District 3
Denver
Republic Office Building
370 17th Street, Suite 2900
Denver, CO 80202-5629
Tel: 303-446-3100
Fax: 303-620-9450

Frank Birgfeld, V.P., Director
Arizona, Colorado, New Mexico, Utah, and Wyoming
Seattle
Two Union Square
601 Union Street, Suite 1616
Seattle, WA 98101-2327
Tel: 206-624-0790
Fax: 206-623-2518

James G. Dawson, Director
Alaska, Idaho, Montana, Oregon, and Washington

District 4
12 Wyandotte Plaza
120 West 12th Street, Suite 900
Kansas City, MO 64105
Tel: 816-421-5700
Fax: 816-421-5029

Jack Rosenfield, V.P., Director
Iowa, Kansas, Minnesota, Missouri, Nebraska, North Dakota, and South Dakota

District 5
1100 Poydras Street
Suite 850, Energy Centre
New Orleans, LA 70163
Tel: 504-522-6527
Fax: 504-522-4077

Warren A. Butler, Jr., V.P., Director
Alabama, Arkansas, Kentucky, Louisiana, Mississippi, Oklahoma, and Tennessee

District 6
12801 North Central Expressway, Suite 1050
Dallas, TX 75243
Tel: 972-701-8554
Fax: 972-716-7646

Bernerd Young, Associate Director
Texas

District 7
One Securities Centre, Suite 500
3490 Piedmont Road, NE
Atlanta, GA 30305
Tel: 404-239-6100
Fax: 404-237-9290

Alan M. Wolper, Director
Florida, Georgia, North Carolina, South Carolina, Virginia, Puerto Rico, the
Canal Zone, and the Virgin Islands

District 8
Chicago
10 S. LaSalle St., 20th Floor
Chicago, IL 60603-1002
Tel: 312-899-4400
Fax: 312-236-3025

Carlotta A. Romano, V.P., Director
Illinois, Indiana, Michigan, and Wisconsin
Cleveland
Renaissance on Playhouse Sq.
1350 Euclid Ave., Suite 650
Cleveland, OH 44115
Tel: 216-694-4545
Fax: 216-694-3048

William H. Jackson, Jr., Director
Ohio and part of upstate New York (the counties of Monroe, Livingston, and
Steuben, and the remainder of the state west of such counties)

District 9
Woodbridge
581 Main Street, 7th floor
Woodbridge, NJ 07095
Tel: 732-596-2000
Fax: 732-596-2001

Gary K. Liebowitz, Sr. V.P., Director
New Jersey (except southern New Jersey in the immediate Philadelphia vicinity)
Philadelphia
11 Penn Center
1835 Market Street, 19th Floor
Philadelphia, PA 19103
Tel: 215-665-1180
Fax: 215-496-0434

John P. Nocella, Sr. V.P., Director
Delaware, Pennsylvania, West Virginia, District of Columbia, Maryland, and
the part of southern New Jersey in the immediate Philadelphia vicinity

District 10
33 Whitehall Street
New York, NY 10004-2193
Tel: 212-858-4000
Fax: 212-858-4189

David A. Leibowitz, Sr. V.P., Director
The five boroughs of New York City

District 11
260 Franklin St., 16th Floor
Boston, MA 02110
Tel: 617-261-0800
Fax: 617-951-2337

Willis Riccio, V.P., Director
Connecticut, Maine, Massachusetts, New Hampshire, Rhode Island, Vermont, and New York (except for the counties of Monroe, Livingston, and Steuben; and the five boroughs of New York City)